Paediatrics
at a Glance

RJ
48
M53
2016

Miall, Lawrence

Paediatrics at a glance

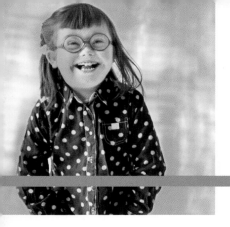

Dedication

To our children: Charlie, Mollie and Rosie, Aaron and Becca, Edward and Daniel and our spouses: Domini, Michael and Kathy and all the patients who have taught us so much over the years.

This title is also available as an e-book.
For more details, please see
www.wiley.com/buy/9781118947838
or scan this QR code

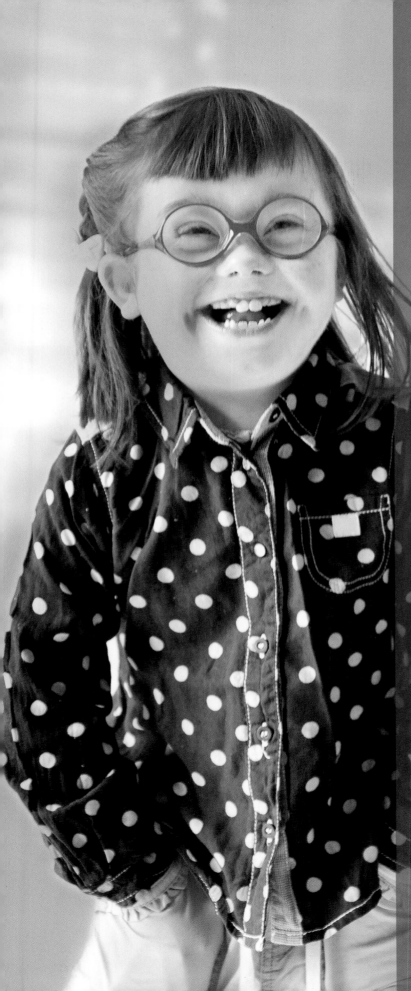

Paediatrics at a Glance

Fourth Edition

Lawrence Miall
MBBS, BSc, MMedSc, MRCP, FRCPCH
Consultant in Neonatal Medicine and
Honorary Senior Lecturer
Leeds Teaching Hospitals NHS Trust and
University of Leeds
Leeds

Mary Rudolf
MBBS, BSc, DCH, FRCPCH, FAAP
Professor of Population Health
Bar Ilan University Faculty of Medicine
in the Galilee, Israel
Visiting Professor of Child Health
University of Leeds, UK

Dominic Smith
MBBS, MMedSc, MRCP, MRCPCH
Consultant Paediatrician
Department of Child Health
York Teaching Hospital and Hull York Medical
School
York

WILEY Blackwell

This edition first published 2016 © 2016 by John Wiley & Sons, Ltd.

Registered office:
John Wiley & Sons, Ltd, The Atrium, Southern Gate, Chichester, West Sussex, PO19 8SQ, UK

Editorial offices:
9600 Garsington Road, Oxford, OX4 2DQ, UK
1606 Golden Aspen Drive, Suites 103 and 104, Ames, Iowa 50010, USA

For details of our global editorial offices, for customer services and for information about how to apply for permission to reuse the copyright material in this book please see our website at www.wiley.com/wiley-blackwell

The right of the author to be identified as the author of this work has been asserted in accordance with the UK Copyright, Designs and Patents Act 1988.

All rights reserved. No part of this publication may be reproduced, stored in a retrieval system, or transmitted, in any form or by any means, electronic, mechanical, photocopying, recording or otherwise, except as permitted by the UK Copyright, Designs and Patents Act 1988, without the prior permission of the publisher.

Designations used by companies to distinguish their products are often claimed as trademarks. All brand names and product names used in this book are trade names, service marks, trademarks or registered trademarks of their respective owners. The publisher is not associated with any product or vendor mentioned in this book. It is sold on the understanding that the publisher is not engaged in rendering professional services. If professional advice or other expert assistance is required, the services of a competent professional should be sought.

The contents of this work are intended to further general scientific research, understanding, and discussion only and are not intended and should not be relied upon as recommending or promoting a specific method, diagnosis, or treatment by health science practitioners for any particular patient. The publisher and the author make no representations or warranties with respect to the accuracy or completeness of the contents of this work and specifically disclaim all warranties, including without limitation any implied warranties of fitness for a particular purpose. In view of ongoing research, equipment modifications, changes in governmental regulations, and the constant flow of information relating to the use of medicines, equipment, and devices, the reader is urged to review and evaluate the information provided in the package insert or instructions for each medicine, equipment, or device for, among other things, any changes in the instructions or indication of usage and for added warnings and precautions. Readers should consult with a specialist where appropriate. The fact that an organization or Website is referred to in this work as a citation and/or a potential source of further information does not mean that the author or the publisher endorses the information the organization or Website may provide or recommendations it may make. Further, readers should be aware that Internet Websites listed in this work may have changed or disappeared between when this work was written and when it is read. No warranty may be created or extended by any promotional statements for this work. Neither the publisher nor the author shall be liable for any damages arising herefrom.

Library of Congress Cataloging-in-Publication Data

Names: Miall, Lawrence, author. | Rudolf, Mary, author. | Smith, Dominic,
    1970- , author.
Title: Paediatrics at a glance / Lawrence Miall, Mary Rudolf, Dominic Smith.
Other titles: At a glance series (Oxford, England)
Description: Fourth edition. | Chicester, West Sussex ; Ames, Iowa : John
    Wiley & Sons, Inc., 2016. | Series: At a glance series | Includes
    bibliographical references and index.
Identifiers: LCCN 2015047744 (print) | LCCN 2015048187 (ebook) | ISBN
    9781118947838 (pbk.) | ISBN 9781118947821 (pdf) | ISBN 9781118947807 (epub)
Subjects: | MESH: Pediatrics–methods | Handbooks
Classification: LCC RJ61 (print) | LCC RJ61 (ebook) | NLM WS 39 | DDC
    618.92—dc23
LC record available at http://lccn.loc.gov/2015047744

A catalogue record for this book is available from the British Library.

Wiley also publishes its books in a variety of electronic formats. Some content that appears in print may not be available in electronic books.

Cover image: © TrevOC/gettyimages

Set in 9.5/11.5pt, MinionPro by SPi Global, Chennai, India.
Printed and bound in Singapore by Markono Print Media Pte Ltd
1   2016

Contents

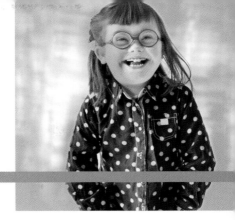

LIBRARY
NSCC, WATERFRONT CAMPUS
80 MAWIOMI PLACE
DARTMOUTH, NS B2Y 0A5 CANADA

Part 13 **Emergency paediatrics** **145**

Part 14 **Child health in the community** **161**

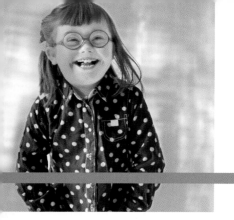

Preface

"'What is the use of a book,' thought Alice, 'without pictures or conversations?'" Lewis Carroll, Alice in Wonderland.

Paediatric medicine requires an understanding of developing anatomy, physiology and psychology as well as a holistic family-orientated approach. There are a wide range of professional challenges: from the technical aspects of intensive care to the ethical and sociological questions relating to issues of autonomy, independence and children's rights. The paediatric environment is very different to the world of adult medicine. This can all be daunting to those who are new to the specialty, but developing the skills and confidence in successfully managing these challenges can enable professionals to make significant differences to the lives of children and families. This makes paediatric medicine amongst the most rewarding of all the medical specialties.

In preparing the fourth edition, we have updated the text to reflect changes in understanding of childhood illness over the last 5 years. The new edition includes advances in genetics, screening and therapy of childhood illness. Multiple choice questions to test and expand on knowledge from the text are included on the companion website. Video clips highlighting clinical signs and examination techniques are available on the companion website.

Children have complex needs that require medical staff to work together with other professionals in child health, psychology, education and social care. There is increasing recognition of the need for all health professionals to have a good understanding of their role in safeguarding vulnerable people. New chapters have been added to expand on psychological issues and ethics in child health. There is a new chapter on Palliative Care, which is an emerging area in the specialty.

We hope that this edition will continue to educate and inspire students and trainees in taking the first steps towards an understanding of children, their illnesses, their resilience in the face of adversity and amazing capacity for recovery. It is a book with many pictures to aid the introduction and revision of the key topics. We hope this will help as students begin their all-important conversations with young patients.

Lawrence Miall
Mary Rudolf
Dominic Smith
Leeds, United Kingdom
February 2016

Acknowledgements

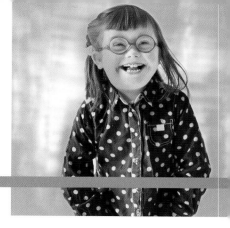

We would like to acknowledge Dr Tim Lee, Dr Adam Glaser, Dr Michael Harari, Dr Claire Wensley and Dr Jemma Cleminson for their contributions to chapters.

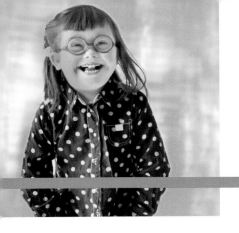

Abbreviations

AABR	automated auditory brainstem response
ACTH	adrenocorticotropic hormone
ADD	attention deficit disorder
ADH	anti-diuretic hormone
ADPKD	autosomal dominant polycystic kidney disease
AFP	alpha-fetoprotein
AIDS	acquired immunodeficiency syndrome
ALL	acute lymphoblastic leukaemia
ALT	alanine transaminase
ALTE	acute life-threatening event
AML	acute myeloid leukaemia
ANA	antinuclear antibody
APTT	activated partial thromboplastin time
ARPKD	autosomal recessive polycystic kidney disease
ASD	atrial septal defect
ASOT	antistreptolysin O titre
AVPU	alert, voice, pain, unresponsive
AVSD	atrioventricular septal defect
AXR	abdominal radiograph
AZT	zidovudine (azidothymidine)
BCG	bacille Calmette–Guérin
BMI	body mass index
BP	blood pressure
BSER	brainstem evoked responses
CDH	congenital dislocation of the hip
CF	cystic fibrosis
CFTR	cystic fibrosis transmembrane regulator
CFU	colony-forming unit
CHARGE	coloboma, heart defects, choanal atresia, retarded growth and development, genital hypoplasia, ear anomalies
CHD	congenital heart disease
CMV	cytomegalovirus
CNS	central nervous system
CONI	care of the next infant
CPAP	continuous positive airway pressure
CPR	cardiopulmonary resuscitation
CRP	C-reactive protein
CRT	capillary refill time
CSF	cerebrospinal fluid
CSII	continuous subcutaneous insulin infusion
CT	computed tomography
CXR	chest radiograph
DDH	developmental dysplasia of the hip
DIC	disseminated intravascular coagulation
DIDMOAD	diabetes insipidus, diabetes mellitus, optic atrophy and deafness
DKA	diabetic ketoacidosis
DM	diabetes mellitus
DMD	Duchenne muscular dystrophy
DMSA	dimercaptosuccinic acid
DTPA	diethylenetriamine penta-acetate
EBV	Epstein–Barr virus
ECG	electrocardiogram
EDD	expected due date
EEG	electroencephalogram
ENT	ear, nose and throat
ESR	erythrocyte sedimentation rate
FBC	full blood count
FDP	fibrin degradation product
FSGS	focal segment glomerulosclerosis
FTT	failure to thrive
G6PD	glucose 6-phosphate dehydrogenase
GCS	Glasgow Coma Scale
GH	growth hormone
GI	gastrointestinal
GOR	gastro-oesophageal reflux
GP	general practitioner
GTT	glucose tolerance test
HAART	highly active antiretroviral therapy
Hb	haemoglobin
HbF	fetal haemoglobin
HbS	sickle-cell haemoglobin
HIE	hypoxic-ischaemic encephalopathy
HIV	human immunodeficiency virus
HPLC	high-performance liquid chromatography
HSP	Henoch–Schönlein purpura
HSV	herpes simplex virus
HUS	haemolytic uraemic syndrome
ICP	intracranial pressure
Ig	immunoglobulin
IM	intramuscular
INR	international normalized ratio
IO	intraosseous
IRT	immunoreactive trypsin
ITP	idiopathic thrombocytopenic purpura
IUGR	intrauterine growth retardation
IV	intravenous
IVC	inferior vena cava
IVF	in vitro fertilization
IVH	intraventricular haemorrhage
IVU	intravenous urogram
JCA	juvenile chronic arthritis
LFT	liver function test

LIP	lymphocytic interstitial pneumonitis	**RBC**	red blood cell
LMN	lower motor neuron	**RDS**	respiratory distress syndrome
LP	lumbar puncture	**RNIB**	Royal National Institute for the Blind
Mag-3	radioisotope technetium ^{99m}Tc mertiatide	**ROP**	retinopathy of prematurity
MCAD	medium-chain acyl-carnitine deficiency	**RSV**	respiratory syncytial virus
MCGN	minimal change glomerulonephritis	**SCBU**	special care baby unit
MCH	mean cell haemoglobin	**SCID**	severe combined immunodeficiency
MCUG	micturating cystourethrogram	**SGA**	small for gestational age
MCV	mean cell volume	**SIADH**	syndrome of inappropriate antidiuretic hormone secretion
MDI	metered dose inhaler	**SIDS**	sudden infant death syndrome
MLD	mild learning difficulty	**SLD**	severe learning difficulty
MMR	measles, mumps, rubella	**SSPE**	subacute sclerosing encephalitis
MRI	magnetic resonance imaging	**STD**	sexually transmitted disease
MUAC	mid-upper arm circumference	**SUDI**	sudden unexpected death in infancy
NEC	necrotizing enterocolitis	**T4**	thyroxine
NF	neurofibromatosis	**TAPVD**	total anomalous pulmonary venous drainage
NHL	non-Hodgkin's lymphoma	**TB**	tuberculosis
NICU	neonatal intensive care unit	**TGA**	transposition of the great arteries
NPA	nasopharyngeal aspirate	**TNF**	tumour necrosis factor
NSAID	non-steroidal anti-inflammatory drug	**TORCH**	toxoplasmosis, other (syphilis), rubella, cytomegalovirus, hepatitis, HIV
OAE	otoacoustic emissions	**TS**	tuberous sclerosis
OFC	occipitofrontal circumference	**TSH**	thyroid stimulating hormone
ORS	oral rehydration solution	**tTG**	tissue transglutaminase
P$_{CO_2}$	partial pressure of carbon dioxide	**U&E**	urea and electrolytes
PCP	pneumocystis pneumonia	**UMN**	upper motor neuron
PCR	polymerase chain reaction	**URTI**	upper respiratory tract infection
PCV	packed cell volume	**UTI**	urinary tract infection
PDA	patent ductus arteriosus	**UV**	ultraviolet
PEFR	peak expiratory flow rate	**VACTERL**	vertebral anomalies, anal atresia, cardiac anomalies, tracheo-oesophageal fistula, renal anomalies, limb defects
PKU	phenylketonuria		
PNET	primitive neuroectodermal tumour	**VER**	visual evoked response
PR	per rectum	**VKDB**	vitamin K deficiency bleeding
PT	prothrombin time	**VSD**	ventricular septal defect
PTT	partial thromboplastin time	**VUR**	vesicoureteric reflux
PUJ	pelviureteric junction	**WCC**	white cell count
PUO	pyrexia of unknown origin		
PVL	periventricular leucomalacia		
RAST	radio-allergosorbent test		

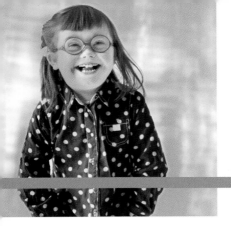

How to use your textbook

Features contained within your textbook

Each topic is presented in a double-page spread with clear, easy-to-follow diagrams supported by succinct explanatory text.

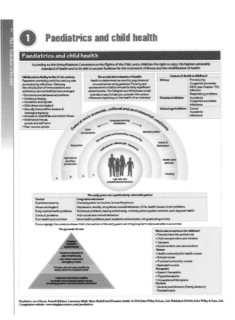

Key point boxes give a summary of the topics covered in a topic.

KEY POINTS

Non-organic pain is characteristically:
- Periodic pain with intervening good health
- Periumbilical
- May be related to school hours.
    Consider organic pain if there is
- Pain occurring at night
- Weight loss, reduced appetite, lack of energy or recurrent fever
- Organ-specific symptoms, e.g. change in bowel habit, polyuria, menstrual problems, vomiting, occult or frank bleeding
- Ill appearance, growth failure or swollen joints.

Your textbook is full of photographs, illustrations and tables.

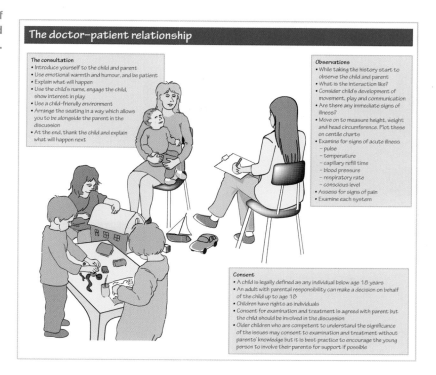

The doctor–patient relationship

The consultation
- Introduce yourself to the child and parent
- Use emotional warmth and humour, and be patient
- Explain what will happen
- Use the child's name, engage the child, show interest in play
- Use a child-friendly environment
- Arrange the seating in a way which allows you to be alongside the parent in the discussion
- At the end, thank the child and explain what will happen next

Observations
- While taking the history start to observe the child and parent
- What is the interaction like?
- Consider child's development of movement, play and communication
- Are there any immediate signs of illness?
- Move on to measure height, weight and head circumference. Plot these on centile charts
- Examine for signs of acute illness
  - pulse
  - temperature
  - capillary refill time
  - blood pressure
  - respiratory rate
  - conscious level
- Assess for signs of pain
- Examine each system

Consent
- A child is legally defined as any individual below age 18 years
- An adult with parental responsibility can make a decision on behalf of the child up to age 18
- Children have rights as individuals
- Consent for examination and treatment is agreed with parent but the child should be involved in the discussion
- Older children who are competent to understand the significance of the issues may consent to examination and treatment without parents' knowledge but it is best practice to encourage the young person to involve their parents for support if possible

Self-assessment review questions and interactive case studies, available on the book's companion website, help you test yourself after each chapter.

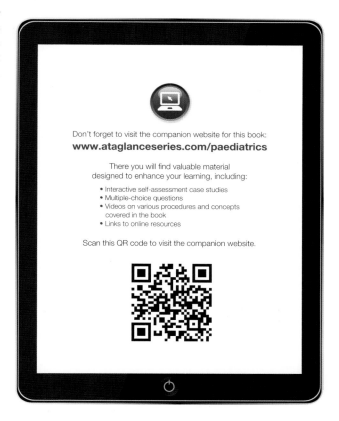

Don't forget to visit the companion website for this book:

www.ataglanceseries.com/paediatrics

There you will find valuable material designed to enhance your learning, including:

- Interactive self-assessment case studies
- Multiple-choice questions
- Videos on various procedures and concepts covered in the book
- Links to online resources

Scan this QR code to visit the companion website.

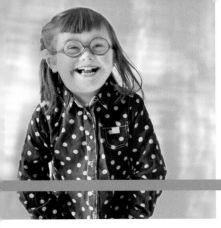

About the companion website

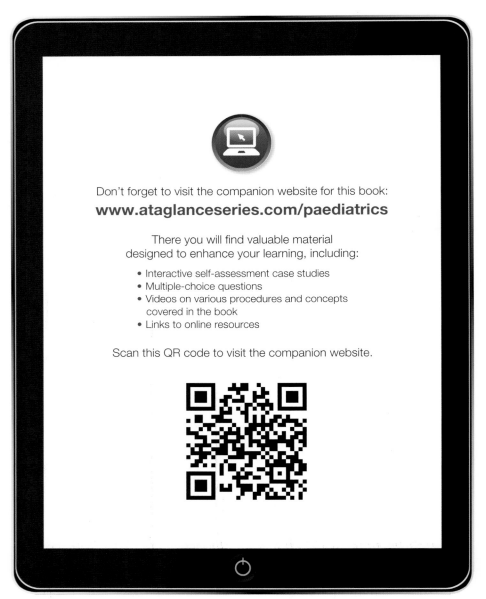

Don't forget to visit the companion website for this book:

www.ataglanceseries.com/paediatrics

There you will find valuable material
designed to enhance your learning, including:

- Interactive self-assessment case studies
- Multiple-choice questions
- Videos on various procedures and concepts
  covered in the book
- Links to online resources

Scan this QR code to visit the companion website.

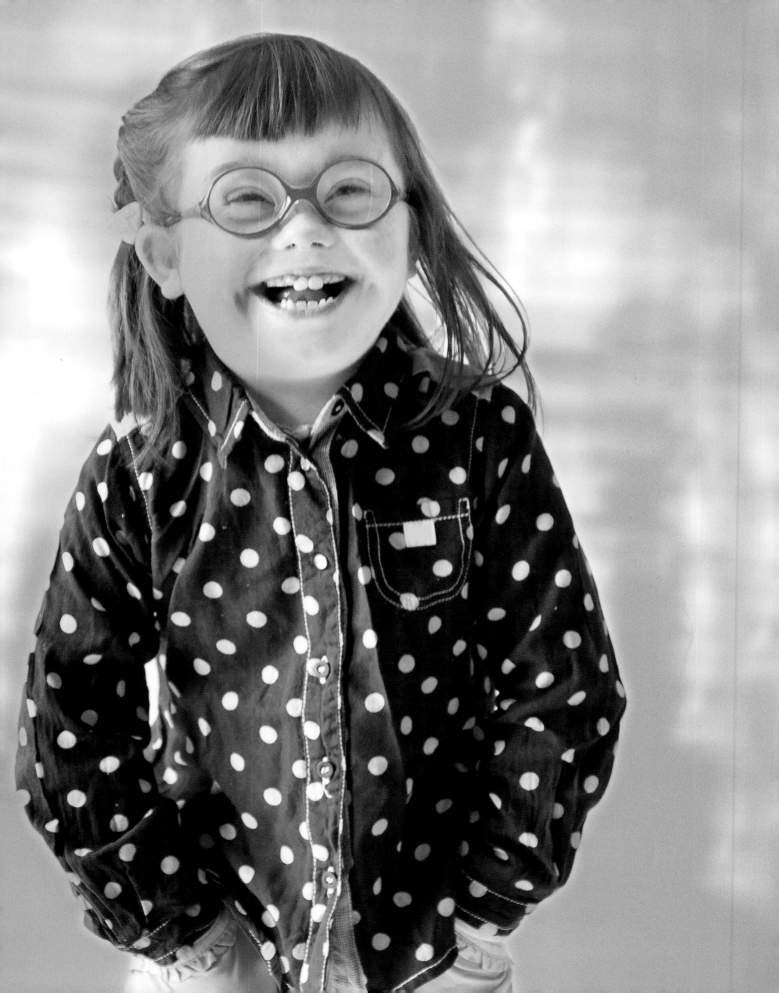

Evaluation of the child

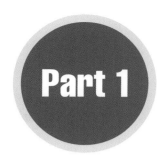
Part 1

Chapters

1 Paediatrics and child health

Paediatrics and child health

According to the United Nations Convention on the Rights of the Child, every child has the right to enjoy the highest attainable standard of health and to be able to access facilities for the treatment of illness and the rehabilitation of health.

Childhood morbidity in the 21st century

Paediatric morbidity until this century was dominated by infections. Following the introduction of immunisations and antibiotics new morbidities have emerged:
- Emotional and behavioural problems
- Childhood obesity
- Accidents and injuries
- Child abuse and neglect
- Sexually transmitted disease & teenage pregnancy
- Increase in disabilities and chronic illness
- Substance misuse, suicide and self harm
- Poor vaccine uptake

The social determinants of health

Health is determined as much by psychosocial circumstances as by genetics. Poverty and socioeconomic status are particularly significant determinants. The Dahlgren and Whitehead model provides a way to help you consider the various influences impacting on the health of an individual

Causes of death in childhood

Infancy	Prematurity
	Congenital anomalies
	SIDS (see Chapter 70)
	Infection
	Respiratory problems
Preschool children	Accidents
	Congenital anomalies
	Infections
School aged children	Cancer
	Accidents
	Infections

General socio economic, cultural and environmental conditions

Living and working conditions

Work environment

Unemployment

Social and community networks

Education

Individual lifestyle factors

Water & Sanitation

Agriculture and food production

Health care services

Housing

4   3   2   1

Age, sex and constitutional factors

The early years are a particularly vulnerable period

Factor	Long term outcomes
Sustained poverty	Unemployment, low income, low working hours
Abuse and neglect	Depression, anxiety, drug abuse, suicidal behaviour, STIs, health issues, trust problems
Early mental health problems	Emotional problems, leaving school early, criminal justice system contact, poor physical health
Conduct problems	Anti-social and criminal behaviour
Poor health and nutrition	More health problems; poor academic achievement, not graduating on time

Encouragingly the evidence shows that intervention in the early years can bring long term improvements in outcomes

The pyramid of care

Hospital inpatient departments

Hospital outpatients departments/day case observation and emergency rooms

Primary care services staffed by family doctors or pediatricians

Maternal child clinics staffed by health visitors/public health nurses providing guidance and child health promotion

Who's who in services for children?
- Parents have the central role
- Child care providers and minders
- Teachers
- Social workers and care workers

Nurses
- Health visitors/public health nurses
- School nurses
- Practice/community nurses
- Specialist nurses

Therapists
- Speech therapists
- Physiotherapists
- Occupational therapists

Doctors
- General practitioners (Family doctors)
- Paediatricians

Paediatrics at a Glance, Fourth Edition. Lawrence Miall, Mary Rudolf and Dominic Smith. © 2016 John Wiley & Sons, Ltd. Published 2016 by John Wiley & Sons, Ltd.
Companion website: www.ataglanceseries.com/paediatrics

Paediatrics is not just about the recognition and treatment of children's illness. It also encompasses child health, covering all aspects of growth and development, promotion of children's health and the prevention of disease. It includes every aspect of life from birth through adulthood. In many countries, such as the UK, paediatric care extends up to the age of 18 and covers all children from the very premature infant to teenagers in the workforce.

All aspects of paediatrics are coloured by the fact that the child is growing and developing both physically and emotionally. Anyone involved in the medical care of children needs to have an understanding of children's normal development and a realization that children must not be considered as mini adults. In paediatrics, more than in any other branch of medicine, the needs of the family and carers must also be taken into consideration. At the end of childhood, a smooth transition of care to adult services is needed, especially for those with chronic conditions.

The changing face of paediatrics and child health

One hundred years ago, infection was the major cause of morbidity and mortality in childhood. Improvements in the environment, sanitation and housing began the trend for advancement in population health, and this was accelerated by the introduction of immunizations and antibiotics. Changes have occurred in society too, many of which are beneficial to children and their health and well-being. Children are better and more widely protected than was the case a century ago. Educational standards, social support, medical care and knowledge about child development have all improved, and child abuse has become unacceptable.

However, inequalities in both wealth and health are increasing, and the 'gap' between the richest and poorest has a profound impact on children's lives. Referrals for emotional and behavioural problems are rising dramatically, and childhood obesity is seen as the major public health problem of our time. A relatively new aspect of paediatrics is the understanding that many determinants of adult health have their origins antenatally, in infancy and in the early years of childhood.

Health care has also changed in paediatrics. Over the last 40 years, we have seen more children admitted to hospital, but the experience of hospitalization has changed. Once visiting hours for parents were limited to 30 minutes per day, but now the normal expectation is that parents will stay with their child. Where possible every effort is made to keep children out of hospital, and many aspects of specialized complex care have become available in the community. Even for the acutely ill child, short-stay observation wards now allow serious causes of illness to be excluded and children to be discharged to recover at home. A significant proportion of admissions are for social reasons, for example, if there are concerns that the family is unable to cope or they live too far away to safely send the child home.

The determinants of health

The way health is considered has also changed over the decades. In the early part of the 20th century, health was considered to be the absence of disease. However, in 1948, the World Health Organization changed the way we look at health when it declared that 'health is a state of complete physical, mental, and social well-being,

and not merely the absence of disease and infirmity'. In paediatrics, this has been accompanied by a more holistic approach to children, with greater emphasis on well-being especially for those coping with chronic conditions and disabilities.

Two major factors have changed priorities in the care of children and their services. The first is the understanding that socioeconomic status has a powerful influence over many aspects of children's health. Poverty is now known to be a significant predictor of a number of major measures of health, including:

- Birth weight
- Perinatal morbidity
- Sudden infant death syndrome (SIDS)
- Admission to hospital
- Obesity.

The other factor that has changed the way we view disease arises from the 'Barker hypothesis'. Barker and his colleagues brought to light how events in pregnancy and infancy can have a long-term effect on health. Exploring infant growth records from the last century, they showed that babies born small for gestational age were at significantly increased risk for hypertension, cardiovascular disease, diabetes and obesity in adult life, particularly if they showed rapid catch-up growth in the first year of life. Their findings demonstrated how critical the early years are in programming later health outcomes.

Rather reassuringly, economists have shown that although the preschool years are a vulnerable period, they are also a critical period amenable to intervention. The evidence clearly shows that when society invests in the early childhood years and provide support, community programmes, guidance for parents and education, there are profound benefits on many later outcomes such as physical health, academic achievement, mental health, antisocial behaviour and substance abuse.

Types of paediatric problems

With the changing face of childhood disease, health professionals need to be competent at managing a broad variety of conditions. These conditions include the following broad categories:

- Acute illnesses such as bronchiolitis, respiratory infections and anaphylaxis
- Chronic illnesses such as asthma, epilepsy, diabetes and cancer
- Disabilities—both physical and intellectual
- Injury: accidental and non-accidental
- Disorders of eating and nutrition, including weight faltering, obesity and anorexia
- Mental health disorders such as attention deficit disorder, challenging behaviour, depression and anxiety.

Some of the particular challenges we need to face are emotional and behavioural problems, childhood obesity, child abuse and neglect, accidents and injuries, sexually transmitted disease and teenage pregnancy, increase in disabilities and chronic illness, substance misuse, suicide and self-harm and poor vaccine uptake.

By directly treating childhood conditions, by ensuring effective screening and prevention programmes and by advocating for better public health interventions, paediatricians and all those working in child health have a fantastic opportunity to influence the long-term outcome of their patients. Paediatrics is a challenging specialty but a very rewarding one.

2 The paediatric consultation

The doctor–patient relationship

The consultation
- Introduce yourself to the child and parent
- Use emotional warmth and humour, and be patient
- Explain what will happen
- Use the child's name, engage the child, show interest in play
- Use a child-friendly environment
- Arrange the seating in a way which allows you to be alongside the parent in the discussion
- At the end, thank the child and explain what will happen next

Observations
- While taking the history start to observe the child and parent
- What is the interaction like?
- Consider child's development of movement, play and communication
- Are there any immediate signs of illness?
- Move on to measure height, weight and head circumference. Plot these on centile charts
- Examine for signs of acute illness
  - pulse
  - temperature
  - capillary refill time
  - blood pressure
  - respiratory rate
  - conscious level
- Assess for signs of pain
- Examine each system

Consent
- A child is legally defined as any individual below age 18 years
- An adult with parental responsibility can make a decision on behalf of the child up to age 18
- Children have rights as individuals
- Consent for examination and treatment is agreed with parent but the child should be involved in the discussion
- Older children who are competent to understand the significance of the issues may consent to examination and treatment without parents' knowledge but it is best practice to encourage the young person to involve their parents for support if possible

Communication skills in paediatrics

Paediatricians need to be happy with informality, enjoy humour and appreciate the unpredictability that children bring to consultations! Young children do not have a full understanding of the role of health professionals. Children will naturally be anxious and uncertain in an unfamiliar environment. They may not understand all of the language in the consultation, but they quickly detect a sense of personal warmth, friendliness and relaxed mood in adults around them. It helps to have pictures, toys and videos to help children understand that the room is a good place for children.

In paediatrics, the focus of the consultation changes with the age and understanding of the child. In a young baby, the discussion is entirely with the carers (usually parents) who act as advocates for the child's needs. As children mature, they need to be included in the discussion. It is important to understand children's concerns and their right to be involved in decisions. Paediatricians need also to consider the concerns of the family and communicate sensitively with all family members.

Approaching the consultation

- Try to be friendly, confident and non-threatening. It may be best to examine an exposed part of the body first before undressing the child, or do a pretend examination on their teddy bear.
- Try to get down to the child's level—kneel on the floor or sit on the bed. Look at the child as you examine them. Use a style and

Paediatrics at a Glance, Fourth Edition. Lawrence Miall, Mary Rudolf and Dominic Smith. © 2016 John Wiley & Sons, Ltd. Published 2016 by John Wiley & Sons, Ltd.
Companion website: www.ataglanceseries.com/paediatrics

language that is appropriate to their age—*'I'm going to feel your tummy'* is good for a small child but not for an adolescent.

- Explain what you are going to do, but be careful of saying *'can I listen to your chest'* as they may refuse!
- Babies are best examined on a couch with the parent nearby; toddlers may need to be examined on the parent's lap.
- In order to perform a proper examination, the child needs to be undressed, but this is often best done by the parent and only the region that is being examined needs to be undressed at any one time.
- Older children and adolescents should always be examined with a chaperone—usually a parent but, if the child prefers, a nurse. Allow as much privacy as possible when the child is undressing and dressing.
- Sometimes, you may need to be opportunistic and perform whatever examination you can when you can. Always leave unpleasant things until the end—for example, looking in the throat and ears can often cause distress.
- Hygiene is important both for the patient and the paediatrician to prevent the spread of infection to other patients. Always wash your hands before and after each examination.
- Always sterilize or dispose of equipment that has been in contact with a patient, such as tongue depressors or auroscope tips.

History taking

The history often indicates the diagnosis before examination or investigations. The history can be taken from a parent, a carer or from the child. Record who gave the history and in what context. Use an independent interpreter if there are language difficulties.

Beginning the examination—observation

Much information can be gained by careful observation of the child. This starts while you are first talking to the parents.

- Signs of acute severe illness (need urgent intervention):
  - shock
  - severe respiratory distress
  - altered consciousness level
- Signs of pain or anxiety
- Growth and nutrition
- Features of syndromic disorders
- Developmental progress:
  - gross motor and fine motor movement
  - social interaction
  - speech and understanding
- Interaction with carers
- Hygiene and clothing
- Mood and behaviour.

The examination of individual systems is discussed in detail in the following chapters.

Presenting complaint	Record the main problems in the family's own words
History of presenting complaint	Try to get an exact chronology from the time the child was last completely well
	Allow the family to describe events themselves; use questions to direct them and probe for specific information
	Try to use open questions—*'tell me about the cough'* rather than *'is the cough worse in the mornings?'* Use direct questions to try to confirm or refute possible diagnoses
Past medical history	In young children and infants, this should start from the pregnancy and include details of the delivery and neonatal period, including any feeding, growth or early development problems
	Ask about all illnesses and hospital attendances, including accidents
Developmental history	Milestones during infancy and school performance
	Are there any areas of concern?
	Do the parents feel the child's development is comparable to their peer group?
	School performance—any academic or behavioural problems?
Immunizations	Review immunizations against national schedule
	Are there any missed or extra vaccinations?
Drugs and allergies	What medication is the child taking? Include over-the-counter preparations
	Does the child have any allergies to drugs or foods?
Systems enquiry	Ask a series of screening questions for symptoms within systems other than the presenting system
Family and social history	What is the family make-up and who lives at home?
	Draw a genogram with the family to discuss extended family history
	Consanguinity—first-cousin parents increase the risk of genetic disorders
	Illnesses or developmental problems in the family
	Any family members with long-term conditions
	Contact with infection or recent travel
Social history	Which school or nursery does the child attend?
	Parents' education background, jobs, physical and mental health
	Home environment—adults who smoke, housing problems and family stresses
Problem list	At the end of the history, prepare a clear problem list to guide further management

Systems examination

Respiratory system

▶ Observation
- Is there respiratory distress?
  – nasal flaring, recession
  – use of accessory muscles
- Count the respiratory rate
- Is there wheeze, stridor or grunting?
- Is the child restless or drowsy?
- Is there cyanosis or pallor?
- Is there finger clubbing?
  – cystic fibrosis, bronchiectasis

Chest wall palpation
- Assess expansion
- Check trachea is central
- Feel apex beat
- Is there chest deformity?
  – Harrison's sulcus: asthma
  – barrel chest: air-trapping
  – pectus excavatum: usually isolated abnormality, can be associated with mitral valve prolapse or Marfan's syndrome
  – pectus carinatum (pigeon chest): idiopathic or associated with severe asthma
- May 'feel' crackles

Ear, nose and throat
- Examine eardrums using an auroscope
  – grey and shiny: normal
  – red and bulging: suggests otitis media
  – dull and retracted: chronic secretory otitis media (glue ear)
- Examine nostrils for inflammation, obstruction and polyps
- Examine pharynx using tongue depressor (leave this until last!)
  – Are the tonsils acutely inflamed (red ± pustules or ulcers) or chronically hypertrophied (enlarged but not red)
- Feel for cervical lymphadenopathy

▶ Auscultation
- Use an appropriately sized stethoscope!
- Listen in all areas for air entry, breath sounds and added sounds
- Absent breath sounds in one area suggests pleural effusion, pneumothorax or dense consolidation
- With consolidation (e.g. pneumonia) there is often bronchial breathing with crackles heard just above the area of consolidation
- In asthma and bronchiolitis expiratory wheeze is heard throughout the lung fields
- In young children upper airway sounds are often transmitted over the whole chest. Asking the child to cough may clear them

Percussion note

Resonant	Normal
Hyper-resonant	Pneumothorax or air-trapping
Dull	Consolidation (or normal liver in right lower zone)
Stony dull	Pleural effusions

Age	Respiratory rate at rest (breaths/min)
<1	30–40
1–2	25–35
2–5	25–30
5–12	20–25
>12	15–20

KEY QUESTIONS FROM THE HISTORY

Breathlessness
- Breathless at rest or with activity?
- Poor weight gain in infancy (a sign of respiratory distress)

Cough
- Chronology—any link to time of day/activity/environment
- Nature of cough: dry (viral), loose (productive), barking (croup), paradoxical (forced repetitive cough with difficult inspiration, seen in whooping cough)

Feeding in infancy
- Choking (gastro-oesophageal reflux)
- Symptoms with introduction of formula milk (cow's milk protein allergy)

Fever

Noisy breathing
- Noise in expiration (wheeze = lower airway obstruction)
- Noise in inspiration (stridor = upper airway obstruction)

Cough, wheeze or stridor in a young child
- If sudden onset, is there a history of inhaled foreign body or choking?

Ear, nose and throat
- Child pulling at their ears (middle ear infection)
- Difficulty in swallowing (tonsillitis or epiglottitis)
- Offensive odour breath (bacterial infection)
- Nasal secretions, bleeding

Family history
- Family history of respiratory problems (asthma, cystic fibrosis)
- Asthma, eczema, hay fever in close relative (atopy)
- Any smokers or pet animals in household?
- Travel to area of high tuberculosis prevalence, or contact with infected relative?

Paediatrics at a Glance, Fourth Edition. Lawrence Miall, Mary Rudolf and Dominic Smith. © 2016 John Wiley & Sons, Ltd. Published 2016 by John Wiley & Sons, Ltd.
Companion website: www.ataglanceseries.com/paediatrics

Cardiovascular system

▶ Observation

- Is there central cyanosis? Peripheral cyanosis can be normal in young babies and those with cold peripheries
- If the child is breathless, pale or sweating this may indicate heart failure
- Is there finger clubbing?—cyanotic heart disease
- Is there failure to thrive?—suggests heart failure

Palpation

- Feel apex beat (position and character), reflects left ventricular function
- Feel for right ventricular heave over sternum (pulmonary hypertension)
- Feel for thrills (palpable murmurs)
- Hepatomegaly suggests heart failure. Peripheral oedema and raised JVP are rarely seen in children

▶ Auscultation

- On the basis of the child's age, pulse, colour and signs of failure try to think what heart lesion may be likely, then confirm this by auscultation
- Listen for murmurs over the valve areas and the back (see Chapter 23). Diastolic murmurs are always pathological
- Listen to the heart sounds: are they normal, increased (pulmonary hypertension), fixed and split (ASD) or are there added sounds (gallop rhythm in heart failure or ejection click in aortic stenosis)?

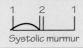

Systolic murmur

Age	Systolic BP (mmHg)
<1	70–90
1–2	80–95
2–5	80–100
5–12	90–110
>12	100–120

Circulation

- Measure blood pressure with age-appropriate cuff, which should cover 2/3 of the upper arm
- Check capillary refill time (CRT) by pressing on the skin for 5 seconds—the time taken for the blanching to fade is the CRT. Normal is ≤2 s. A prolonged CRT >2 s may be a sign of shock. If the child is in a cold room peripheral CRT may be delayed, so always check centrally (e.g. over the sternum)

Pulse

- Rate: fast, slow or normal?

Age (years)	Normal pulse (beats/min)
<1	110–160
2–5	95–140
5–12	80–120
>12	60–100

- Rhythm: regular or irregular? Occasional ventricular ectopic beats are normal in children
- Volume: full or thready (shock)
- Character: collapsing pulse is most commonly due to patent arterial duct. Slow rising pulse suggests left ventricular outflow tract obstruction
- Always check femoral pulses in infants—coarctation of the aorta leads to reduced or delayed femoral pulses

KEY QUESTIONS FROM THE HISTORY

Breathlessness
- Breathing difficulties without signs of acute infection (consider cardiac disease)

Exercise
- Exercise limited by shortness of breath, palpitations or chest pain
- Competitive sports—rarely these may need to be limited with some cardiac defects

Colour change
- Cyanosis—central (tongue) or peripheral (hands and feet)
- Pale and sweaty, poor perfusion (sign of cardiac failure or an arrhythmia)

Growth
- Feeding problems in babies (breathlessness impairs feeding)
- Poor weight gain on growth chart

Syncope
- Unexplained collapse or fainting
- Collapse linked with exercise
- Palpitations
- Ask the parents to demonstrate rate/rhythm by tapping with their hand

Murmurs
- Previously noted heart murmur (physiological flow murmurs sometimes audible only at times of illness or after exercise)

Family history
- Family history of congenital heart disease
- Sudden death in early adulthood (congenital cardiomyopathy)

Medical condition associated with cardiovascular problems
- Genetic syndromes involving structural heart defects (e.g. Down's, Turner's or Marfan's syndromes)
- Renal problems (hypertension)
- Chemotherapy (some drugs cardiotoxic)

Abdominal system and nutritional status

Observation
- Make sure the child is relaxed
  - small children can be examined on a parent's lap, older children should lie on bed or couch
- Assess nutritional status
  - body mass index or mid-upper arm circumference
- Jaundice—yellow colour at skin and sclerae
- Pale if anaemic, most noticeable at palmar creases and conjunctivae
- Abdominal distension or oedema
- Wasting of buttocks (coeliac disease)

Palpation
- Check whether there is any pain before palpating
- Examiner should warm hands and get down to child's level
- Palpate 4 quadrants gently, check for tenderness
- Deeper palpation for organomegaly spleen, liver, kidneys
- Feel for any other masses, any palpable faecal loading in colon

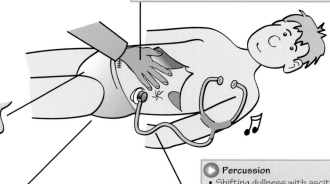

Genitalia and anus
- Intimate examination should not be performed without senior staff supervision and chaperone
- Examine boys for hypospadias, undescended testes, hydrocoele, hernia

Percussion
- Shifting dullness with ascites
- Tympanic percussion with gaseous distension

Rectal examination
- This is very rarely indicated, but examine the anus for fissures or trauma

Auscultation
- Increased bowel sounds in obstruction
- Reduced in ileus

KEY QUESTIONS FROM THE HISTORY

Nutrition
- Infant feeding pattern—duration of breastfeeding
- Note any breastfeeding problems
- Is there a key professional to give support to breastfeeding?
- If formula milk fed, review type and volume (note: 1 fluid ounce = 28 mL)
- Review intake—typical infant intake is 100–150 mL/kg in 24 hours
- Age at weaning on to semi-solids, any choking problems, foods taken
- Detail what the child eats in a typical day
- Review calorie intake and nutritional balance
- Level of appetite, any difficult feeding behaviours
- Pattern of weight gain
- Review the parent-held health record (UK Red Book) growth pattern

Vomiting
- Vomiting frequency, colour
- Green vomit in infancy suggests bile (gastrointestinal obstruction)
- Posseting (small vomits of milk in mouth) in infancy suggests gastro-oesophageal reflux
- Blood in vomit in infancy suggests maternal blood swallowed with breastfeeding
- Blood in vomit in older children suggests oesophageal bleeding due to vomiting

Bowel habit
- Faeces—frequency, consistency, colour, any mucus, blood, greasy faeces
- Diarrhoea—frequency, consistency, urgency, blood, link with diet
- In newborn, meconium should be passed in first 24 hours after birth
- Age of potty training (child develops awareness and can control bowel movement to use potty)
- Constipation—straining, pain, reduced frequency, hard faeces
- Soiling of faeces in underwear (seen with overflow in constipation)
- Encopresis (behavioural problem of passing faeces in inappropriate place)

Pain
- Abdominal pain—site, radiation, chronology, nature, exacerbating and relieving factors

Family history
- Family history of liver, kidney, bowel disease

Genito-urinary symptoms
- Urinary frequency, dysuria, haematuria
- Enuresis (childhood urinary incontinence) by day and night
- Age at menarche, cycle frequency, regularity
- Menstrual bleeding flow, duration, pain symptoms

Neurological assessment

Observation

Conscious level

- AVPU scale = Alert/responds to voice/responds to pain/unresponsive
- Glasgow coma scale

General observations

- Posture, movement and gait
- Limb deformity, contractures, hypertonicity
- Postural abnormalities in cerebral palsy:
  – diplegia, hemiplegia, quadriplegia
  – choreoathetoid movement
- Growth and head circumference
- Skin signs linked with neurological disorders (pigmentation, vascular birth marks)
- Dysmorphic features
- Equipment to aid neurological problems (e.g. hearing aid, limb splints, Pedro boots)

▶ Tone

- Hypotonia suggests LMN lesion
- Spasticity suggests UMN lesion and is seen in cerebral palsy, especially in thigh adductors and calf muscles (may cause toe walking)

Power

- Describe in upper and lower limbs
- Describe whether movement is possible against resistance or against gravity

Peripheral exam

- Limbs—tone, power, coordination, muscle bulk, reflexes
- Gait (diplegia, hemiplegia, ataxia)
- Examine shoes for signs of unequal wear
- Sensation

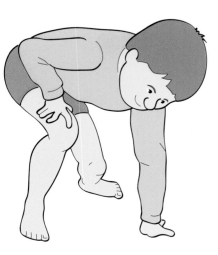

▶ Cranial nerves

- Examine as in adults
- Drooping mouth or expressionless face may be a sign of myopathy (e.g. myotonic dystrophy)

Facial exam

- Cranial nerves
- Eye exam, pupil reactions and fundoscopy

▶ Coordination

- Finger–nose test and heel–shin test, and observe gait
  – Very important if considering CNS tumours as cerebellar signs are common

Developmental exam

- Part of complete neurological exam in children
  See Chapter 4

Reflexes

- Assess at knee, ankle, biceps, triceps and supinator tendons
- Clonus may be seen in UMN lesions
- Plantar reflex is upwards until 8 months of age, then downwards

---

KEY QUESTIONS FROM THE HISTORY

- Problems during pregnancy or neonatal period
- Review development:
  – loss of developmental milestone skills (regression, a sign of serious problems)
  – pattern of delay—global or limited (e.g. isolated speech and language delay)
- Headache symptoms
- Early morning vomiting (raised intracranial pressure)
- Involuntary movement, convulsion, unexplained collapse, altered consciousness level
- Sensory symptoms
- Urinary and faecal continence
- Hearing or vision problems, squint
- School performance
- Behaviour, mood, empathy, concentration
- Coordination, clumsiness, gait problems
- Function—how is the child limited by any neurological impairment?
- Home environment—any adaptations to assist care?
- Extra support received:
  – who assists with care of the child?
  – respite to parents
  – financial support to assist with care and mobility
- Family history of neurological problems:
  – epilepsy, blindness, deafness, learning difficulty, genetic disorder

▶ The visual system

Observation of eyes
- Look at the iris, sclera and pupil
- Check pupils are equal and react to light, both directly and indirectly
- Look for red reflex to exclude cataract, especially in the newborn
- Look at reflection of light on the cornea—is it symmetrical or is one eye squinting? (see box opposite)
- Look at the inner epicanthic folds—if very prominent they may cause a pseudosquint

Normal symmetrical light reflex

Pseudosquint due to prominent inner epicanthic folds

Visual acuity
- Does the child fix and follow an object through 180 degrees?
- Can they see small objects (e.g. hundreds and thousands, small rolling Stycar balls)
- Older children can perform a modified Snellen chart with objects

Left convergent squint
—note asymmetrical light reflex

Ocular movements and visual fields
- Test full range of movements, looking for paralytic muscle or nerve lesions
- Look for and describe any nystagmus
- Check visual fields by using a 'wiggling' finger

When the good eye is covered the squinting eye straightens (fixates)

Assessment of a squint
- Any squint in an infant beyond the age of 6 weeks needs referral to an ophthalmologist. A squinting eye that is left untreated may cause amblyopia (cortical blindness) on that side
- Some 'latent' squints are present only when the child is tired; the history is important
- Check the corneal light reflex at different angles of gaze
- Check ocular movements—is there a fixed angle between the eyes or a paralytic squint, where the squint increases with eye movement?
- Check visual acuity
- Perform fundoscopy and red reflex
- Perform the **cover test** by asking the child to fix on an object. Cover the 'good' eye and watch the squinting eye flick to fix on the object. Latent squints may also become apparent when that eye is covered
- Divergent squints are usually more pathological

Fundoscopy
- An essential but difficult skill—practise on every child you see!
- Look at the anterior chamber of the eye Cloudiness of the cornea suggests a cataract
- Examine the red reflex by looking through the ophthalmoscope held at a distance from the patient's eye. If the red reflex is absent this suggests cataract. A white reflex is suggestive of retinoblastoma
- Complete the examination by carefully examining the optic disc and retina

▶ Neurological examination in infants

Young children cannot cooperate with a formal neurological examination so observation becomes more important: watch what the child is doing while you play with them

- How does the infant move spontaneously? Reduced movement suggests muscle weakness
- What position are they lying in? A severely hypotonic baby adopts a 'frog's leg' position (see below)
- Palpate anterior fontanelle to assess intracranial pressure and check head circumference
- Assess tone by posture and handling: a very floppy hypotonic baby tends to slip through your hands like a rag doll. Put your hand under the abdomen and lift the baby up in the ventral position: a hypotonic infant will droop over your hand. Pull the baby to sit by holding the baby's arms: observe the degree of head lag. Hypertonia is suggested by resistance to passive extension of the limbs and by scissoring (crossing-over) of the lower limbs when the infant is lifted up (see below)

Moro reflex	Symmetrical abduction and then adduction of the arms when the baby's head is dropped back quickly into your hand (see below). Usually disappears by 4 months
Palmar grasp	Stroking the palm causes hand to grasp. Usually disappears by 3 months
Asymmetrical tonic neck reflex	When the head is turned to one side the baby extends the arm on that side and flexes the contralateral arm ('fencing posture', see below). Disappears by 6–7 months

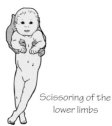

Scissoring of the lower limbs

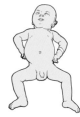

'Frog's leg' position

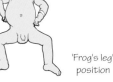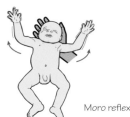

Moro reflex

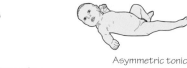

Asymmetric tonic neck reflex

Musculoskeletal system

Individual joint problems are discussed in Chapters 46 and 47

Observation
- Growth
- Joint inflammation
  - swelling, redness, heat, pain
- Limp or other functional impairment
- Signs of diagnosis linked to musculoskeletal problems
  - neurological (e.g. cerebral palsy, spina bifida)
  - genetic (e.g. neurofibromatosis, Marfan's syndrome)
- Skin signs (e.g. Henoch-Schönlein purpura, dermatomyositis)
- Skeletal deformity (e.g. spinal scoliosis)
- Ligamentous hyperlaxity

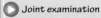 Joint examination
- Compare 2 sides
- Palpate all joints for swelling (effusion) and heat
- Test range of movement for all joints
- Observe for any pain during movement
- Examine for hip stability in newborn
- Check lengths are equal

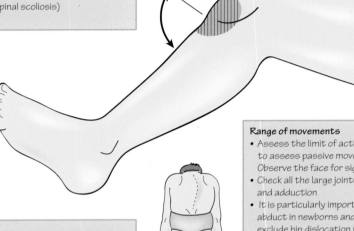

Range of movements
- Assess the limit of active movements, then move the child's limb to assess passive movements.
  Observe the face for signs of pain, and stop before this occurs
- Check all the large joints in flexion, extension, rotation, abduction and adduction
- It is particularly important to check that the hip joints fully abduct in newborns and in children with cerebral palsy in order to exclude hip dislocation (see Chapter 45)

Scoliosis
- Observe the child standing—is there any asymmetry?
- Ask the child to flex their spine to touch their toes—scoliosis causes chest asymmetry with this movement
- Scoliosis can be part of a syndromic diagnosis or develop spontaneously through childhood or adolescence

Gait analysis
- Some centres use video gait analysis to measure gait anomalies and response to treatment (e.g. following botulinum toxin injections to leg muscles to reduce hypertonicity in cerebral palsy)

KEY QUESTIONS FROM THE HISTORY

Newborn
- Risk factors for congenital hip dysplasia—female gender, breech, family history

Older children
- Inflammation—joint pain, swelling, heat, restricted movement
- Limitation to activities (sports, walking distance)

- Gait problems:
  - limp with pain, hemiplegia
  - waddling gait with diplegia, muscle weakness, congenital dislocation of the hip
  - tip-toe walking—often behavioural but may also be a sign of diplegic cerebral palsy
- Fever or skin rash (autoimmune disorders, septic arthritis)

4 Development and developmental assessment

- Parents are usually concerned if development is delayed but may not be aware of normal milestones so development should be reviewed by a trained health professional at critical stages in preschool years and at other health contacts such as attendance for immunization
- Development is an important indicator of a child's wellbeing. Delay or abnormal development may have serious consequences for later life
- Development problems can be a strong indicator of significant condition such as genetic disorder, structural neuroanatomical malformation or inborn error of metabolism

Tips on performing a developmental assessment
- Young children will not often immediately cooperate so use early opportunities to observe them informally
- You may have to rely heavily on parental report but, whenever possible, verify this through observation and testing with the child
- It is hard to remember all the milestones, so make sure you learn the essential points for key ages.
- Present the tasks one at a time
- Correct for prematurity until the child is 2 years old
- Measure milestones against a validated score, e.g. schedule of growing skills
- Define any delay as global or specific to a limited number of developmental areas, e.g. isolated speech and language delay
- Repeat assessments over months to measure the rate of development of new skills

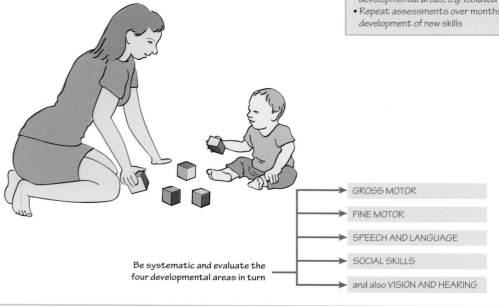

Be systematic and evaluate the four developmental areas in turn

| GROSS MOTOR |
| FINE MOTOR |
| SPEECH AND LANGUAGE |
| SOCIAL SKILLS |
| and also VISION AND HEARING |

Standing and walking

6 months
Stands with support

7–10 months
Crawling/ bottom shuffling

10 months
Pulls to standing and stands holding on

12 months
Stands, and walks with one hand held

15 months
Walks independently and stoops to pick up objects

Gross motor development

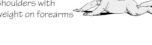

Prone position

Birth
Generally flexed posture

6 weeks
Pelvis flatter

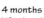

4 months
Lifts head and shoulders with weight on forearms

6 months
Arms extended supporting chest off couch

Pull to sit

Birth
Complete head lag

6 weeks
Head control developing

4 months
No head lag

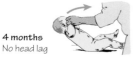

Sitting

6 weeks
Curved back, needs support from adult

6–7 months
Sits with self-propping

9 months
Gets into sitting position alone

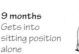
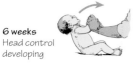

Paediatrics at a Glance, Fourth Edition. Lawrence Miall, Mary Rudolf and Dominic Smith. © 2016 John Wiley & Sons, Ltd. Published 2016 by John Wiley & Sons, Ltd.
Companion website: www.ataglanceseries.com/paediatrics

Fine motor development

Grasping and reaching

4 months
Holds a rattle and shakes purposefully

5 months
Reaches for object

 6 months
Transfers object from hand to hand

7 months
Finger feeds

Building bricks

12 months
Gives bricks to examiner
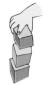

15 months
Builds a tower of two cubes

18 months
Builds a tower of three to four cubes
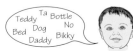

Manipulation

5 months
Whole hand grasp

 9 months
Immature pincer grasp
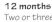

10 months
Points at bead

12 months
Mature pincer grasp

Pencil skills

18 months
Scribbles with a pencil

3 years
Draws a circle

4 years
Draws a cross

5 years
Draws a triangle
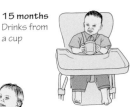

Speech and language development

Speech

3 months
Vocalizes
ooh, aah

8 months
Double babble
dada baba mama

12 months
Two or three words with meaning
Mummy

18 months
10 words
Teddy Ta Bottle Bed Dog No Daddy Bikky

24 months
Linking two words
Daddy gone

3 years
Full sentences, talks incessantly
Teddy goes to sleep Teddy's tired Good night Teddy
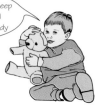

Social development

6 weeks
Smiles responsively

16 weeks
Laughing out loud

7 months
Stranger anxiety

9 months
Peek a boo, waves bye bye

15 months
Drinks from a cup
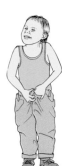

18 months
Spoon-feeding self
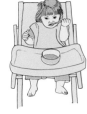

About 2½ years
(very variable)
Toilet trained by day
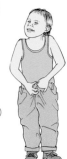

3 years
Dresses self
(except buttons)
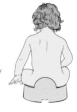

An assessment of developmental progress is important at every clinical encounter with children. It is important to understand the normal progression of development in the early years and to develop skills in examination to assess development in babies and children of different ages.

Milestones

It is hard to remember all the milestones, so learn the essential ones given in the table.

Milestones that are essential to remember

Age	Milestone
4–6 weeks	Fixes to faces with eyes
	Smiles responsively
6–7 months	Sits up unsupported
9 months	Gets to a sitting position
10 months	Pincer grasp
	Waves bye-bye
12 months	Walks unsupported
	Two or three words with meaning
18 months	Feeds self with spoon
	Points to things
	Tower of three to four cubes
	Throws a ball without falling
24 months	Sentences of two to three words
	Running
	Kicks a ball

Developmental warning signs

There is a wide variation in the age at which milestones are met. Key warning signs of significant developmental problems are listed in the following table.

Key developmental warning signs

Age	Warning sign
At any age	Maternal concern
	Regression in previously acquired skills
10 weeks	No smiling
6 months	Persistent primitive reflexes
	Persistent squint
	Hand preference
	Little interest in people, toys and noises
10–12 months	No sitting
	No double-syllable babble
	No pincer grasp
	Not chewing
18 months	Not walking independently
	Less than six words
	Persistent mouthing and drooling
2.5 years	No two- to three-word sentences
	Not responding to one-word commands
	Not turning single pages
	No symbolic play
4 years	Unintelligible speech

KEY POINTS

- Develop your examination skills by assessing the development of any preschool child you encounter.
- Correct for prematurity, but remember premature babies are at increased risk of developmental delay.
- Early recognition aids diagnosis of underlying disorders and allows the child to access targeted developmental therapy.
- See Chapter 41 for causes of delayed development.

5 Growth and puberty

Growth

Accurate measurement of growth is a vital part of the assessment of children. In order to interpret a child's growth, measurements must be plotted on a growth chart. If there is concern about growth, the *rate* of growth must be assessed by measuring the child on two occasions at least 4–6 months apart.

▶ Height
- Use a properly calibrated standing frame
- The child should be measured barefoot with knees straight and feet flat on the floor
- Stretch the child gently and read the measurement

Length
- The child should be measured lying down until 2 years of age
- Measuring the length of infants requires skill
- Use proper equipment and two people to hold the child

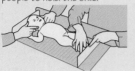

Weight
- Scales must be calibrated accurately
- Babies should be weighed naked (no nappy!)
- Older children should be weighed in underwear only

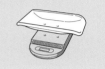

Head circumference
- Use flexible non-stretchable tape
- Obtain three successive measurements and take the largest to be the occipito frontal circumference (OFC)

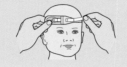

GROWTH CHART

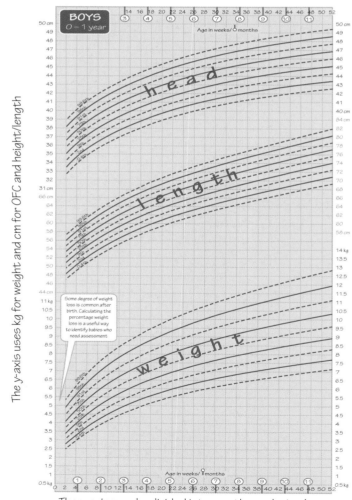

The y-axis uses kg for weight and cm for OFC and height/length

Some degree of weight loss is common after birth. Calculating the percentage weight loss is a useful way to identify babies who need assessment

The x-axis may be divided into months or decimal age

Source: WHO Growth Charts. 2010. http://www.cdc.gov/growthcharts/who_charts.htm

Plot on a growth chart

In the UK the UK-WHO charts are used for children aged 0–4 years. Charts for older children combine UK 1990 growth reference data with the WHO growth standards

- Nine equidistant centile lines are marked
- The weight centiles are splayed as the population is skewed towards being overweight
- The 50th centile is the median for the population
- A measurement on the 98th centile means only 2% of the population are taller or heavier than the child
- A measurement on the 2nd centile means that only 2% of the population are lighter or shorter than the child

Principles of plotting

- The child's measurement should be marked with a dot (not a cross or circle)
- Correct for prematurity up to the age of 1 year at least
- Height should follow one centile between 2 years and puberty
- Infants may normally cross centiles in the first year or two, but consider whether failure to thrive is a problem (see Chapter 18)
- A child's final height is expected to fall midway between the parents' centile positions

Paediatrics at a Glance, Fourth Edition. Lawrence Miall, Mary Rudolf and Dominic Smith. © 2016 John Wiley & Sons, Ltd. Published 2016 by John Wiley & Sons, Ltd.
Companion website: www.ataglanceseries.com/paediatrics

Examples of growth charts

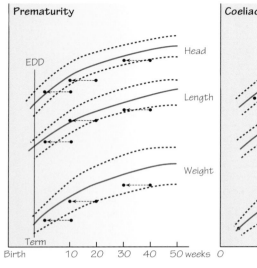

Prematurity

Head

Length

Weight

EDD

Term

Birth   10   20   30   40   50 weeks

Premature baby
- This child was born at 30 weeks gestation. He is now 40 weeks old (30 weeks corrected age). Horizontal arrows show the correction for prematurity for all three clinic visits.

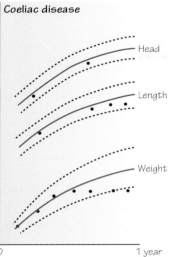

Coeliac disease

Head

Length

Weight

0   1 year

Coeliac disease
- Note fall-off in weight at time of weaning when wheat was introduced
- The fall-off in length follows later

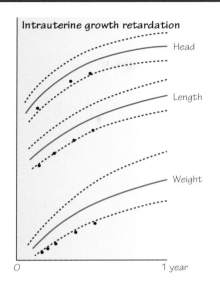

Intrauterine growth retardation

Head

Length

Weight

0   1 year

Intrauterine growth retardation (IUGR)
- Low birthweight baby
- Many IUGR babies show catch-up but this baby clearly has not, and may have reduced growth potential
- The IUGR probably started early in pregnancy because head circumference and length are also affected

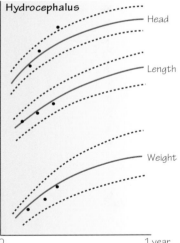

Hydrocephalus

Head

Length

Weight

0   1 year

Hydrocephalus
- The head circumference is crossing centile lines upwards
- A normal but large head would grow above but parallel to the centile lines

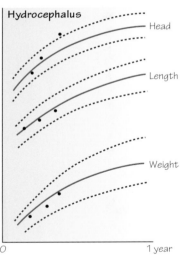

Turner's syndrome

Height

0   18 years

Turner's syndrome
- There is poor growth from a young age
- Absence of pubertal growth spurt
- The child should have been referred for growth-promoting treatment when young

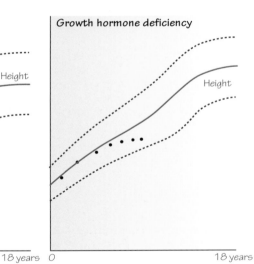

Growth hormone deficiency

Height

0   18 years

Growth hormone deficiency
- Note the fall-off in height
- GH deficiency is rare
- It can be congenital, but as growth has plateaued at the age of 6 years, pituitary deficiency due to a brain tumour must be considered
- Acquired hypothyroidism has a similar growth pattern

Puberty

Puberty is evaluated by clinical examination of the genitalia, breasts and secondary sexual characteristics. The scale used is known as Tanner staging.

Boys

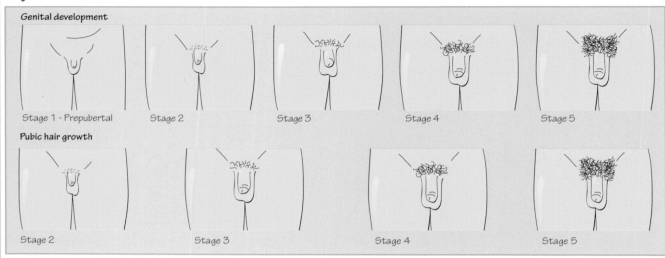

Girls

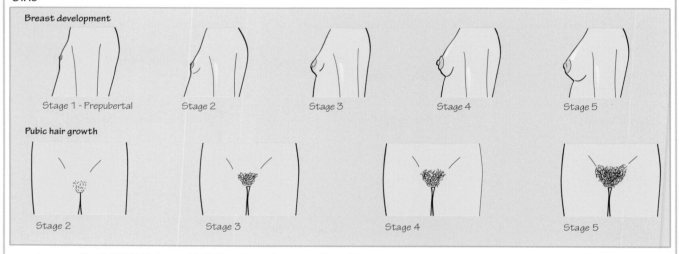

Source: Heffner, L.J. (2010) Chapter 12, *The Reproductive System at a Glance*, 3rd edition, Blackwell Publishing Ltd., Oxford.

Principles of puberty

- The first signs of puberty are usually testicular enlargement in boys, and breast budding in girls.
- Puberty is precocious if it starts before the age of 8.5 years in girls and 9.5 years in boys.
- Puberty is delayed if onset is after 13 years in girls and 14 years in boys.
- A growth spurt occurs early in puberty for girls, but at the end of puberty for boys.
- Menarche occurs at the end of puberty. Delay is defined as no periods by 16 years of age.

6 Understanding investigations

I: Haematology and Clinical Chemistry

Haematology

Normal values

Haemoglobin	110–140 g/dL
Haematocrit	30–45%
White cell count	6–15 × 10⁹/L
Reticulocytes	0–2%
Platelets	150–450 × 10⁹/L
MCV	76–88 fL
MCH	24–30 pg
ESR	10–20 mm/h

Normal values:
Haemoglobin 110–140 g/dL
White cell count $6-15 \times 10^9$/L
Platelets $150-450 \times 10^9$/L
MCV 76–88 fL

Blood film

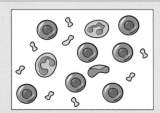

This blood film shows erythrocytes, leucocytes and platelets. The blood film can be useful to identify abnormally shaped cells (e.g. spherocytosis) or primitive cells (e.g. lymphoblasts in leukaemia). It may show pale (hypochromatic) red cells in iron deficiency

Red blood cells

- Low numbers of red cells or low haemoglobin within them represents anaemia. Too many red cells causes polycythemia red cell mass falls in the first 6 weeks of life

Coombs test

- Detects the presence of IgG antibodies bound to the surface of RBCs leading to agglutination
- Useful in the diagnosis of immune mediated haemolytic anaemia (HA) such as autoimmune HA or haemolytic disease of the newborn

Mean cell volume (MCV)

- Measures the size of RBCs
- Microcytic anaemia (MCV < 76 fL) is usually due to iron deficiency, thalassaemia trait or lead poisoning
- Macrocytosis may reflect folate deficiency

Mean cell haemoglobin (MCH)

- Reflects the amount of haemoglobin in each red cell. Is usually low (hypochromic) in iron deficiency

Flow diagram to show the investigation of anaemia

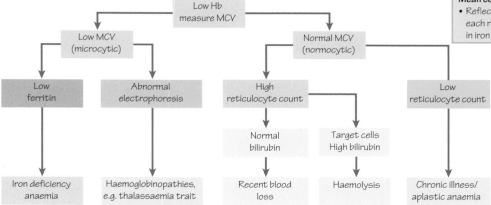

Flow diagram to show the investigation of anaemia

Low Hb measure MCV →

- Low MCV (microcytic)
  - Low ferritin → Iron deficiency anaemia
  - Abnormal electrophoresis → Haemoglobinopathies, e.g. thalassaemia trait
- Normal MCV (normocytic)
  - High reticulocyte count
    - Normal bilirubin → Recent blood loss
    - Target cells High bilirubin → Haemolysis
  - Low reticulocyte count → Chronic illness/ aplastic anaemia

Platelets

- High platelet count usually reflects bleeding or inflammation (e.g. Kawasaki disease)
- Low platelet count is commonly seen with idiopathic thrombocytopenic purpura (ITP) when there is a risk of spontaneous bruising and bleeding. In the newborn it may be low due to maternal IgG-mediated immune thrombocytopenia
- Platelets may sometimes be functionally abnormal (e.g. von Willebrand disease, Glanzmann disease or Bernard–Soulier disease) which requires further investigation

Clotting

- Prothrombin time (PT) compared with a control is used to calculate the INR: normal is 1.0. Principally assesses extrinsic pathway. Prolonged in vitamin K deficiency, liver disease and disseminated intravascular coagulation (DIC)
- Activated partial thromboplastin time (APTT) reflects the intrinsic pathway. Prolonged in heparin excess, DIC and haemophilia A
- Fibrin degradation products (FDPs) are increased in DIC
- Bleeding time: literally the time a wound bleeds for. Prolonged in von Willebrand disease and thrombocytopenia
- Specific clotting factor assays are performed in the investigation of haemophilia and other bleeding disorders

White blood cells

- Leucocytosis usually reflects infection—neutrophilia and 'left shift' (i.e. immature neutrophils) implies bacterial infection. Lymphocytosis is more common in viral infections, atypical bacterial infection and whooping cough
- Neutropenia (neutrophils < 1.0 × 10⁹/L) can occur in severe infection or due to immunosuppression. There is a high risk of spontaneous infection
- Leukaemia: There is usually a very high (or occasionally low) WCC with blast cells seen. Bone marrow aspirate is required (see Chapter 52)

Paediatrics at a Glance, Fourth Edition. Lawrence Miall, Mary Rudolf and Dominic Smith. © 2016 John Wiley & Sons, Ltd. Published 2016 by John Wiley & Sons, Ltd.
Companion website: www.ataglanceseries.com/paediatrics

Interpretation of blood gases

The acidity of the blood is measured by pH. Ideally blood gases should be measured on an arterial sample, but in babies capillary samples are sometimes used, which makes the PO_2 unreliable. A high pH refers to an alkalosis and a low pH to an acidosis. The pH is a logarithmic scale, so a small change in pH can represent a large change in hydrogen ion concentration. Once the blood becomes profoundly acidotic (pH < 7.0), normal cellular function becomes impossible. There are metabolic and respiratory causes of both acidosis and alkalosis (see below). The pattern pH and PCO_2 can be used to determine the type of abnormality.

Metabolic acidosis
- Severe gastroenteritis
- Perinatal asphyxia (build-up of lactic acid)
- Shock
- Diabetic ketoacidosis
- Inborn errors of metabolism
- Loss of bicarbonate (renal tubular acidosis)

Respiratory acidosis
- Respiratory failure and underventilation

Metabolic alkalosis
- Usually due to vomiting, e.g. pyloric stenosis

Respiratory alkalosis
- Hyperventilation (e.g. anxiety)
- Salicylate poisoning: causes initial hyperventilation and then metabolic acidosis due to acid load

$$CO_2 + H_2O \rightleftharpoons H_2CO_3 \rightleftharpoons H^+ + HCO_3^-$$

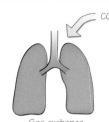

Control of acid–base balance

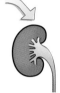

Gas exchange   Renal adaptation

Compensation can occur by the kidneys, which can vary the amount of bicarbonate excreted. A persistent respiratory acidosis will lead to retention of bicarbonate ions to buffer the acid produced by CO_2 retention. Hence, a **compensated respiratory acidosis** will have a low–normal pH, a high PCO_2 and a very high bicarbonate level

Normal arterial blood gas values

pH	7.35 – 7.42
PCO_2	4.0 – 5.5 kPa
PO_2	11 – 14 kPa (children)
	8 – 10 kPa (neonatal period)
HCO_3^-	17 – 27 mmol/L

Determining the type of blood gas abnormality (N = normal)

	pH	PCO_2	PO_2	HCO_3^-
Metabolic acidosis	Low	N	N	Low
Respiratory acidosis	Low	High	N/low	N
Metabolic alkalosis	High	N	N	High
Respiratory alkalosis	High	Low	N/high	N
Compensated respiratory acidosis	N	High	N	High

Electrolytes and clinical chemistry

Normal ranges

Sodium	135 – 145	mmol/L
Potassium	3.5 – 5.0	mmol/L
Chloride	96 – 110	mmol/L
Bicarbonate	17 – 27	mmol/L
Creatinine	20 – 80	µmol/L
Urea	2.5 – 6.5	mmol/L
Glucose	3.0 – 6.0	mmol/L
Calcium	2.15 – 2.70	mmol/L

Characteristic patterns of serum electrolyte abnormality sometimes suggest particular diagnoses:
- **Pyloric stenosis:**
  There is often a metabolic alkalosis, a low chloride and low potassium concentration (due to repeated vomiting and loss of stomach acid) and a low sodium concentration
- **Diabetic ketoacidosis:**
  There is a metabolic acidosis with a very low bicarbonate, a high potassium, high urea and creatinine and a very high glucose concentration
- **Gastroenteritis:**
  Urea concentration is high, but the sodium may be either high or low depending on the sodium content of the diarrhoea, and on the type of rehydration fluid that has been administered

Causes of abnormal sodium balance

Hypernatraemia (Na+ >145 mmo/L)
- Dehydration – fluid deprivation or diarrhoea
- Excessive sodium intake
  - inappropriate formula feed preparation
  - deliberate salt poisoning (very rare)

Hyponatraemia (Na <135 mmol/L)
- Sodium loss
  - diarrhoea (especially if replacement fluids hypotonic)
  - renal loss (renal failure)
  - cystic fibrosis (loss in sweat)
- Water excess
  - excessive intravenous fluid administration
  - SIADH (inappropriate antidiuretic hormone secretion)

Potassium
- **Hyperkalaemia:** High potassium levels can cause serious cardiac arrhythmias and need to be controlled rapidly. Check for a wide QRS complex and peaked T waves on ECG.
  Treatment includes salbutamol infusion, insulin and dextrose infusion (to drive potassium into cells) and rectal calcium resonium
- **Causes of hyperkaleamia (>5.5 mmol/L):**
  - renal failure or sudden oliguria
  - massive haemolysis or tissue necrosis
  - congenital adrenal hyperplasia
- **Hypokalaemia (<3.5 mmol/L):** A low potassium causes muscle weakness, ileus and lethargy
- **Causes of hypokalaemia:**
  - diarrhoea and vomiting,
  - diuretic therapy,
  - inadequate intake (e.g. starvation).

Calcium
- Hypocalcaemia is commonly caused by vitamin D deficiency and can present with weakness, tetany, cardiac arrhythmias and convulsions. Congenital hypocalcaemia is caused by hypoparathyroidism in DiGeorge syndrome
- Hypercalcaemia is rare in childhood. Various types of hyperparathyroidism may be present. Congenital hypercalcaemia may be seen in Williams syndrome or subcutaneous fat necrosis

Understanding investigations II—Radiology

Features to look for on a chest radiograph

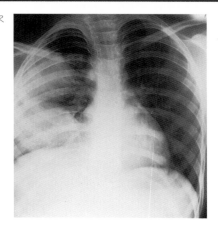

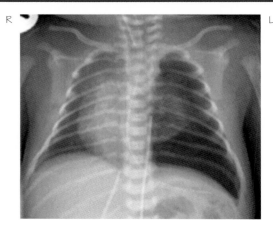

Radiograph of right middle and upper lobe pneumonia

Radiograph showing left sided tension pneumothorax with mediastinal shift to the right

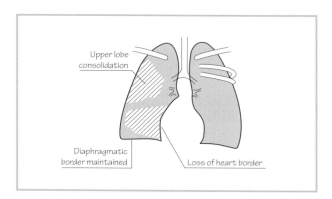

Upper lobe consolidation

Diaphragmatic border maintained

Loss of heart border

Chest radiography

As respiratory disorders are so common in paediatric practice, it is very important to be able to accurately interpret chest radiographs. If there is uncertainty, the film should be discussed with an experienced radiologist.

- Identify the patient name, date and orientation (left and right).
- Check the penetration—the vertebrae should just be visible behind the heart shadow.
- Check that the alignment is central by looking at the head of the clavicles and the shape of the ribs on each side.
- Comment on any foreign objects such as central lines.
- Examine the bony structures, looking for fractures, asymmetry and abnormalities (e.g. hemivertebrae). Rib fractures are best seen by placing the radiograph on its side.
- Check both diaphragms and costophrenic angles are clear. The right diaphragm is higher than the left because of the liver. Check there is no air beneath the diaphragm (indicates intestinal perforation).
- Look at the cardiac outline. At its widest, it should be less than half the width of the ribcage (cardiothoracic ratio < 0.5), although in infants it can be wider due to the anteroposterior way the radiograph is taken.

- Look at the mediastinum—note that in infants the thymus gland can give a 'sail'-like shadow just above the heart.
- Check lung expansion—if there is air trapping the lung fields will cover more than nine ribs posteriorly, and the heart will look long and thin.
- Examine the lung fields looking for signs of consolidation, vascular markings, abnormal masses or foreign bodies.
- Check that the lung markings extend right to the edge of the lung—if not, consider a pneumothorax (dark) or a pleural effusion (opaque).
- Consolidation may be patchy or dense lobar consolidation. A lateral radiograph may be required to determine exactly which lobe is affected. A rule of thumb is that consolidation in the right middle lobe causes loss of the right heart border shadow and right lower lobe consolidation causes loss of the right diaphragmatic shadow.
- Always look at the area 'behind' the heart shadow for infection in the lingula. If the mediastinum is pulled towards an area of opacity, consider collapse rather than consolidation as the pathology.

Magnetic resonance imaging scans

Magnetic resonance imaging (MRI) uses radio waves and powerful electromagnetic fields to obtain detailed images, which can highlight different tissues. Images can be obtained in any plane. MRI has the great advantage of being free of ionizing radiation. The scanners are often claustrophobic and can be noisy, so young children may require a general anaesthetic.

MRI is very good at delineating tissues with high water content from those with high fat content. MRI can distinguish white matter from grey matter within the brain. It is the imaging of choice for the investigation of CNS abnormalities including spinal abnormalities. Increasingly, it is being used for complex cardiac and joint imaging also. On a standard T2 weighted image, water (e.g. CSF or oedema) shows up white. On a T1-weighted image, it shows dark (Figures 6.1–6.3).

Figure 6.1 Axial T2-weighted MRI of an infant brain. The dark grey cortex is clearly distinguished from the deeper white matter (light grey). The lateral ventricles are filled with CSF. There are bilateral haemorrhages (black) within the subependyma (just outside the wall of the lateral ventricles—arrowed).

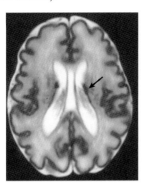

Figure 6.2 A sagittal T1-weighted image showing cerebral atrophy with increased CSF (dark) spaces around the brain. The corpus callosum, brainstem structures and cerebellum are clearly identified.

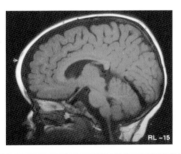

Figure 6.3 T1-weighted sagittal MRI scan showing a large optic glioma. Note the heterogeneous nature with solid and cystic areas. This tumour is characteristically associated with neurofibromatosis type 1.

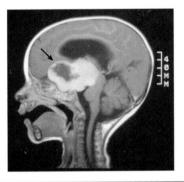

Figure 6.4 CT scan showing a large extradural haematoma secondary to a left parieto-occipital skull fracture. Note the midline shift and compression of the left lateral ventricle.

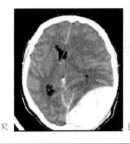

Figure 6.5 CT scan showing collapse and bronchiectasis in the right upper lobe.

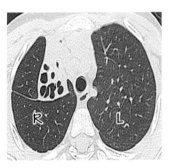

images of the abdominal and pelvic organs, and in newborn infants can be used to image the brain and the lower spinal cord. The examination is best performed in real time. Increasingly, congenital abnormalities are detected antenatally by ultrasound examination, usually performed at 18–20 weeks gestation (Figures 6.6 and 6.7).

Figure 6.6 Coronal ultrasound examination of the brain, performed in a preterm infant via the anterior fontanelle. The lateral ventricles are dilated and there is haemorrhage within the right ventricle, with a large right-sided parietal venous infarction.

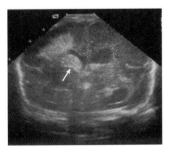

Figure 6.7 Ultrasound scan of kidney showing gross hydronephrosis.

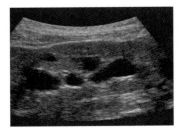

Computed tomography scans

Computed tomography (CT) scans also give axial images ('slices' through the body). They have the advantage of being significantly faster to perform than MRI scans, and the machines are quieter and less claustrophobic, so children can be scanned while awake. CT is predominant in assessing traumatic brain injury and in imaging the lungs and is particularly good at detecting acute haemorrhage. The disadvantage is there is a significant radiation exposure (Figures 6.4 and 6.5).

Ultrasound

Ultrasound is an excellent investigation for children, since it is safe and non-invasive, and the ultrasound machine can often be brought to the patient's bedside. It is used extensively to obtain

Understanding investigations III—Microbiology

Different methods are available to detect infection. Some are non-specific, such as changes in blood inflammatory markers, and others give specific information about the exact infection. Proof of infection includes direct detection (e.g. microscopy, antigen detection, PCR), detection of an antibody response (serology) or culture of an organism from a normally sterile site.

Non-specific markers of infection	
Leucocytosis	High white count ($>15 \times 10^9$/L) suggests inflammation or infection High neutrophil count suggests bacterial infection Lymphocytosis is seen in viral or some atypical bacterial infection (e.g. whooping cough)
C-reactive protein (CRP)	An acute phase protein that normally rises within 24 hours of infection
Erythrocyte sedimentation rate (ESR)	A non-specific marker of inflammation. Rarely used

Blood culture

Culture of a pure growth of a bacterium (or occasionally a fungus) from blood is usually definitive proof of infection. However, if the culture is of several different organisms, or if low pathogenic bacteria normally found on the skin (such as coagulase-negative *Staphylococci*) are isolated, then the result should be interpreted with caution. The way the blood sample is taken is crucial—the skin must be thoroughly cleaned with antiseptic and an aseptic technique used. Very small blood samples (<1 mL) reduce the chances of a positive culture. Blood cultures usually take 24–48 hours to show evidence of infection and so are usually used to confirm a clinical suspicion of infection retrospectively. Cultures will provide information about the sensitivity of the organism, which can be used to rationalize antibiotic therapy. Most modern blood culture systems are able to detect significant bacteraemia in children with a single medium, which is designed specifically for this purpose. Unusual results should always be discussed with a microbiologist.

Serological evidence of infection

Measurement of antibody response to specific infectious agents can be useful. This is important to check for prior immunity (e.g. in an at-risk child vaccinated against hepatitis B) or to confirm prior infection (e.g. cytomegalovirus (CMV)). IgG antibody tends to persist after infection, whereas IgM antibody reflects recent infection. This can be important in the newborn period for distinguishing congenital infection (e.g. syphilis) from maternal infection since IgG antibody readily crosses the placenta. Antibody responses to infection are often described as 'titres'. The titre is the reciprocal of the highest dilution of the patient's serum in which antibody was detected, e.g. a titre of 1024 means that antibody was detected in a 1:1024 dilution of serum. The higher the titre, the more the antibody is present. The anti-streptolysin-O titre (ASOT) is sometimes used as a marker of streptococcal infection in rheumatic fever.

Direct detection methods

Molecular biology techniques can now identify certain organisms, such as viruses, that have traditionally been difficult to culture. These tests can either use immunofluorescence, e.g. to identify respiratory syncytial virus (RSV) in pharyngeal secretions in a child with bronchiolitis, or polymerase chain reaction (PCR) to amplify bacterial or viral DNA using specific primers. PCR methods are available for many important paediatric infectious agents, including herpes simplex virus (HSV), *Neisseria meningitidis* groups B and C, and HIV. They are particularly useful in confirming infection after antibiotics have already been given and in detecting viral CNS infection.

Lumbar puncture and CSF analysis

Lumbar puncture is usually performed to diagnose or exclude meningitis. It should not be performed if there is evidence of raised intracranial pressure, if the child is haemodynamically unstable (e.g. septic shock) or if there is a low platelet count or coagulopathy. A fine spinal needle with a stylet is passed between the vertebral spines into the subdural space. A few drops of CSF are collected for microbiological examination and for analysis of protein and glucose concentrations. Examination of CSF includes microscopy and culture and may also include other direct detection techniques (e.g. DNA detection with PCR). Normal CSF is usually 'crystal clear'. If it is cloudy, this suggests infection or bleeding. Fresh blood that clears usually indicates a traumatic tap, but a massive intracranial haemorrhage must be considered if the CSF remains bloodstained. Old blood gives a yellow 'xanthochromic' appearance. A manometer can be used to measure the CSF pressure, though this is not routinely performed.

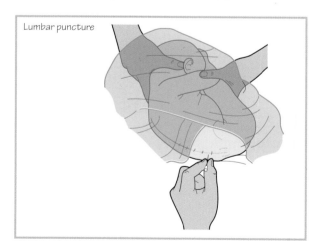

Lumbar puncture

Analysis of CSF

	Normal	Bacterial meningitis	Viral meningitis
Appearance	Crystal clear	Turbid, organisms seen	Clear
White cells	$<5/mm^3$	$\uparrow\uparrow\uparrow$ (polymorphs)	$\uparrow$ (lymphocytes)
Protein	0.15–0.4 g/L	$\uparrow\uparrow$	Normal
Glucose	>50% blood	$\downarrow$	Normal

Although these are typical CSF findings for the organisms indicated, partially treated infection and infection with specific microorganisms may result in alternative profiles. For example, meningitis caused by *Listeria monocytogenes* usually presents with a CSF lymphocytosis.

Urinalysis

Fresh urine should be collected into a sterile container from a midstream sample if possible. Urine bags applied over the genitalia may be used in infants, but often become contaminated with perineal bacteria. Catheter specimens and supra pubic aspirate are alternatives.

- Observe the urine—is it cloudy (suggests infection) or clear?
- What is the colour?—pink or red suggests haematuria from the lower urinary tract; brown ('cola'-coloured) urine suggests renal haematuria or haemolytic disease (haemoglobinuria).
- Smell the urine for ketones and for the smell of infection. Unusual-smelling urine may suggest an inborn error of metabolism.
- Test the urine using commercial dipsticks. This may reveal the following:
  - protein—infection, renal damage or nephrotic syndrome
  - glucose—diabetes
  - ketones—diabetic ketoacidosis (DKA)
  - white cells or nitrites—suggestive of infection
- These sticks are very sensitive to the presence of blood and may detect haematuria even if the urine looks clear.
- Examine the urine under the microscope for white cells, red cells, casts and the presence of organisms. A sample should also be sent for culture. A pure growth of $>10^5$ colony-forming units of a single organism and >50 white cells/mm^3 confirms infection. Infection is extremely unlikely in the absence of pyuria.

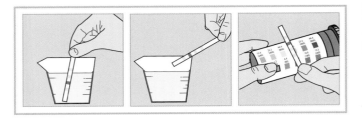

Immunology

Immunological investigations may be needed to investigate a child with suspected immunodeficiency (severe, recurrent or unusual infections—see Chapter 25) or with an autoimmune disorder such as juvenile rheumatoid arthritis (see Chapter 47) or systemic lupus erythematosus or renal disease.

Basic immunological investigations include the following:

WBC	To ascertain the total number of white blood cells including neutrophils and lymphocytes (e.g. cyclical neutropenia)
T-cell subsets	To examine the number of CD4 and CD8 T cells (e.g. HIV infection)
Immunoglobulins (IgG, IgM, IgA and IgE)	To investigate immunodeficiency with recurrent infections such as X-linked agammaglobulinaemia or severe combined immunodeficiency (SCID)
Functional antibodies	To detect specific IgG to confirm an adequate immune response to a trigger, such as *Haemophilus influenzae* immunization
Complement	May be low in certain immune-mediated kidney disorders (e.g. mesangiocapillary glomerulonephritis). Complement deficiency (e.g. C3 deficiency) is associated with recurrent infection of encapsulated organisms (e.g. *Neisseria meningitidis*)
Specific IgE antibodies	Used to investigate allergic disorders (see Chapter 57)
Specific antibody markers	Anti-tissue transglutaminase type 2 (tTGA$_2$) antibodies in coeliac disease (see Chapter 34) Antinuclear antibody (ANA) in juvenile idiopathic arthritis (see Chapter 47)

Investigations should only be requested to confirm a clinical diagnosis, or if indicated following a thorough history and examination. Sometimes, they are performed to rule out more serious but less likely conditions. Blindly performing investigations as a 'fishing' exercise in the hope of throwing up an abnormality is usually counterproductive, often leading to increased anxiety and further investigations when unexpected results are obtained.

KEY POINTS

- Before ordering an investigation, consider how the result might alter the management.
- Try to focus investigations on the differential diagnosis based on clinical assessment.
- Sometimes, investigations can be used to quickly rule out important or serious diagnoses (e.g. urine dipstix, CSF microscopy).
- Anyone who initiates a test request should ensure that the results are seen and dealt with appropriately.

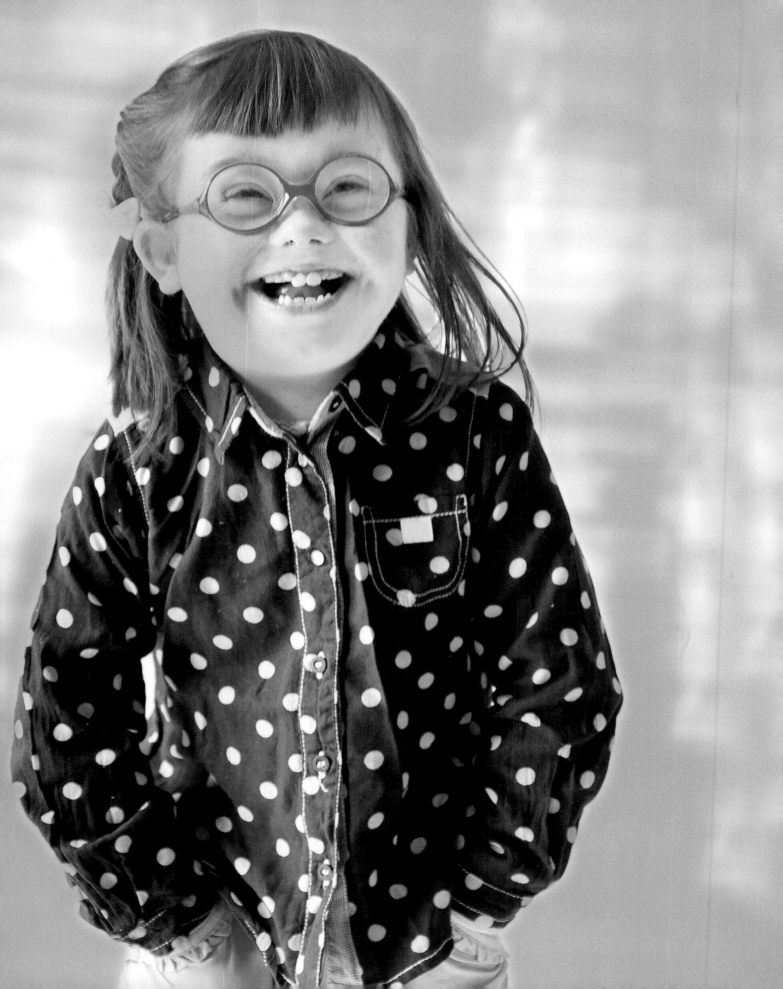

Moving through childhood

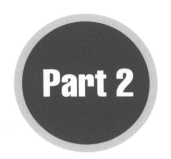

Part 2

Chapters

7 Screening

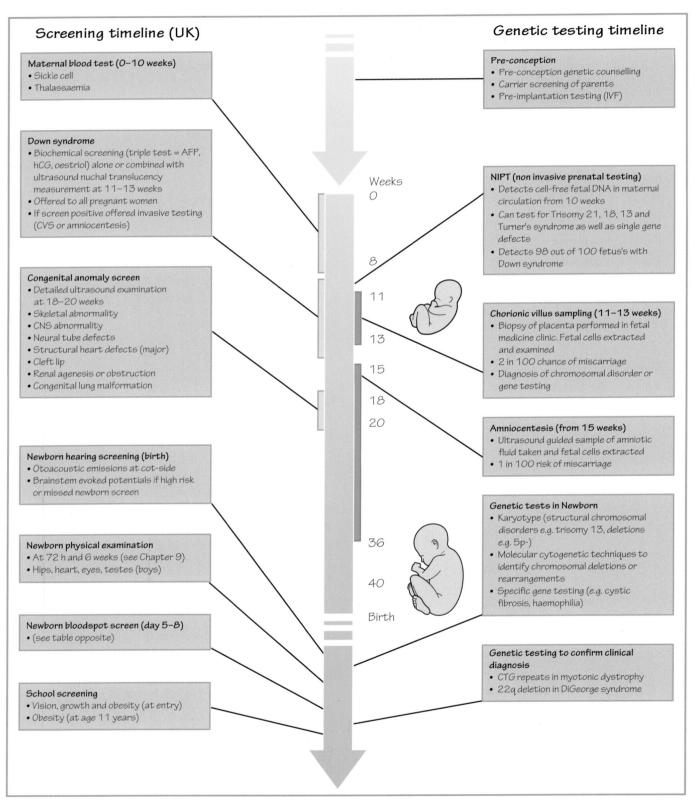

Screening timeline (UK)

Maternal blood test (0–10 weeks)
- Sickle cell
- Thalassaemia

Down syndrome
- Biochemical screening (triple test = AFP, hCG, oestriol) alone or combined with ultrasound nuchal translucency measurement at 11–13 weeks
- Offered to all pregnant women
- If screen positive offered invasive testing (CVS or amniocentesis)

Congenital anomaly screen
- Detailed ultrasound examination at 18–20 weeks
- Skeletal abnormality
- CNS abnormality
- Neural tube defects
- Structural heart defects (major)
- Cleft lip
- Renal agenesis or obstruction
- Congenital lung malformation

Newborn hearing screening (birth)
- Otoacoustic emissions at cot-side
- Brainstem evoked potentials if high risk or missed newborn screen

Newborn physical examination
- At 72 h and 6 weeks (see Chapter 9)
- Hips, heart, eyes, testes (boys)

Newborn bloodspot screen (day 5–8)
- (see table opposite)

School screening
- Vision, growth and obesity (at entry)
- Obesity (at age 11 years)

Genetic testing timeline

Pre-conception
- Pre-conception genetic counselling
- Carrier screening of parents
- Pre-implantation testing (IVF)

NIPT (non invasive prenatal testing)
- Detects cell-free fetal DNA in maternal circulation from 10 weeks
- Can test for Trisomy 21, 18, 13 and Turner's syndrome as well as single gene defects
- Detects 98 out of 100 fetus's with Down syndrome

Chorionic villus sampling (11–13 weeks)
- Biopsy of placenta performed in fetal medicine clinic. Fetal cells extracted and examined
- 2 in 100 chance of miscarriage
- Diagnosis of chromosomal disorder or gene testing

Amniocentesis (from 15 weeks)
- Ultrasound guided sample of amniotic fluid taken and fetal cells extracted
- 1 in 100 risk of miscarriage

Genetic tests in Newborn
- Karyotype (structural chromosomal disorders e.g. trisomy 13, deletions e.g. 5p-)
- Molecular cytogenetic techniques to identify chromosomal deletions or rearrangements
- Specific gene testing (e.g. cystic fibrosis, haemophilia)

Genetic testing to confirm clinical diagnosis
- CTG repeats in myotonic dystrophy
- 22q deletion in DiGeorge syndrome

Weeks
0
8
11
13
15
18
20
36
40
Birth

Screening

Screening aims to identify unrecognized disease in apparently well people. The cost must be considered and balanced against that of treatment if the problem presents later. Conditions suitable for screening should:

- Be identifiable at a latent or early symptomatic stage
- Be treatable
- Have a better prognosis if treated early.

Screening programs vary around the world. Screening of pregnant women, newborns and children in the UK is described at http://www.screening.nhs.uk/england.

Screening in pregnancy

Pregnancy is an ideal time to screen for inherited disorders and for vertically transmitted infections as the mothers are engaged with health services (often for the first time since childhood) and are usually very motivated. All pregnant women in the UK are screened at booking for syphilis and hepatitis B infection and rubella susceptibility. All are offered HIV screening, with a >98% uptake. Mothers are offered testing for sickle cell disease and thalassaemia (and other haemoglobin variants depending on ethnicity). If positive, then partners are tested and if they are also positive (or untraceable), then antenatal diagnosis of the fetus is offered. Sickle cell disease is also screened for after birth using the newborn bloodspot (see below). All pregnant women have an anomaly ultrasound scan at 18–20 weeks that is designed to detect serious malformations of the major organs. This is sometimes followed by more detailed tests such as MRI, fetal echocardiography or amniocentesis. If there is a strong family history of inherited serious disorders in the parents, then pre-conception genetic screening of embryos can be offered.

Screening for Down's syndrome

Down's syndrome affects 1 in 1000 live births (1 in 600 fetuses). There is an association with increased maternal age (1 in 880 at 30 years rising to 1 in 100 at age 40 years). 95% are due to non-disjunction during meiosis and 3% to an unbalanced translocation; 1% are mosaics, with only a proportion of cells within the body having trisomy 21. About 55% of affected fetuses are detected antenatally through screening. In those diagnosed before birth, only 5% of couples choose to continue with the pregnancy. Antenatal screening for Down's syndrome is offered to all mothers regardless of age. In the first trimester, a 'combined test' of nuchal fold thickness (subcutaneous tissue at back of the neck) and measurement of serum beta-hCG and pregnancy-associated plasma protein A (PAPP-A) is used. In the second trimester, the 'quadruple test' is offered (measurement of serum beta-hCG, alpha-fetoprotein, inhibin A and unconjugated estriol). These tests give a calculated risk, which if high may prompt diagnostic testing via chorionic villus sampling or amniocentesis. Recent studies show that cell-free fetal DNA fragments circulating in the maternal plasma can be used to detect trisomy 13, 18 and 21 with a very low (<1%) false-positive rate.

Newborn blood spot screening

Midwives collect bloodspots from the heel of every newborn baby on day 5–8 of life on to an absorbent card. Formally called the 'Guthrie card', but now the bloodspots are analysed for a variety of disorders and stored for further diagnostic tests. Disorders screened for the UK include congenital hypothyroidism, phenylketonuria (PKU), medium-chain acylcarnitine deficiency (MCAD), cystic fibrosis (CF) and sickle cell disease. From 2015, the bloodspot screening will also test for maple syrup urine disease (MSUD), isovaleric academia (IVA), glutaric aciduria type I (GA1)

Newborn heel prick test (in the UK)

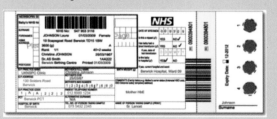

Congenital hypothyroidism	Screen detects high TSH level but will miss hypothyroidism secondary to pituitary dysfunction. Thyroid replacement allows normal development
Sickle cell disease	Universal screening to all pregnant women aims to identify at-risk couples. Newborn bloodspots are analysed by High-Performance Liquid Chromatography for all sickle cell variants
Phenylketonuria (PKU)	A phenylalanine assay has replaced the original 'Guthrie' test. Babies PKU need urgent advice on starting a low-phenylalanine diet and long-term follow-up to prevent learning disability from phenylalanine metabolites
Cystic fibrosis (CF)	A high immunoreactive trypsin (IRT) on the newborn blood spot is followed up with DNA testing for common CF mutations
Medium-chain acylcarnitine deficiency (MCAD)	A fatty acid oxidation defect that can lead to significant hypoglycaemia during periods of illness. Acylcarnitine abnormalities can be detected by tandem mass spectrometry. MCAD is a preventable cause of sudden death in infancy. Frequent feeds prevent the need for breakdown of fatty acids
MSUD, IVA, GA1 and HCU	These four additional metabolic disorders will be screened for in the UK from 2015

and homocystinuria (HCU). In very premature babies, the test should be repeated at 28 days of life, and in sick neonates, it is important to obtain at least one additional blood spot prior to any blood transfusions.

Newborn hearing screening

All newborn babies in the UK now receive a hearing test, prior to discharge or within the first few days of life. This test uses a small probe placed in the ear to detect otoacoustic emissions—vibrations from the cochlear in the inner ear which show that the pathway between the external auditory meatus and the cochlear is intact. In equivocal cases, brainstem evoked responses to sounds are also measured. This screening program has dramatically reduced the age at which congenitally deaf children receive hearing aids, allowing them to hear at a critical phase of their language development. Cochlear implants are implanted in children whose hearing is not amenable to external aids.

Newborn infant physical examination (NIPE)

This examination, conducted within the first 72 hours of life and repeated at 8 weeks, aims to screen for congenital heart disease (CHD), developmental dysplasia of the hip, congenital cataract and (in boys) undescended testes. Oxygen saturation screening for CHD is also undertaken in some areas. NIPE is described in Chapter 13.

Screening in later childhood

The child health screening program continues in the community in the pre-school and school years. In the UK, this includes tests of vision and monitoring of height (for growth disorders) at school entry and BMI (for obesity) at primary school entry and exit.

8 Genetics and inherited disorders

Patterns of genetic inheritance

Our genes control most aspects of our organ development and it is not surprising that if mutations or deletions occur in our genome these can lead to the development of diseases or to changes in our appearance (phenotype). Many disorders are due to an interaction between genes and the environment or between several different genes (polygenic inheritance). Epigenetics refers to changes in gene expression due to chemical interactions (e.g. methylation of DNA) which do not actually change the genome sequence. Other genetic disorders are due to a single gene defect such as a change in one of the nucleotide base pairs in the DNA and these are often inherited in predictable patterns such as autosomal recessive and dominant. Some genetic disorders are due to errors in the mitochondrial DNA. Some are due to large scale changes in the chromosomes such as duplications (triploidy), deletions or translocations.

Polygenic (multifactorial) disorders

- Due to abnormalities in several different genes and environmental factors
- Incidence can be higher in certain populations or cluster in families, but do not show a clear pattern of inheritance
- The chance of recurrence depends on how many genes the child shares with the affected person- ie how closely related to them they are. Cousins will have a lower recurrence risk than siblings
- Examples include diabetes mellitus, neural tube defects (see below), developmental dysplasia of the hip and schizophrenia

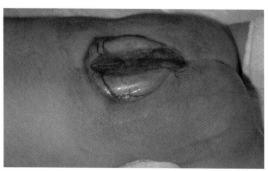

Myelomeningocele (neural tube defect)

Source : Photograph courtesy of Mr Paul Chumas.

X-linked recessive

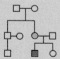

- Due to mutations in genes on the X chromosome
- Males are generally affected, females are usually carriers and can occasionally be affected. Inheritance cannot occur
- Examples include Haemophilia, Colour blindness, Duchenne muscular dystrophy

X-linked dominant

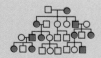

- Due to mutation of genes on X chromosome
- Females are more frequently affected than males (often lethal in males as no normal allele to counterbalance)
- Often both males and females affected in one generation
- Examples include Fragile X syndrome, incontinentia pigmenti, Rett's syndrome

Autosomal dominant (AD)

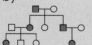

- Only one copy of the abnormal gene is needed to express the disorder
- Usually there will be someone affected in every generation although many AD conditions are 'new mutations'
- On average 1 in 2 of the children of an affected person will inherit the disorder
- Examples include neurofibromatosis (NF1) and hereditary spherocytosis

Autosomal recessive (AR)

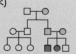

- To express the disorder two copies of the abnormal gene required (homozygous).
- If you have one normal copy and one abnormal copy of the gene (heterozygote) you are a carrier.
- If two carriers of the same gene defect have children, there is a 1 in 4 chance of each child being affected. There is a 1 in 2 chance of each child being a carrier.
- Examples include cystic fibrosis, sickle cell disease and congenital adrenal hyperplasia.
- Sometimes an affected person can inherit two different mutations of the same gene—compound heterozygote. This can occur in some people with cystic fibrosis

Co-dominant inheritance

- Two different versions of a gene can be expressed. Both alleles contribute to the phenotype
- Examples include blood group antigens-For example if father is blood group A (carries A and O alleles) and mother is blood group B (carried B and O allele) then 1 in 4 of their children will be blood group AB (codominant), with both A and B antigens expressed on their red cells. On average one child will be blood group O (OO), one A (AO) and one B (BO)

Mitochondrial inheritance

- Mitochondria within the egg cells contain a small amount of DNA that can sometimes contain mutations
- Affected mothers can pass on mitochondrial disorders to their children (males and females) but affected fathers cannot pass it on to their children
- Phenotype can vary as each egg cell contains variable amounts of the abnormal mitochondrial DNA
- Examples include mitochondrial myopathies, diabetes insipidus with deafness and some forms of optic atrophy

Paediatrics at a Glance, Fourth Edition. Lawrence Miall, Mary Rudolf and Dominic Smith. © 2016 John Wiley & Sons, Ltd. Published 2016 by John Wiley & Sons, Ltd.
Companion website: www.ataglanceseries.com/paediatrics

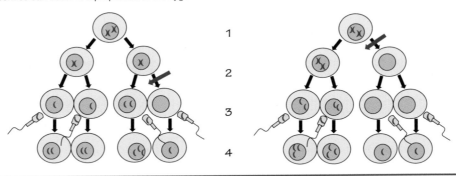

Figure 8.1 Non-dysjunction trisomy occurring at first meiosis (green arrow) or second meiosis (blue arrow) in oocyte gamete production. With fertilization (stage 4) trisomies can occur in a proportion of the zygotes.

Unusual patterns of inheritance

Imprinting: Certain genetic disorders show a phenomenon called imprinting—where the expression of the allele depends on which parent it is inherited from. For example, in Angelman's syndrome, the abnormal deleted genes are on the maternally derived chromosome 15, but the normal paternal copy is imprinted (silenced) and so the child develops features of the disease including neurodegenerative disease, seizures, hand-flapping and an unusually happy demeanour. The same genetic material, if deleted from the paternal chromosome 15, with the maternal genes imprinted, leads to Prader–Willi syndrome, with neonatal hypotonia and feeding difficulties, developmental delay and later onset obesity and delayed sexual development.

In Beckwith–Wiedermann syndrome (neonatal hyperinsulinism, macroglossia and macrosomia), there is often **uniparental disomy** of Chromosome 11, with the maternally derived chromosome 11 replaced with an extra paternal copy. This leads to abnormal expression of IGF2 (insulin like growth factor) gene. About 85% of Beckwith–Wiedermann cases are sporadic.

Some autosomal dominant disorders such as congenital myotonic dystrophy (type 1) show a phenomenon called **genetic anticipation**. That is, the disease tends to present earlier, or with a more severe phenotype, in each successive generation. In the case of myotonic dystrophy, this is due to increasing numbers of abnormal CTG base triplet repeats in a gene on chromosome 19. Many hundreds of repeats of this sequence can be found.

Chromosomal disorders

Chromosomal disorders are usually sporadic due to non-disjunction of chromosomes during the first or second meiosis (trisomy 21, 18 or 13) of gamete formation (Figure 8.1). This means there are two copies of a chromosome in some eggs and with a third from the sperm triploidy results. Triploidy of the larger chromosomes is usually lethal but 13, 18 and 21 can survive. Chromosome 21 is actually the smallest chromosome (number 22 was mislabelled!) and so there is less disruption of genetic material and people with trisomy 21 (Down syndrome) can survive into adulthood. The extra chromosome is seen in a karyotype test (Figure 8.2). Trisomies are more common with advanced maternal age. As well as occurring by non-dysjunction, trisomy can occur due to a 'balanced translocation', where material from one chromosome is attached to another, so that with fertilization an

Figure 8.2 Karyotype showing 47, XY + 21 (trisomy 21).

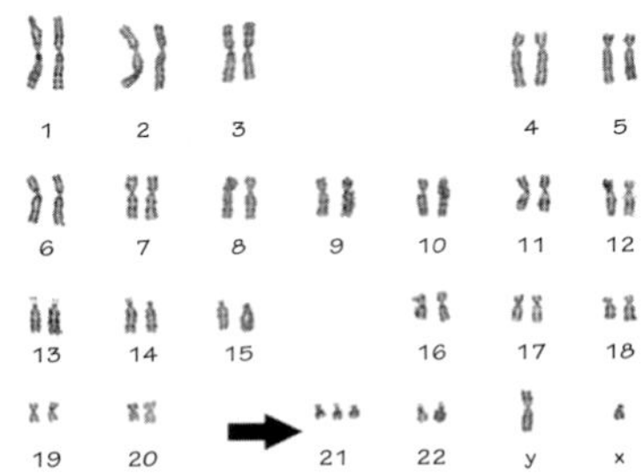

embryo can end up with three copies of the same part of one of the chromosomes. This can be inherited and so if found it is important to check parental karyotype also.

Chromosomal disorders can also be due to deletion of an entire chromosome—e.g. loss of an X chromosome leads to 45 XO (Turner's syndrome) with short stature, webbed neck, as risk of coarctation of the aorta and infertility due to ovarian dysgenesis. Other sex chromosome anomalies include 47XXY (Klinefelter's syndrome with tall stature and hypogonadism). Sometimes, only part of a chromosome is deleted, for example, 5p-, where the short arm of chromosome 5 is missing, leads to cri-du-chat syndrome with a characteristic cat-like cry as a baby, cognitive delay and behavioural problems.

Testing for genetic disorders

Most disorders that are screened for in newborns have a genetic basis. Molecular genetic techniques are increasingly used to identify abnormal genes or chromosomes. It is vital that families receive appropriate counselling so that they understand the implications of an abnormal result. Genetic tests can be performed at various times (see Chapter 7):

- **Pre-implantation testing** is only available with in vitro fertilization techniques but can allow screening prior to implantation.
- **Antenatal genetic testing** via chorionic villus sampling or amniocentesis allows the possibility of termination of pregnancy. Some families choose to continue the pregnancy despite a positive result and this allows them time to come to terms with the diagnosis.

Genetic diagnostic tests

Karyotype	Uses microscopy to analyse the number and character of the chromosomes. Requires cell culture and can take up to 5 days to process
FISH	Fluorescent *in situ* hybridization—a probe targets DNA sequences—the number of copies (bright spots) is then analysed with a microscope. Used to diagnose trisomy 13, 18 or 21 with a result in <24 hours (see Figure 8.3)
QF-PCR	Quantitative fluorescent polymerase chain reaction uses fluorescent labelled primers and automated PCR methodology to measure the number of copies of a sequence of DNA. Used to rapidly screen for trisomy 13, 18, 21 and 45XO
Comparative genomic hybridization (CGH) array	Uses molecular fluorescent *in situ* hybridization to compare the number of copies of DNA in a sample compared with a standard sample. This automated analysis can detect duplications and deletions in small areas of the genome (5–10 M base pairs). It is a good way to 'screen' for genetic abnormality when there is a strong suspicion, but analyses the whole genome so can sometimes identify abnormalities for which we do not have clear prognostic information
Sequencing	The nucleotide base pair order for a specific area of interest is 'read' and known mutations can be detected
Direct gene testing	If the exact gene mutation is known, an RNA probe can be designed to bind to the abnormal gene sequence and identify it
Linkage testing	When genetic material is available from other affected family members, but there isn't a specific gene test available, this technique can be used for prenatal testing

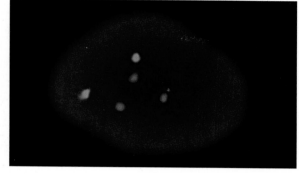

Figure 8.3 Fluorescent *in situ* hybridization (FISH) showing three copies of the probe for chromosome 18 (red) and only two copies of chromosome 13 (green), confirming the diagnosis of Edward's syndrome (trisomy 18).

- **Newborn genetic testing** may be performed to confirm a clinical diagnosis (e.g. Down's syndrome or congenital myotonic dystrophy) or following a positive screening test (e.g. CF gene testing following an abnormal IRT result on the newborn blood spot screen).
- **Genetic testing of older children** may be needed to confirm a diagnosis presenting later in childhood (e.g. fragile X or Duchenne muscular dystrophy). In general, children should not be tested for adult-onset genetic disorders without their own informed consent unless it is going to alter their treatment during childhood.

9 The newborn baby

Gestation
- Full-term: born between 37 and 42 weeks gestation
- Preterm: born before 37 weeks gestation
- Post-term: born after 42 weeks gestation

Vernix
- A white waxy substance that is often present, especially in preterm infants. Thought to provide insulation and lubrication

Mortality definitions
- Stillbirth: a baby (>24 weeks' gestation) who shows no signs of life after delivery (including no heart beat)
- Perinatal mortality rate: Stillbirths and deaths within the first week of life per 1000 births. Approximately 7/1000 in the UK
- Infant mortality rate: Number of deaths in the first year of life per 1000 live-born infants; approximately 5 per 1000

Breast-feeding
- A healthy baby can be put straight to the breast and will suckle soon after birth (see Chapter 13)

Birthweight
- Small for gestational age: birthweight <10th centile
- Very low birthweight: <1500 g
- Extremely low birthweight: <1000 g

The first breath
- Interruption to umbilical blood flow and response to cold stimulates the baby to take its first breath within a minute of birth
- Lung fluid is actively reabsorbed as well as being expelled during delivery
- Surfactant in the alveoli helps them to expand and fill with air
- Most babies can be dried, covered and given straight to the mother. Occasionally, the onset of breathing may be delayed and the baby requires resuscitation

Umbilical cord
- Normally has two arteries and one vein
- After clamping it dries up and usually separates from the baby within the first week. It can be a site of infection

Resuscitation
- Usually, simple stimulation, drying and warming is sufficient but resuscitation may be needed in some babies
- Air or oxygen (if required) can be given by a pressure limiting device and mask and the baby placed under a warmer
- Intubation may sometimes be needed, especially if the baby has aspirated meconium or needs ongoing ventilation

Meconium
- Green–black stool passed by babies in the first days after birth
- Fresh meconium-stained liquor can be a sign of fetal distress but can be normal in full-term infants
- The asphyxiated gasping baby can aspirate meconium into the lungs, causing respiratory distress

Vitamin K
- Babies can sometimes be deficient in vitamin K, leading to severe bleeding disorders
- Vitamin K is routinely offered to all babies, either orally or by intramuscular injection. Breast-fed babies require three oral doses as breast milk contains less vitamin K than formula milks

The Apgar score

Score	0	1	2
Heart rate	Absent	<100	>100
Respiration	Absent	Irregular	Strong cry
Tone	Limp	Some flexion	Good flexion
Reflex to suction	None	Grimace	Cough or sneeze
Colour	White	Blue periphery	Pink

- The Apgar score is often used to describe the infant's condition at birth
- The score (0–10) is recorded at 1 min and 5 min of life
- A normal score at 1 min is 7–10
- Babies with a score of 0–3 at 1 min require rapid resuscitation or they will die

The normal newborn

The vast majority of babies are born in good condition at full term and do not require any medical involvement. Most babies in the UK are born in hospital, where a paediatrician is usually available to attend 'high-risk' deliveries, where it is anticipated that resuscitation will be required. A healthy newborn infant should cry soon after birth, have pink mucous membranes, good muscle tone, a normal heart rate and regular respiration. They can be dried and placed on the mother's chest. The cord is clamped after a minute or two. Skin-to-skin care helps establish breastfeeding. Newborn babies, especially premature babies, are covered in a waxy material called vernix. Post-term infants may have very dry, cracked skin. Babies pass a green–black stool called meconium that changes to a normal yellow–brown seedy stool after a few days. It is recommended that infants be given vitamin K at birth to prevent potentially catastrophic bleeding. Newborn infants are

Paediatrics at a Glance, Fourth Edition. Lawrence Miall, Mary Rudolf and Dominic Smith. © 2016 John Wiley & Sons, Ltd. Published 2016 by John Wiley & Sons, Ltd.
Companion website: www.ataglanceseries.com/paediatrics

routinely examined within the first few days to exclude congenital abnormalities (see Chapter 10) and have blood taken from a heel prick around day 5 to screen for hypothyroidism and metabolic disorders (see Chapter 7).

Asphyxia and resuscitation

The perinatal mortality rate (currently 7 per 1000) has halved in the UK over the last 20 years, largely due to improvements in obstetric care. The reduction in neonatal mortality rate (now less than 3 per 1000 live births) is due to improvements in the management of babies with complex congenital abnormalities and to improved care of preterm infants. Some babies still require immediate resuscitation after birth, and personnel attending deliveries must be trained in effective and rapid resuscitation. The need for resuscitation can often be anticipated and a skilled professional should be in attendance. Such situations include the following:

- Prematurity
- Fetal distress
- Thick meconium staining of the liquor
- Emergency caesarean section
- Instrumental delivery
- Known congenital abnormality
- Multiple births.

Apgar score

The condition of the infant after birth is described by the Apgar score (see opposite). Five parameters are scored from 0 to 2. A total Apgar score of 7–10 at 1 min of age is normal. A score of 4–6 is a moderately ill baby and 0–3 represents a severely compromised infant who may die without urgent resuscitation. Such babies will often require intubation and may require cardiac massage. In the most depressed babies IV drugs such as adrenaline (epinephrine) and bicarbonate may be necessary to re-establish cardiac output. The outcome for these infants may be poor.

Hypoxic-ischaemic encephalopathy (HIE)

Some infants in poor condition at birth may have suffered a hypoxic or ischaemic insult during pregnancy or labour. A healthy fetus can withstand brief physiological hypoxia, but an already compromised fetus may become exhausted and decompensate with build-up of lactic acid. These infants may develop irreversible organ damage, in particular to the brain. Umbilical cord blood gas samples should be assessed. Evidence of severe asphyxia includes a cord blood pH < 7.0, Apgar score of <5 at 10 mins, a delay in spontaneous respiration beyond 10 mins and development of a characteristic encephalopathy with abnormal neurological signs including convulsions. Death or severe handicap occurs in more than 75% of the most severely asphyxiated term infants. Therapeutic hypothermia (cooling to 33.5 °C) for 72 h can prevent secondary neuronal damage in moderate-to-severe HIE. However, for normal, well babies, it is important to prevent hypothermia by careful drying and early skin-to-skin contact after birth. Preterm babies are at particular risk of hypothermia, and they should be delivered in a warm room and enclosed in clean plastic wrap before stabilization under a heater to help maintain normothermia.

Intrauterine growth retardation

A baby with a birth weight below the 10th centile is small for gestational age (SGA). This may be familial or may be due to intrauterine growth retardation (IUGR). The pattern of growth retardation gives some indication of the cause. An insult in early pregnancy, such as infection, will cause symmetrical growth retardation, where the head and length are also affected. A later insult, usually placental insufficiency, can cause asymmetric growth retardation with relative sparing of head growth due to selective shunting of blood to the developing brain. Abnormalities of blood flow in the umbilical or fetal vessels can now be detected using Doppler ultrasound; these can be used to plan when to intervene and deliver the baby.

Causes of IUGR include the following:

- Multiple pregnancy
- Placental insufficiency
- Maternal smoking
- Congenital infections (e.g. toxoplasmosis and rubella)
- Genetic syndromes (e.g. Down's syndrome).

Babies with severe IUGR should be screened for congenital infection—'TORCH' screen (Toxoplasmosis, Other [syphilis], Rubella, Cytomegalovirus, Hepatitis and HIV). In the first few days of life, babies with IUGR are at risk of hypoglycaemia and hypothermia due to low glycogen stores and lack of subcutaneous fat. Symptomatic hypoglycaemia can cause neurodevelopmental injury. If there has been poor head growth during pregnancy, intellect may be impaired. Babies with IUGR must not be overfed during infancy as there is evidence that excessive weight gain leads to hypertension, ischaemic heart disease and diabetes in later life.

Vitamin K

Vitamin K deficiency or persistent obstructive jaundice can lead to poor synthesis of vitamin K-dependent clotting factors and subsequent bleeding. The bleeding may be minor bruising or significant intracranial haemorrhage. This used to be known as haemorrhagic disease of the newborn but is now referred to as vitamin K deficiency bleeding (VKDB). Breast milk is low in vitamin K, unlike formula milk, which is supplemented. For this reason, vitamin K should be given routinely to all newborn infants, either as a single intramuscular injection or by mouth at birth, 1 and 6 weeks. Babies with persistent jaundice should receive further doses (see Chapter 51).

KEY POINTS

- Most babies are born healthy and do not require any resuscitation.
- The Apgar score is used to describe the condition after birth.
- Vitamin K is recommended for all babies.
- Babies with severe IUGR are at increased risk of asphyxia, hypoglycaemia and hypothermia and may be at risk of intellectual impairment.

10 Congenital abnormalities

▶ The newborn examination

All newborn babies are carefully examined in the first 24 h of life to check they are healthy and to screen for congenital abnormalities, some of which may not be obvious to the parents. The baby should be fully undressed in a warm room and examined from head to toe. Ask the mother if she has any concerns and whether there is any family history of note, for example of deafness or congenital dislocation of the hips

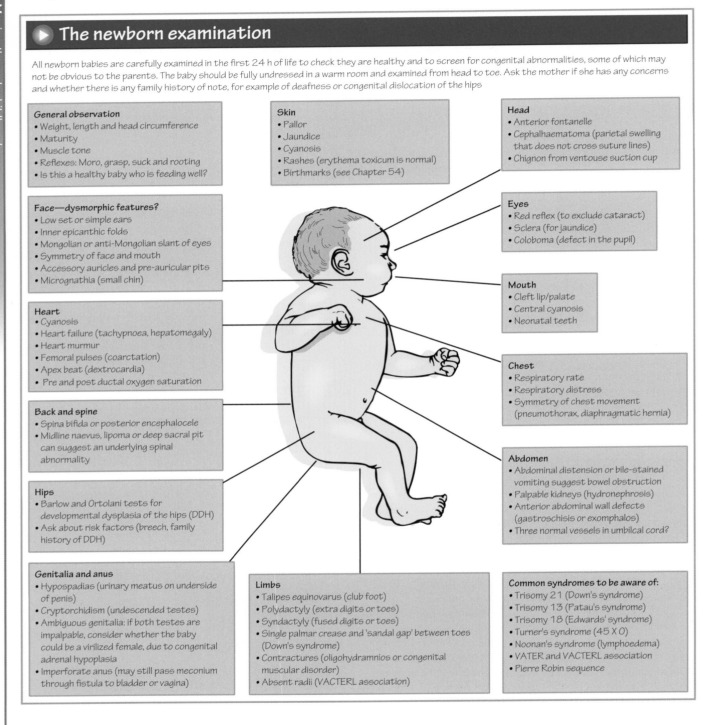

General observation
- Weight, length and head circumference
- Maturity
- Muscle tone
- Reflexes: Moro, grasp, suck and rooting
- Is this a healthy baby who is feeding well?

Face—dysmorphic features?
- Low set or simple ears
- Inner epicanthic folds
- Mongolian or anti-Mongolian slant of eyes
- Symmetry of face and mouth
- Accessory auricles and pre-auricular pits
- Micrognathia (small chin)

Heart
- Cyanosis
- Heart failure (tachypnoea, hepatomegaly)
- Heart murmur
- Femoral pulses (coarctation)
- Apex beat (dextrocardia)
- Pre and post ductal oxygen saturation

Back and spine
- Spina bifida or posterior encephalocele
- Midline naevus, lipoma or deep sacral pit can suggest an underlying spinal abnormality

Hips
- Barlow and Ortolani tests for developmental dysplasia of the hips (DDH)
- Ask about risk factors (breech, family history of DDH)

Genitalia and anus
- Hypospadias (urinary meatus on underside of penis)
- Cryptorchidism (undescended testes)
- Ambiguous genitalia: if both testes are impalpable, consider whether the baby could be a virilized female, due to congenital adrenal hypoplasia
- Imperforate anus (may still pass meconium through fistula to bladder or vagina)

Skin
- Pallor
- Jaundice
- Cyanosis
- Rashes (erythema toxicum is normal)
- Birthmarks (see Chapter 54)

Limbs
- Talipes equinovarus (club foot)
- Polydactyly (extra digits or toes)
- Syndactyly (fused digits or toes)
- Single palmar crease and 'sandal gap' between toes (Down's syndrome)
- Contractures (oligohydramnios or congenital muscular disorder)
- Absent radii (VACTERL association)

Head
- Anterior fontanelle
- Cephalhaematoma (parietal swelling that does not cross suture lines)
- Chignon from ventouse suction cup

Eyes
- Red reflex (to exclude cataract)
- Sclera (for jaundice)
- Coloboma (defect in the pupil)

Mouth
- Cleft lip/palate
- Central cyanosis
- Neonatal teeth

Chest
- Respiratory rate
- Respiratory distress
- Symmetry of chest movement (pneumothorax, diaphragmatic hernia)

Abdomen
- Abdominal distension or bile-stained vomiting suggest bowel obstruction
- Palpable kidneys (hydronephrosis)
- Anterior abdominal wall defects (gastroschisis or exomphalos)
- Three normal vessels in umbilcal cord?

Common syndromes to be aware of:
- Trisomy 21 (Down's syndrome)
- Trisomy 13 (Patau's syndrome)
- Trisomy 18 (Edwards' syndrome)
- Turner's syndrome (45 X O)
- Noonan's syndrome (lymphoedema)
- VATER and VACTERL association
- Pierre Robin sequence

Patterns of congenital abnormality

The incidence of congenital abnormalities is 10–15 per 1000 births. The commonest are congenital heart defects (8 per 1000) (see Chapter 22). Abnormalities range from a trivial birthmark to a syndrome diagnosis. The majority of congenital abnormalities are genetically determined, but some may be due to a combination of genetics and environment (e.g. spina bifida) or due entirely to environment (e.g. fetal alcohol syndrome).

A *syndrome* is a consistent pattern of dysmorphic features seen together and suggests a genetic origin. A *sequence* is where one abnormality leads to another—for example, the

Paediatrics at a Glance, Fourth Edition. Lawrence Miall, Mary Rudolf and Dominic Smith. © 2016 John Wiley & Sons, Ltd. Published 2016 by John Wiley & Sons, Ltd.
Companion website: www.ataglanceseries.com/paediatrics

small mandible (micrognathia) in Pierre Robin sequence causes posterior displacement of the tongue, which prevents the palate forming correctly, leading to cleft palate. An *association* is a non-random collection of abnormalities (see the following table).

Syndromes and associations	
Syndromes	
Down's syndrome	Trisomy 21: see Chapters 7 and 66
Patau's syndrome	Trisomy 13 midline defects, cleft lip and palate, cutis aplasia, holoprosencephaly, polydactyly, heart defects (VSD, PDA, ASD)
Edward's syndrome	Trisomy 18 IUGR, polyhydramnios, rocker-bottom feet, clenched hands, prominent occiput, heart defects (VSD, PDA, ASD), apnoea
Turner's syndrome	(45XO) see Chapter 19
Noonan's syndrome	Phenotypically similar to Turner's but occurs in both sexes. Short stature, oedema, pulmonary stenosis
Associations	
VACTERL	**V**ertebral, **a**nal atresia, **c**ardiac, **t**racheo-oesophageal fistula, **r**enal, **l**imb (absent radii)
CHARGE	**C**oloboma, **h**eart defects, choanal **a**tresia, **r**etarded growth and development, **g**enital hypoplasia and **e**ar anomalies

Cleft lip and palate

Cleft lip occurs in 1 in 1000 infants. Seventy percent have a cleft palate as well. Cleft lip may be diagnosed antenatally, allowing the parents to receive counselling. After birth, a cleft palate is confirmed by palpating <u>and</u> observing the defect in the palate. A submucosal cleft is palpable but not visible. Cleft palate is best managed by a multidisciplinary team including cleft surgeon, orthodontist and speech therapist. Repair of the lip is performed at 3 months and the palate at 9 months. The cosmetic appearance following surgery is excellent. Showing the parents 'before and after' photographs (see Figure 10.1) can help allay anxiety. Expected difficulties include feeding difficulty, milk aspiration, conductive hearing loss and speech and dental problems. Regular audiological assessments are essential.

Neural tube defects (spina bifida)

Failure of the neural tube to close normally in early pregnancy causes spina bifida. It used to be a major cause of disability, but folic acid supplementation in early pregnancy has reduced the incidence by 75%. Antenatal ultrasound screening and selective termination has made open spina bifida a rare condition. Neural tube defects are always midline. The severity depends on the extent to which the neural tube has failed to develop:

- **Anencephaly**. The cranial part of the neural tube does not exist and the brain cortex does not develop. Infants die soon after birth.

- **Myelomeningocele**. It is an open lesion where the spinal cord is covered by a thin membrane of meninges. There is severe weakness of the lower limbs with bladder and anal denervation and an associated hydrocephalus. Survivors have severe disability.
- **Meningocele**. The spinal cord is intact, but there is an exposed sac of meninges, which can rupture, with the risk of meningitis.
- **Spina bifida occulta**. It is a 'hidden' neural tube defect where the vertebral bodies fail to fuse posteriorly. Some degree may be present in 5–10% of normal infants. The only clue may be a tuft of hair, naevus, lipoma or deep sacral pit in the midline over the lower back. A spinal ultrasound is indicated.

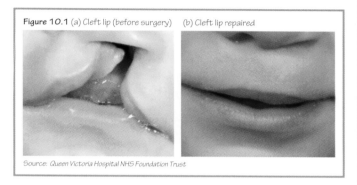

Figure 10.1 (a) Cleft lip (before surgery)   (b) Cleft lip repaired

Source: Queen Victoria Hospital NHS Foundation Trust

Developmental dysplasia of the hip

Developmental dysplasia of the hip (DDH) occurs in 1% of infants. The acetabulum is shallow and does not adequately cover the femoral head, leading to the hip joint being dislocatable or dislocated. Risk factors are breech position, family history, female sex and impaired limb movement. There is an association with talipes. True congenital dislocation of the hip (CDH) occurs in 2 per 1000 infants. Examination includes observation of symmetrical skin creases and leg length, the Ortolani test (a *dislocated* hip will not abduct fully, and 'clunks' as it relocates into the acetabulum) and the Barlow test (feeling a clunk as a *dislocatable* hip slips out of the acetabulum). Babies with risk factors or abnormal examination should have an ultrasound of the hip joint at 6 weeks post-term. Treatment involves wearing a harness or splint for several months, to hold the joint in flexion and abduction.

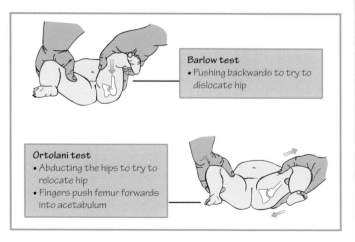

Barlow test
- Pushing backwards to try to dislocate hip

Ortolani test
- Abducting the hips to try to relocate hip
- Fingers push femur forwards into acetabulum

(11) Common neonatal problems

Common neonatal problems

It is important to remember that most newborn babies are perfectly healthy, but around 1 in 10 will need some additional neonatal care, due to either prematurity (see Ch 12), congenital abnormality (see Ch 10) or perinatal illness including respiratory disorders, infection and jaundice. Babies who develop problems in the first weeks after birth may be in a variety of care settings and with varying amounts of parental support- both family and professional. It is vital that parental concerns are taken seriously by health professionals- sometimes they can be quickly reassured, but sometimes a parents sense that "something is not right" is the first clue of serious, even life threatening sepsis.

Meconium aspiration
- Can occur before or during birth
- More common after 40 weeks
- May reflect fetal distress
- Usually presents immediately after birth
- Can cause pneumonitis and is a risk for pneumothorax
- Can delay normal physiological transition leading to persistent pulmonary hypertension of newborn (PPHN)

Umbilical and skin disorders
- Umbilical cord usually dried and detaches by 7–10 days
- Failure to detach by 6 weeks may reflect poor phagocyte function
- Bowel present in the cord (exompholos minor) needs surgery, but umbilical hernias almost always resolve without surgery
- Umbilical granuloma is a fleshy overgrowth of the stump that bleed. If needed treat with sclerosants or silver nitrate (but protect the skin with petroleum jelly)
- Infection around the umbilicus must be treated urgently
- Erythema toxicum and milia are very common (see Chapter 54)
- Other skin rashes need investigation as may be serious

Weight loss
- Most babies, especially breastfed, lose up to 10% of birth weight in first week of life.
- Extensive weight loss needs investigation and may need top up or nasogastric feeds (with breast feeding support)
- If due to failure of lactation may be associated with severe hypernatremia which can mask signs of dehydration (e.g. fontanelle may not be sunken, baby may be quiet and appear settled)

Early onset sepsis
- Defined as sepsis within first 7 days.
- Up to 10% of infants may be investigated, but incidence of culture positive sepsis is 1.5/1000 births
- E.Coli and Group B streptococcus are main pathogens, but can also be viral (e.g. Herpes)
- Presents with lethargy, feeding difficulties and pyrexia, or respiratory distress and shock.
- Early recognition and treatment is vital

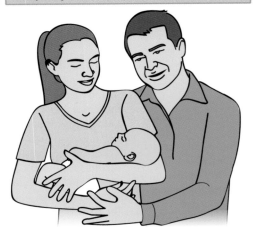

Parental anxiety/depression
- New parents are often anxious, especially if they are young, first time parents or are unsupported.
- Parents often worry about breathing pattern (can be very irregular) or movements (can be very exaggerated startle reflexes) but concerns must always be taken seriously
- Mothers commonly tearful (baby blues) due to extreme tiredness and hormonal changes.
- Postnatal depression (including psychosis) is much more serious and needs urgent psychiatric assessment and may need safeguarding of baby

Jaundice
- Physiological jaundice occurs in up to 50% of newborn babies
- High RBC mass and delayed conjugation by the liver lead to transient rise in unconjugated bilirubin and clinical jaundice
- Babies may be sleepy and less interested in feeding
- Many pathological causes (see Chapter 51) including blood group incompatibility, sepsis and congenital viral hepatitis
- All jaundice <24 h or >14 days needs investigation

Feeding difficulties
- Not uncommon, especially with first time mothers.
- Breast feeding advice must be available from day 1
- Can lead to hypoglycemia
- Tongue-tie can sometimes interfere with feeding-most do not need intervention but if severe feeding can improve after division
- Can sometimes be an indication of early onset sepsis or congenital malformations such as cleft palate

Late onset sepsis
- Sepsis beyond 7 days of life
- Often presents with meningitis
- Baby may be irritable and difficult to feed or to settle
- Grunting or gasping respiration is always an emergency in a previously well baby
- All neonates with possible signs of sepsis should be investigated including blood culture and LP
- Group B streptococcus, Listeria and Herpes virus can al present late despite being vertically acquired

Parents, especially first-time parents, can be understandably anxious about minor symptoms that may just require reassurance; however, a small proportion of babies may present with life-threatening illness in the first days and weeks after birth such as seizures or sepsis and so it is always important to listen to concerns and to assess babies carefully at this age.

Respiratory disorders presenting from birth

Respiratory distress syndrome due to prematurity is discussed in Chapter 12, but term babies can also commonly develop respiratory distress after birth and a number of causes should be considered (see the following table).

Paediatrics at a Glance, Fourth Edition. Lawrence Miall, Mary Rudolf and Dominic Smith. © 2016 John Wiley & Sons, Ltd. Published 2016 by John Wiley & Sons, Ltd.
Companion website: www.ataglanceseries.com/paediatrics

Common causes of respiratory distress after birth in term babies	
Meconium aspiration	History of meconium-stained liquor. Chest X-ray shows patchy opacities throughout. A pneumonitis occurs with tachypnoea and often a prolonged oxygen requirement for several days. Mechanical ventilation may be necessary. Often associated with persistent pulmonary hypertension, when there is right-to-left shunting across the patent duct and hence cyanosis.
Pneumothorax	About 1 in 100 babies may have a small spontaneous pneumothorax. Other risk factors include over-aggressive lung inflation during resuscitation, meconium aspiration (a ball-valve effect of the meconium in the small airways) or pulmonary hypoplasia.
Congenital lung malformations	Pulmonary hypoplasia (secondary to oligohydramnios due to very early rupture of membranes or fetal kidney failure or urinary obstruction). Congenital cystic adenomatous malformation (CCAM). Congenital diaphragmatic hernia.
Congenital pneumonia	Bacterial or viral pneumonia. Commonly group B streptococcus
Transient tachypnoea of newborn (TTN)	Usually in babies born by caesarean section, especially if the mother was not in labour. Chest X-ray shows plethoric lung fields with streaky peri-hilar shadowing and fluid in the transverse fissure. Resolves completely within 24 h but may require oxygen or respiratory support.
Aspiration of milk or airway obstruction	Babies can occasionally aspirate milk—especially if they are not neurologically normal. Babies may have a congenital airway obstruction (e.g. choanal atresia—occluded nostrils) or suffer accidental suffocation when put to the breast or if asleep in bed with the mother (rare but important cause of postnatal collapse).

Early onset neonatal sepsis

The birth canal is not sterile and babies can be colonized with bacteria before or during birth. Infection prior to birth is usually due to ascending infection with chorioamnionitis (infected amniotic fluid), and this is much more likely if there is prolonged rupture of the membranes for >18–24 h before birth. The overall risk of early onset sepsis is small (1–2 per 1000 births), but the consequences can be severe if it is not recognized and treated early.

Common causes of sepsis at this time are

- Group B haemolytic streptococcal disease
- *Escherichia coli* sepsis
- Other gram-negative infections
- Listeria
- *Staph aureus*
- Viral—herpes simplex virus (I or II), enteroviruses, parechovirus.

Group B streptococcal (GBS) sepsis

About 20–30% of women are colonized by GBS, and there is about a 10% chance of the baby becoming colonized and a 1% chance of the baby developing sepsis, which carries a high mortality. In the United States, women are screened for GBS at 36 weeks and if present prophylactic antibiotics are given. In the UK, there is a risk factor–based approach and i.v. penicillin is given during labour if there has been GBS infection (e.g. a UTI) or a positive high vaginal swab in this pregnancy or a previously affected child with GBS sepsis. Babies with GBS sepsis usually present within the first 12 h of life with pneumonia, PPHN or septic shock. They will often require respiratory support and if GBS is confirmed, they should receive a prolonged course of antibiotics, especially if there is meningitis.

Late onset sepsis

This by definition means sepsis after the first 7 days of life. It may still be vertically acquired or may be acquired horizontally from the environment (e.g. nosocomial infection in a neonatal unit), visitors (e.g. herpes simplex) or maternal breast milk (e.g. GBS). The crucial thing is early recognition. Late onset sepsis is more often associated with meningitis or encephalitis and the neurodevelopmental outcome may be poor if not treated early.

Weight loss and feeding problems

Whilst breastfeeding is undoubtedly best for babies, it is not always as easy and natural as it is sometimes portrayed. It is vital that new mothers are supported to breastfeed and receive good advice in the first days of feeding. Specialist breastfeeding advisors should be available.

It is not unusual for babies to lose 5–10% of their birth weight after birth. Some of this is due to loss of extracellular water, and there is some evidence of a long-term protection against diabetes and heart disease in those that do lose weight, but excessive weight loss >10% can be due to failure of maternal lactation—the baby becomes gradually more lethargic and less interested in feeding, so the maternal milk supply may dwindle further, creating a vicious cycle. In some cases, this can lead to extreme hypernatremic dehydration—with serum sodium as high as 160–170 mmol/L. This should be corrected extremely carefully over several days; the safest method is by giving additional milk (expressed breast milk or formula) via a nasogastric tube. Too rapid correction can lead to seizures.

Feeding difficulties can also be of infant origin—there may be neurological incoordination (e.g. Down syndrome), a mechanical problem such as severe micrognathia, tongue-tie or cleft palate (typically milk can come down the nose). Minor tongue ties do not need dividing. There is evidence that more severe degrees (where the tongue is tethered) can cause feeding problems and respond to division of the frenulum.

Jaundice

Jaundice is discussed in detail in Chapter 51. Many babies develop a degree of hyperbilirubinaemia after birth as the liver has to conjugate a large amount of bilirubin generated from fetal red blood cells that was previously cleared by the placenta. Unconjugated bilirubin is neurotoxic and can make babies sleepy and less interested in feeds. If babies are visibly jaundice <24 h of age, they should be thoroughly investigated as there may be a pathological cause such as ABO blood group incompatibility or infection. Mild jaundice on day 2–4 will usually respond to good hydration, but it is notoriously hard to estimate the level by eye and all jaundiced babies should have their bilirubin measured, either using a transcutaneous bilrubinometer or with a serum sample. If the total bilirubin concentration is above a treatment line (which depends on age and gestation—see http://www.nice.org.uk/guidance/cg98/chapter/appendix-d-the-treatment-threshold-graphs) then the baby should receive phototherapy (blue wavelength light), which converts bilirubin into a water-soluble form that is excreted easily.

12 The premature baby

Complications of prematurity

Eyes
- Retinopathy of prematurity due to abnormal vascularization of the developing retina
- Requires–screening and possible laser treatment to prevent retinal detachment and blindness

Respiratory
- Respiratory distress syndrome (surfactant deficiency)
- Apnoea and bradycardia
- Pneumothorax
- Chronic lung disease

Cardiovascular (see Chapter 22)
- Hypotension
- Patent ductus arteriosus

Thermoregulation
- Increased surface area to volume ratio leads to loss of heat
- Immature skin cannot retain heat and fluids efficiently
- Reduced subcutaneous fat reduces insulation

Metabolic
- Hypoglycaemia is common. Symptomatic hypoglycaemia must be treated promptly. Blood glucose should be maintained above 2.6 mmol/L to prevent neurological damage
- Hypocalcaemia
- Electrolyte imbalance
- Osteopenia of prematurity (with risk of fractures)

Brain
- Intraventricular haemorrhage
- Posthaemorrhagic hydrocephalus
- Periventricular leucomalacia
- Increased risk of cerebral palsy

Nutrition
- May require parenteral nutrition
- Nasogastric feeds until sucking reflex develops at 32–34 weeks
- Difficult to achieve in-utero growth rates

Gastrointestinal
- Necrotizing enterocolitis: a life-threatening inflammation of the bowel wall due to ischaemia and infection and which can lead to bowel perforation
- Gastro-oesophageal reflux
- Inguinal hernias (with high risk of strangulation)

Infection
- Increased risk of sepsis, especially group B streptococcus and coliforms
- Pneumonia is common
- Infection is a potential complication of central venous lines required for feeding

95%

Blood
- Anaemia of prematurity
- Neonatal jaundice (see Chapter 51)

What you need from your evaluation

History

- **Risk factors for prematurity:** young maternal age, multiple pregnancy, infection, maternal illness (e.g. pregnancy-induced hypertension), cervical incompetence, antepartum haemorrhage, smoking, alcohol and infection
- **Full obstetric history**
- **Condition at birth:** Apgar score, resuscitation required?
- **Birthweight:** appropriate for gestational age?
- **Gestation:** must be known to give accurate prognosis. Calculate from menstrual period, by early dating ultrasound scan or by assessment of gestation after birth (Dubowitz score)
  Associated problems such as twin pregnancy (much higher risk of poor neurological outcome), congenital abnormalities or infection (chorioamnionitis may have been trigger for preterm labour)
- **Antenatal steroids:** if given, these reduce the incidence of respiratory distress syndrome and intraventricular haemorrhage

Long-term complications

- **Survival:** about 45% of infants born alive at 24 weeks gestation survive (see figure opposite). By 27 weeks this rises to 80% and after 32 weeks the chances of survival are excellent
- **Chronic lung disease** (bronchopulmonary dysplasia): this is a consequence of disrupted lung development and may require long-term oxygen treatment for months or sometimes years
- **Neurological sequelae:** there is a significant risk of hydrocephalus developing secondary to an intraventricular haemorrhage. A shunt may need to be inserted to relieve pressure. Hypotension may have been sustained, leading to periventricular leucomalacia. This carries the risk of cerebral palsy, particularly of the diplegic type
- **Blindness:** as a consequence of severe retinopathy of prematurity (ROP). This is becoming less common with better prevention, detection and treatment of ROP
- **Poor growth:** especially if catch-up growth is not achieved

Paediatrics at a Glance, Fourth Edition. Lawrence Miall, Mary Rudolf and Dominic Smith. © 2016 John Wiley & Sons, Ltd. Published 2016 by John Wiley & Sons, Ltd.
Companion website: www.ataglanceseries.com/paediatrics

7% of all babies are premature (<37 weeks) and 1% are extremely premature (<28 weeks) or very low birthweight (VLBW < 1500 g). Premature babies can survive from 23 weeks, although mortality is 60–70% and only 25% of those that survive at these gestations will be free of disability. Beyond 30–32 weeks, the prognosis is excellent. Premature infants and IUGR babies are at risk of hypothermia, hypoglycaemia and difficulty feeding.

Premature babies need care on a special care baby unit (SCBU) or neonatal intensive care unit (NICU). Incubators provide warmth and humidity to prevent hypothermia and protect the skin, which is thin, and is a poor barrier to heat and fluid loss. Feeding problems are common. A mature suck–swallow pattern does not develop until 34 weeks, so they need to be fed via a nasogastric tube. Very sick premature babies, or those with IUGR or asphyxia, may be at increased risk of necrotizing enterocolitis (NEC) and are given intravenous parenteral nutrition. Premature babies are at risk of brain injury and also infection, either vertically acquired from the mother or from the hospital environment.

Respiratory distress syndrome

Pneumonia, pneumothorax, cardiac failure and congenital lung malformation can all cause respiratory distress in preterm infants but by far the commonest cause is respiratory distress syndrome (RDS) due to surfactant deficiency.

Signs of RDS include tachypnoea, intercostal recession, cyanosis and expiratory 'grunting'. CXR shows a 'ground glass' appearance due to alveolar collapse. Surfactant is a phospholipid that reduces alveolar surface tension. Production is not mature until about 35–36 weeks, although the stress of labour stimulates production, and RDS is therefore usually self-limiting, lasting 5–7 days. Corticosteroids administered antenatally reduce RDS. IUGR babies are physiologically 'stressed' and get less severe RDS due to endogenous corticosteroid release.

Management involves optimizing oxygenation and supporting respiration, either with continuous positive airway pressure (CPAP) or high flow air/oxygen via nasal prongs, or ventilation. Surfactant can be administered via an endotracheal tube. 20% of babies with RDS develop chronic lung disease of prematurity (bronchopulmonary dysplasia), which if severe may require home-oxygen therapy.

Necrotizing enterocolitis

This serious complication is due to impaired blood flow to the bowel. Mucosal ischaemia allows gut microorganisms to penetrate the bowel wall, causing a severe haemorrhagic colitis. Breast milk and probiotics (healthy bacteria) are protective, but increasing milk feeds (especially formula feeds) too rapidly is a risk, as is a patent arterial duct (PDA). NEC presents with abdominal distension, bile-stained vomiting, bloody diarrhoea and sometimes collapse. An abdominal radiograph may show gas in the bowel wall or portal veins. Management involves stopping feeds, supporting the circulation and antibiotics. Laparotomy is required if perforation occurs. Complications include intestinal stricture and short bowel syndrome.

Retinopathy of prematurity

Retinopathy of prematurity (ROP) is common in very premature infants, occurring in up to 35%. In most cases, it requires no treatment, but in about 1% of these babies, it causes blindness. ROP is caused by proliferation of new blood vessels in an area of

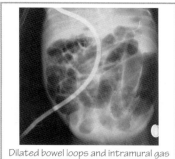

Dilated bowel loops and intramural gas typical of NEC.

relative ischaemia in the developing retina. Oxygen toxicity is one cause although there may also be a genetic predisposition. At-risk infants should be screened for ROP by an ophthalmologist. If detected, laser ablation can be used to prevent retinal detachment and blindness.

Brain injury

Preterm infants are at risk of brain injury, and this is the most important factor affecting their long-term prognosis.

- **Intraventricular haemorrhage** (IVH) occurs in up to 30% of VLBW. Haemorrhage develops in the floor of the lateral ventricle (germinal matrix) and ruptures into the ventricle. In a small minority, the haemorrhage involves the white matter around the ventricle by a process of obstructive venous infarction. This carries a high risk of hemiplegic cerebral palsy (see Chapter 45). IVH may be asymptomatic and is diagnosed by ultrasound scan.
- **Posthaemorrhagic hydrocephalus** occurs in 15% of severe IVH and may require insertion of a ventriculo-peritoneal shunt.
- **Periventricular leucomalacia** (PVL) is caused by ischaemic damage to the periventricular white matter. It is less common than IVH but is the commonest cause of cerebral palsy in surviving infants. PVL is particularly likely where there has been chorioamnionitis, severe hypotension or in monozygotic twins. If cystic change develops, 80% develop cerebral palsy.
- **Neurodevelopmental consequences of prematurity**

Even with a normal ultrasound scan, there is an increased incidence of learning difficulties in extremely preterm infants. Attention difficulties are common, and subtle problems in higher functioning (e.g. mathematics) may not manifest until school age. Outcome in survivors is shown below.

Outcome at 3 years for all babies born in the UK at 22–26 weeks gestation in 2006 (based on Epicure 2 data).

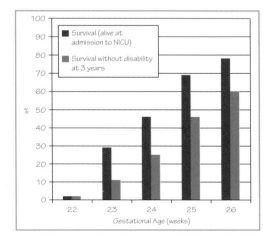

(13) Nutrition in childhood

Breast-feeding

Ways to encourage successful breast-feeding
- Introduce concept of breast-feeding to both parents antenatally
- Put the baby to the breast immediately after delivery
- Allow the baby to feed on demand, especially in the early days
- Avoid offering any formula feeds
- Ensure mother receives good nutrition and plenty of rest
- Provide skilled breast-feeding advisors to help mother through any initial problems with breast-feeding
- Ensure correct 'latching on' with the baby's mouth wide open and good positioning

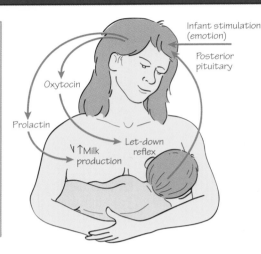

Infant stimulation (emotion)
Posterior pituitary
Oxytocin
Prolactin
Let-down reflex
↓↑Milk production

Lactation
- At birth, prolactin levels rise sharply and this is further stimulated by the infant sucking at the breast. Prolactin determines milk production from the breast alveoli, and is increased by the frequency, duration and intensity of sucking
- The actual flow of milk is aided by the 'let-down' reflex. Rooting at the nipple causes afferent pathways to stimulate the posterior pituitary to secrete oxytocin, which stimulates the smooth muscle around the alveolar ducts to express the milk from the breast. The let-down reflex can be stimulated by hearing the baby cry or by contact with the baby, and can be inhibited by stress or embarrassment
- The majority of the milk is taken from the breast in the first 5 min and this may be followed by non-nutritive sucking

Advantages of breast-feeding
- Perfect balance of milk constituents
- Little risk of bacterial contamination
- Anti-infective properties (IgA, macrophages, etc.)
- Ideal food for brain growth and development
- Convenient
- No expense of purchasing milk
- Psychologically satisfying
- Reduces risk of atopic disorders

Possible problems with breast-feeding (rare)
- Can transmit infection (e.g. HIV, although in developing countries the best advice is still to exclusively breast-feed)
- Some drugs can be excreted in breast milk (e.g. warfarin)
- Can initially be tiring for the mother

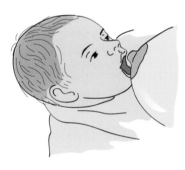

Weaning
- 0–6 months: breast or formula milk only
- 6 months: puréed or liquidized foods
- 7–9 months: finger foods, juice in a cup
- 9–12 months: 3 meals a day with family and 3 snacktimes
- >1 year: cow's milk in a beaker or cup; adult-type food chopped up

Formula milk feeds

- Formula milks are based on cow's milk, but are carefully adjusted to meet the basic nutritional requirements of growing infants. The fat component is generally replaced with polyunsaturated vegetable oils to provide the correct essential fatty acids. Minerals, vitamins and trace elements are then added
- Formula milk is usually made up from a dry powder, by adding one level measure of powder to each 30 mL (1 fl.oz) of cooled boiled water. Great care must be taken to sterilize the bottles and teats carefully to avoid introducing infection. The milk is then re-warmed prior to feeding. Ensure the milk is at a safe comfortable temperature before feeding. Never re-warm in a microwave. Each feed should be made freshly.

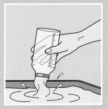

1. Sterilize the feeding bottle

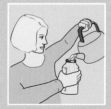

2. Add the appropriate volume of cooled boiled water to the bottle

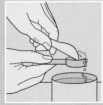

3. Add 1 level scoop of milk powder to each 30 mL of water

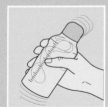

4. Shake bottle well

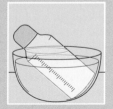

5. Ensure the milk is at a safe comfortable temperature before feeding

Infant nutrition

Milk provides all the nutrients needed by newborn infants for the first 6 months of life. Breast milk is the ideal milk for human babies, but formula milk may be needed as an alternative in some cases. The newborn infant has high calorie and fluid requirements and to achieve optimal growth requires approximately 150 mL/kg per day of fluid and 110 kcal/kg per day (462 kJ/kg per day). About 40% of this energy comes from carbohydrate (mostly lactose) and 50% from fat. Milk also contains protein in the form of casein, lactalbumin and lactoferrin. Colostrum is the yellow concentrated milk produced in the first few days, which is high in immunoglobulins.

Infants also require adequate amounts of minerals such as calcium and phosphate, as well as vitamins and trace elements. All newborn infants are given vitamin K at birth to prevent haemorrhagic disease of the newborn. Weaning on to solids usually starts around 6 months, and infants should not have cow's milk until they are over a year.

The stool pattern of breastfed babies differs from that of bottle-fed babies. They have non-offensive, porridge-consistency, yellow stools, initially after each feed. The frequency then reduces so they may have only one per week without being constipated.

Technique of breast-feeding

Mothers should be encouraged to put their babies to the breast soon after delivery. Little milk is produced but the suckling stimulates lactation. It is important that the baby is taught to 'latch on' to the breast properly with a widely open mouth, so that the areola and not just the nipple is within the baby's mouth. The majority of the milk is taken by the baby in the first 5 min, and time after this is spent in non-nutritive suckling. Babies should not be pulled off the breast, but the suck released by inserting a clean finger at the side of the baby's mouth. Each feed should start on the alternate breast.

In the first few days, the breasts may become painfully engorged with milk and the nipples sore, especially if the baby's position is not optimal. Mothers should be encouraged to continue breastfeeding as it relieves the engorgement and ensures the milk supply is maintained.

Formula feeds should only be introduced if breastfeeding is contraindicated or has failed completely. It is not appropriate to 'top up' with formula or use bottles to give the mother a rest. This may help in the short term but leads to tailing off of milk production and breastfeeding failing altogether.

Weaning

Current recommendations are to start weaning at 6 months of age. In the UK, cereals, rusks or rice-based mixtures are generally introduced first, mixed with expressed breast milk or formula milk. This is given by spoon before milk feeds. Puréed fruit or vegetables are also suitable. Modern baby cereals are gluten-free, which may be associated with a fall in the incidence of coeliac disease (see Chapter 34). As the baby grows older, the feeds can become more solid and are given as three meals a day. From 7 to 9 months, they will enjoy finger-feeding themselves. From about 9 months, they can generally eat a mashed or cut-up version of adult food. Undiluted full-fat pasteurized cow's milk can be given from 12 months. Earlier introduction of cow's milk or the persistence of exclusive breastfeeding can lead to iron deficiency. Vitamin supplements may be needed from 6 months in breastfed babies, until they are on a full mixed diet.

Nutrition in the preschool years

As a toddler, the child becomes more adept at holding a spoon and can feed independently and drink from a beaker or cup. Milk is no longer the main source of nutrients although the child should still drink a pint a day. Whole-fat milk should be used until age 5 years to provide plenty of calories, unless the child is overweight. A well-balanced diet should include food from the following four main groups:

- Meat, fish, poultry and eggs
- Dairy products (milk, cheese and yoghurt)
- Fruit and vegetables
- Cereals, grains, potatoes and rice.

In order to avoid dental caries and obesity, it is important to avoid frequent snacking on sugary foods or drinks—three meals and two snacks is recommended although this may be adapted to the individual child. Iron-deficiency anaemia (see Chapter 50) is common at this age, due to high requirements for growth and poor dietary intake, especially in the 'faddy eater'. Vitamin C present in orange juice can enhance iron absorption from the gut. Feeding difficulties are common in the preschool years (see Chapter 14).

Nutrition in the school-age child

At school, children have to learn to eat food outside the family setting. They usually have a midday meal, and fruit or milk may be provided at break times. The principles of healthy eating should be maintained although peer pressure to eat energy-rich foods such as crisps or sugary snacks is often high. Schools have an educational role to play in encouraging healthy eating and a healthy lifestyle. During adolescence, there is a greater energy requirement to allow for increased growth. This may coincide with a lifestyle that leads to snacking and missing meals, or to restrictive dieting or the over-consumption of fast food. Obesity and eating disorders often have their onset around this time.

KEY POINTS

- Breast milk provides ideal nutrition for babies.
- The optimum time for weaning is 6 months.
- Formula feeds need to be made up carefully to avoid infection.
- 'Doorstep' cow's milk should not be used until 1 year.
- Full-fat milk is recommended until 5 years of age.
- Toddlers need to be allowed to explore food and develop independent eating habits.
- Children should be offered a well-balanced diet in proportion to the four main food groups.

14 Common behaviour concerns

The crying baby
- Wet or dirty nappy
- Too hot or too cold
- Hungry
- Wind
- Colic
- Environmental stress
- Reflux oesophagitis
- Teething

If sudden severe crying, consider:
- Any acute illness
- Otitis media
- Intussusception
- Strangulated inguinal hernia

Temper tantrums
- Normal, peak at 18–36 months
- Screaming
- Hitting
- Biting
- Breath-holding attacks (see Chapter 43)

Strategies that may help
- Avoid precipitants such as hunger and tiredness
- Divert the tantrum by distraction
- Stay calm to teach control
- Reward good behaviour
- Try to ignore bad behaviour until calm
- Use time-out

Sleeping problems
- Difficulty getting to sleep
- Waking during the night
- Sleeping in parents' bed
- Nightmares and night terrors

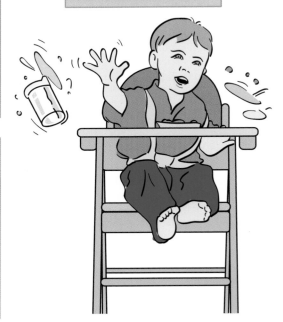

Eating problems in toddlers
- Food refusal
- Fussy eating—only eating a limited variety of foods
- Overeating
- Battles over eating and mealtimes
- Snacking
- Excessive drinking of juice

Unwanted habits
- Thumb sucking
- Nail biting
- Masturbation
- Head banging
- Hair pulling
- Bedwetting
- Encopresis (passing faeces in inappropriate places)

Aggressive behaviour
- Temper tantrums
- Hitting and biting other children
- Destroying toys
- Destroying furniture
- Commoner in boys and in larger families
- May reflect aggression within family
- Requires calm, consistent approach
- Avoid countering with aggression
- Use time-out and star charts

What you need from your evaluation

History
- Ask what is troubling the parents most—is it the child or other stresses in their lives, such as tiredness, problems at work or relationship problems?
- What are the triggers for difficult or unwanted behaviour? Does it occur when the child is hungry or tired, or at any particular time of day?
- Colic tends to occur in the evenings; tantrums may be more common if the child is tired
- Does the behaviour happen consistently in all settings or is it specific to one place, e.g. the toddler may behave well at nursery but show difficult behaviour at home?
- Does the behaviour differ with each parent?
- How do the parents deal with the behaviour—do they get angry or aggressive, are they consistent, do they use bribery or do they give in to the toddler eventually?
- What strategies have the parents already tried to deal with the situation?
- Is there any serious risk of harm? Some behaviour, such as encopresis or deliberate self-harm, may reflect serious emotional upset. Most toddlers who are faddy eaters are growing well and do not suffer any long-term nutritional problems
- Babies with colic are usually less than 3 months old, go red in the face with a tense abdomen and draw up their legs. The episodes start abruptly and end with the passage of flatus or faeces

Examination
- The history usually contributes more than a physical examination
- If the parents are concerned about sudden-onset or severe crying in a baby, it is important to exclude serious infection such as meningitis or urinary tract infection, intussusception, hernias and otitis media

Management
- In most cases the parents can be reassured that the behaviour is very common, often normal and that with time and common sense it can be controlled
- With tantrums it can be helpful to use the **ABC** approach:
  - A What **a**ntecedents were there? What happened to trigger the episode?
  - B What was the **b**ehaviour? Could it be modified, diverted or stopped?
  - C What were the **c**onsequences of the behaviour? Was the child told off, shouted at or given a cuddle?
- Generally, it is best to reward good behaviour (catch the child being good) and ignore bad behaviour. Star charts can be very useful: the child gets a star for good behaviour (staying in bed, etc.) and then a reward after several stars
- Parents should try hard not to be angry or aggressive as this may reinforce attention-seeking behaviour

Paediatrics at a Glance, Fourth Edition. Lawrence Miall, Mary Rudolf and Dominic Smith. © 2016 John Wiley & Sons, Ltd. Published 2016 by John Wiley & Sons, Ltd.
Companion website: www.ataglanceseries.com/paediatrics

Common emotional and behavioural problems

These problems are seen so often that many would regard them as normal, although in a small minority, the behaviour is so disruptive that it causes major family upset. General practitioners and paediatricians should be comfortable giving basic guidance on behaviour management to help parents through what can be a stressful, exasperating and exhausting phase of their child's development.

Crying babies and colic

Crying is usually periodic and related to discomfort, stress or temperament. However, it may indicate a serious problem, particularly if the onset is sudden. In most instances, it is just a case of ensuring that the baby is well fed, warm but not too hot, has a clean nappy, comfortable clothes and a calm and peaceful environment. A persistently crying baby can be very stressful for inexperienced parents. It is important that they recognize when they are no longer coping and are offered support.

Infantile colic is a term used to describe periodic crying affecting infants in the first 3 months of life. The crying is paroxysmal and may be associated with hunger, swallowed air or discomfort from overfeeding. It often occurs in the evenings. Crying can last for several hours, with a flushed face, distended and tense abdomen and drawn-up legs. In between attacks, the child is happy and well. It is important to consider more serious pathology such as intussusception or infection. Colic is managed by giving advice on feeding, winding after feeds and carrying the baby. It is not a reason to stop breastfeeding, but discontinuing cow's milk in the mother's diet can be helpful. Various remedies are available, but there is little evidence for their effectiveness. Infantile colic usually resolves spontaneously by 3 months.

Feeding problems

Once weaned, infants need to gradually move from being fed with a spoon to finger feeding and feeding themselves. This is a messy time, but the infant needs to be allowed to explore their food and not be made to eat or reprimanded for making a mess.

Toddler eating habits can be unpredictable—eating large amounts at one meal and sometimes hardly anything at the next. At this age, mealtimes can easily become a battle, and it is important that they are kept relaxed and the child is not pressurized into eating. Small helpings that the child can finish work best, and second helpings can be given if wanted. Eating together as a family encourages the child to eat in a social context. Feeding at mealtimes should not become a long protracted battle!

Sleeping problems

Babies and children differ in the amount of sleep they need and parents vary in how they tolerate their child waking at night. In most cases, sleeping 'difficulties' are really just habits that have developed through lack of clear bedtime routine. Difficulty sleeping may also reflect conflict in the family or anxieties, for example, about starting school or fear of dying. Successfully tackling sleeping problems requires determination, support and reassurance.

- **Refusal to settle at night.** Difficulty settling may develop if babies are only put to bed once they are asleep. A clear bedtime routine is important for older children—for example a bath, a story and a drink.
- **Waking during the night.** This often causes a lot of stress as the parents become exhausted. It is important to reassure the child, and then put them back to bed quietly. Sometimes, a technique of 'controlled crying' can be helpful—the child is left to cry for a few minutes, then reassured and left again, this time for longer. Taking the child into the parents' bed is understandable, but usually stores up problems for later when it is difficult to break the habit.
- **Nightmares.** The child wakes as the result of a bad dream, quickly becomes lucid and can usually remember the content. The child should be reassured and returned to sleep. If particularly severe or persistent, nightmares may reflect stresses and may need psychological help.
- **Night terrors.** Night terrors occur in preschool years. The child wakes up confused, disorientated and frightened and may not recognize their parent. They take several minutes to become orientated and the dream content cannot be recalled. These episodes should not be confused with epilepsy. They are short-lived and just require reassurance, especially for the parents.

Temper tantrums

Tantrums are very common in the third year of life (the 'terrible twos') and are part of the child learning the boundaries of acceptable behaviour and parental control. They can be extremely challenging, especially when they occur in public!

The key to dealing with toddler tantrums is to try to avoid getting into the situation in the first place. This does not mean giving in to the child's every demand, but ensuring the child does not get overtired or hungry, and setting clear boundaries in a calm, consistent way. It is generally best to ignore the tantrum until the child calms down. If this fails, then 'time out' can be a useful technique. The child is taken to a safe, quiet environment, such as a bedroom, and left for a few minutes (1 minute for each year of age is a good guide) until calm. This is usually very effective as it removes the attention the child desires, and allows the parents time to control their own anger.

Unwanted or aggressive behaviour

Young children often have aggressive outbursts, which may involve biting, hitting or scratching other children. These require consistent firm management, with use of time out and star charts for good behaviour. It is important not to respond with more aggression as this sends conflicting messages. If aggressive behaviour is persistent, it is important to explore other tensions or disturbances within the family. In older children, the school may need to be involved.

Unwanted behaviours such as thumb-sucking, hair-pulling, nail-biting and masturbation are also common in young children. The majority can be ignored and resolve with time. Masturbation can usually be prevented by distracting the child or dressing them in clothes that make it more difficult. Older children should not be reprimanded but informed that it is not acceptable in public.

KEY POINTS

- Emotional and behavioural problems are extremely common, to the point of being part of normal child development.
- Parents need to be encouraged that they can manage most behaviour with a clear strategy.
- A calm, confident and consistent approach to the child's behaviour is recommended.
- Parents should reward good behaviour and try to minimize attention given to undesirable behaviour.

15 Child care and school

Child care
Increasingly, mothers are working outside the home
and need to find care for their children. Options in the UK include:
- A nanny or minder
- A childminder who takes other children into their own
  home and has to be legally approved and registered with
  the social services
- A day nursery staffed by nursery nurses and run either
  privately, by social services departments, or by voluntary
  organizations
- Children's Centres in disadvantaged areas that
  provide a variety of facilities and programmes
  for young families

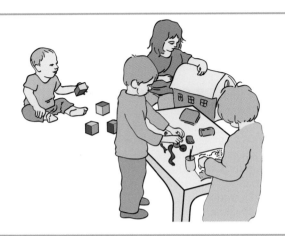

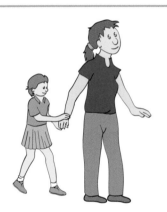

Education
In the UK, compulsory education begins at age 5 and continues to age 16. For younger
children there are opportunities to meet, play and socialize with others
Preschool
- Mother and toddler groups for children accompanied by a carer
- Playgroups run by trained and registered leaders
- A limited availability of nursery school places from 3 years of age
School
- Primary school from 5 to 11 years of age
- Secondary school from 11 to 16 years
- Sixth form, sixth form college or college of further education at age 16 years

School and health
Health promotion
School offers the opportunity to educate children about healthy living
- healthy relationships
- nutrition
- physical activity
- drugs and alcohol abuse
- contraception and safe sex
- smoking
- how to care for babies and young children

The child with medical problems (see Chapter 64)
Doctors have a role in making sure that children who have chronic health
problems are well integrated and that staff understand the child's
medical condition

The child with special educational needs (see Chapter 66)
Where at all possible, children with special educational needs are included
in mainstream education. In the UK one of the teachers in the school is appointed
as a special needs coordinator (SENCO). She has responsibility for children with
educational needs and ensures the child is supported through learning in small
groups or with special needs assistance. When needed, physiotherapy, occupational
therapy and speech and language therapy is provided at school

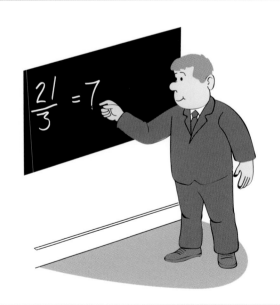

$$\frac{21}{3} = 7$$

Common problems at school age
Attention deficit and hyperactivity disorder (ADHD)

Hyperactivity is characterized by overactivity, difficulty keeping still and restlessness. These children can be impulsive and excitable; learning can be impaired and classes disrupted. Children with *attention deficit disorder* have difficulty concentrating on a task. It may or may not occur with hyperactivity (when it is known as ADHD) and is more common in boys.

A diagnosis of ADHD should only be made following independent reporting by family and school as well as direct observation of the child. The problems need to be pervasive (present in different settings). Management includes strategies to reduce distraction, focus on task, build concentration and provision of a calm regular daily routine with consistent boundaries. Support with teaching assistance may be helpful to help the child focus on tasks. Central nervous system (CNS) stimulant drugs such as methylphenidate can help improve concentration.

Aggressive behaviour

Temper tantrums with shouting and physical outbursts are normal in the toddler years but should settle as children learn to control their anger and frustration through consistent parenting. Aggressive behaviour in children is very rarely caused by medical illness (e.g. precocious puberty and frontal lobe problems). It is the most often behaviour that the child has learned from their home environment by adults showing verbal or physical aggression, for example if children witness domestic violence. Aggressive children may be involved in bullying in school and further social problems beyond. If persistent, then the description 'conduct disorder' is sometimes applied. Maintaining a calm environment with emotional warmth and clear boundaries at home is necessary. School staff should be involved along with parents in order to address peer problems, academic or social problems and to institute behaviour modification.

Teasing and bullying

Bullying is the term used when a child deliberately behaves in a way that upsets or frightens another child. This can be a single episode or repeated over long periods of time and can lead to significant distress. The bullied child may react by becoming withdrawn or aggressive or may develop illness symptoms. In schools where bullying is a problem, a whole-school approach where the bullies are helped as well as the victims is most effective. The bullied child needs to feel safe and supported if they disclose. They need help in handling the situation and to increase social confidence.

Non-attendance at school

Most absences from school occur as a result of acute illness, which is usually minor, but may be prolonged through parental anxiety. School refusal may be due to separation anxiety (common on first starting school) or school phobia (usually triggered by distressing events, such as problems with peers). There may be abnormal attachment affecting the parent–child relationship. The child may have non-specific illness symptoms and social withdrawal. Truancy is most common at secondary school age. Persistent truancy is associated with antisocial behaviour, poor academic achievement and family relationship problems.

Management of non-attendance must involve close collaboration between the parents and teachers. The child should be supported in a gradual return to full attendance through a combined approach involving parents, school, child health and child psychology. Truancy is managed with school or education welfare staff.

Severe educational difficulties

Reasons for severe educational difficulties include the following.

Developmental problems
- Learning difficulties
- ADHD
- Hearing or visual deficit
- Dyslexia
- Dyspraxia
- Autistic spectrum disorder.

Social problems
- Family problems at home
- Emotional, physical, sexual abuse or neglect
- Peer problems
- Absence from school.

School failure is associated with low self-esteem, behavioural difficulties, psychosomatic disorders and has profound effects on adult life. It is important to resolve the problems as early as possible.

Dyslexia

Dyslexia is the most common type of specific learning difficulty. Dyslexic children are unable to process effectively the information required in order to read. The result is a reading ability below that expected for the child's level of intelligence. Children may struggle with spelling and handwriting.

There may be a history of early language delay. If dyslexia is unrecognized, the child is likely to fail at school and may respond by withdrawing or disruptive behaviour. The diagnosis should be confirmed by an educational psychologist, and individual help is required to overcome the difficulties. Strategies to help children with dyslexia include allowing extra time to complete written tasks, use of computers as writing aids and adapting the presentation of information to suit their learning style.

Dyspraxia

Motor incoordination leads to significant problems with handwriting, and difficulty with sports and with practical tasks such as dressing and eating with cutlery. If it is disproportionate to the child's general developmental ability, the term 'dyspraxia' or 'developmental coordination disorder' may be applied. The academic and social difficulties that ensue can cause unhappiness and behaviour problems. Occupational therapists have experience in assessing the level of difficulties and can assist in devising treatment programmes, sometimes using equipment to reduce the functional difficulties.

16 Child health promotion

Child health promotion

What does promoting child health involve?

Child health promotion covers a broad range of activities that aims to ensure that children grow up in a healthy, safe environment, attain their potential and are protected from disease. In the UK the Healthy Child Programme is a comprehensive programme, which has the following goals for babies and preschool children:

- Encouraging a strong bond between parents and child and helping parents enhance their parenting skills
- Protecting children from serious diseases through immunization and screening
- Promoting healthy eating, physical activity and reducing obesity
- Identifying problems in children's health and development (such as learning difficulties) and safety (such as parental neglect), and directing families for help
- Making sure children are ready for school
- Identifying and helping children with problems that might affect their chances later in life.

Information on The Healthy Child Programme is available at *https://www.gov.uk/government/uploads/system/uploads/attachment_data/file/167998/Health_Child_Programme.pdf*

At-risk families

Disadvantage is known to place children at risk for adverse outcomes. Extra support is needed to minimize the impact on the child:

- Poor quality or overcrowded housing
- Both parents unemployed and low income families
- Lack of parental educational
- Parental mental illness
- Long-standing limiting illness or disability in a parent

Protective factors and resilience

Health promotion also involves encouraging protective factors that build resilience and mitigate against adversity. These include authoritative parenting combined with warmth and affectionate attachment between the child and primary caregiver.

Opportunities for promoting child health

Child health promotion should start in pregnancy, and continue with the family through the early years. In the UK routine reviews occur in

- The first trimester of pregnancy
- The neonatal examination
- At the age of 2 weeks
- At 6–8 weeks
- Around the age of 1 year
- Between 2 and 2½ years
- At school entry

Parents and professionals are encouraged to use the parent-held child health record (often referred to as "the red book" in the UK)

Topics to be addressed in promoting child health

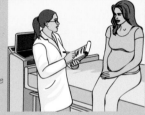

In pregnancy:
- Parental health and well-being
- Smoking cessation
- Folic acid
- Breast feeding
- Attitudes and concerns
- Assessment of risks and protective factors

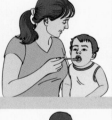

In the child:
- Physical health, growth and development
- Language, vision and hearing
- Development of independence and self-care skills
- Parental attachment
- Immunizations and screening

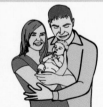

In the family:
- Parenting skills.
- Financial advice, housing and employment
- Safety and dietary issues
- Family relationships and health
- Assessment of risk factors

Who is involved?

In the UK health promotion is primarily the responsibility of health visitors (public health nurses). Other professionals include general practitioners, communit paediatricians and school nurses.

Paediatrics at a Glance, Fourth Edition. Lawrence Miall, Mary Rudolf and Dominic Smith. © 2016 John Wiley & Sons, Ltd. Published 2016 by John Wiley & Sons, Ltd.
Companion website: www.ataglanceseries.com/paediatrics

Child health promotion is of universal and practical importance in supporting young families as they grow up. It is delivered in a number of ways in different countries and generally involves guidance, immunization, screening and identification of children with additional needs. In the UK, a 'package of care' is delivered by health visiting teams through the Healthy Child Programme. Routine contact takes place in the first 2 weeks, at 6–8 weeks, 6–12 months and at 24 to 30 months. In addition, parents can attend drop-in clinics when they choose. Sure Start Children's Centres, a UK government initiative, provide skilled staff and facilities with child health promotion at the core of their work.

The Healthy Child Programme is underpinned by a principle of progressive universalism, where all children receive a basic service with increased input according to a child or family's needs, so ensuring that the most vulnerable families are supported. Alongside identifying children who are at risk because of adverse circumstances in the family, it is important that protective factors are strengthened to promote children's resilience to adversity. These include encouraging bonding between parent and child and authoritative parenting, where parents are able to set boundaries to children's behaviour while remaining warm and responsive.

Parenting support

Many young parents have had little experience of young children before having a baby and lack the support of an extended family. An important component of child health promotion is supporting parents and helping them develop the skills to cope with the challenges of bringing up children. One way is to offer parents the opportunity to participate in a parenting programme, where they are helped to enhance their parenting skills and have the benefit of sharing their concerns with others.

Parental mental health

Parents' ability to provide a quality home life for their families can be profoundly affected by mental health. An important aspect of child health promotion is to recognize when this is an issue and to guide parents towards receiving appropriate help. Postnatal depression is common, and health professionals need to be alert to identifying it and ensuring support is in place.

Baby care

Guidance needs to be offered to parents about all aspects of baby care, including clothing, bathing, handling and positioning a baby. Information is also needed about normal development, what to expect from the child, how to promote learning and how to recognize developmental difficulties. Advice is given about common medical problems and how to manage them.

Child development and behavioural problems

Early intervention is important if a child has developmental delay or a developmental disorder. A key aspect of child health promotion involves the early detection of developmental concerns and directing the family to appropriate evaluation and input (see Chapters 4 and 41).

Behavioural concerns around crying, sleep and temper tantrums are universal. Advice and support in the early stages can avoid them developing into major problems (see Chapter 14).

Nutrition

Addressing nutritional issues is an important component of preventive health care. It includes promotion of breastfeeding, advice about weaning, dealing with toddlers' eating difficulties and education about healthy diets for the entire family. Now that obesity is epidemic in children, an important aspect of child health promotion relates to ensuring that children have a healthy balanced diet and increasing their physical activity (see Chapter 20).

Dental health

Healthy dental development is encouraged by a good diet, which is low in sugar to reduce dental decay. Sugar should not be added to weaning foods and from 1 year of age, feeding from a bottle should be discouraged. Drinks containing sugar, including juice, should be limited. Tooth brushing should start as soon as teeth erupt, and children should be taught to clean their teeth from an early age. Fluorinated toothpaste should be used especially in areas with inadequate levels in the drinking water.

Passive smoking

Children exposed to passive smoking are at increased risk of sudden infant death syndrome, middle ear disease, lower respiratory tract illness and asthma. Avoidance of exposing children to smoke at home and in cars is, therefore, an important health promotion issue.

Injury prevention

Most injuries occur in the home, so education of parents can have an important impact on their prevention. Issues of importance include car seats and belts, road safety and use of cycle helmets, gates on stairs, safety in the kitchen, smoke alarms, protection against fire hazards, covering electric sockets and keeping medicines/poisons out of reach (see Chapters 62 and 63).

Identifying risks and safeguarding children

Raising children is a challenging task, and it is made more so when families live in poverty, when parents lack education, where there are mental health problems or there is domestic violence. Where there are concerns that a child might be the victim of neglect, non-accidental injury or emotional or sexual abuse, social care needs to be informed (see Chapter 68).

Health promotion in school

School provides an invaluable opportunity to educate the young about healthy living, and, hopefully, the school years are a time when adjustments in lifestyle can be made more easily than later on in life. Issues of particular importance that are addressed are:

- Nutrition
- Physical activity
- Reducing risk factors for obesity
- Drugs and alcohol abuse
- Contraception and safe sex
- Sexually transmitted diseases
- Smoking
- Healthy relationships
- Caring for young children.

Screening and immunization

These important aspects of the child health promotion programme are covered in Chapters 7 and 17.

17 The immunization schedule

The immunization schedule

5-in-1 infant vaccine DTaP/IPV/Hib
- Primary immunization given intramuscularly three times in infancy, with boosters preschool and in high school
- Protects against the five following diseases:
  - Diphtheria (D)
  - Tetanus (T)
  - Pertussis (aP)
  - Polio (IPV)
  - Haemophilus influenzae type B (Hib)
- Pertussis should not be given to a child with a progressive neurological condition
- Possible side effects within 12–24 hours include the following:
  - Swelling and redness at site
  - Fever
  - Diarrhoea and/or vomiting
  - Papule at injection site lasting a few weeks
  - Irritability for 48 hours
  - Rarely high fever, febrile convulsions, and anaphylaxis

4-in-1 preschool booster DTaP/IPV
- Protects against diphtheria, tetanus, whooping cough, polio

3-in-1 teenage booster Td/IPV
- Protects against tetanus, diphtheria and polio

Men B and Men C
Given IM. Protects against infection by meningococcal groups B and C bacteria respectively—meningitis and septicaemia. It does not protect against any other form of meningitis

Pneumoccoccal
Given IM. Protects against pneumococcal infection—pneumonia, septicaemia and meningitis

Tetanus
- Given IM in infancy as part of the 5-in-1 infant vaccine, with boosters preschool and in high school
- *Dirty wounds:* Give tetanus immunoglobulin, with booster if last vaccination was >10 years previously (or give full course if not immunized)

NATIONAL IMMUNIZATION SCHEDULE IN THE UK*

Infant

Birth	Hepatitis B and BCG for infants at risk
2 months	5-in-1; pneumococcal; meningitis B; rotavirus
3 months	5-in-1; pneumococcal; rotavirus; meninigitis C
4 months	5-in-1; pneumococcal; meninigitis B
12–13 (months)	Hib/ Men C; MMR; Pneumococcal; meninigitis B

Preschool

2–4 years	Children's flu (annual)
3yrs 4 months	MMR
	4-in1 preschool booster

Secondary school

12–13 years	HPV
13–18 years	3-in-1 teenage booster; Men ACWY

*schedules are similar in USA, Australia.

Rotavirus
- Given orally at 2 and 3 months
- Protects against rotavirus gastro-enteritis
- Side effects: irritability and mild diarrhoea

Men ACWY
Given IM. Recommended for adolescents and students. Protects against infection by 4 strains of Meningococcus — meningitis and septicaemia.

MMR
- Live attenuated vaccine against:
  - Measles
  - Mumps
  - Rubella
- The vaccine is a live attenuated virus given at 12–13 months and at school entry. Children who are severely immunosuppressed should not receive the vaccine, or pregnant girls. Advice is needed if the child is severely allergic to eggs (the vaccine is grown on chick embryo tissue)
- There is no evidence that it is related to autism and bowel disease
- Side effects:
  - Common to have rash and fever 5–10 days later
  - Mild mumps 2 weeks later

BCG (Bacille Calmette–Guérin)
Protects against tuberculosis. Given to babies living in areas with a high rate of TB or to children recently arrived from countries with high levels of TB or who have come into close contact with somebody infected with respiratory TB
  - A live attenuated bacterium strain of *Mycobacterium bovis*
  - Given intradermally
  - Papule forms and often ulcerates
  - Heals over 6–8 weeks with a scar

HPV (human papillomavirus virus)
Given to girls aged 12–13 years 2 injections 6 to 24 months apart Protects against common causes of cervical cancer, and offers some protection for genital warts too

General immunization guidelines
- Immunizations should not be given to a child who:
  - is younger than indicated in the schedule
  - is acutely unwell with fever
  - has had an anaphylactic reaction to a previous dose of the vaccine
- Repeat immunizations should not be given sooner than indicated in the schedule
- If a child misses an immunization, it should be given later. There is no need to restart the course
- Live attenuated vaccines (e.g. measles, mumps, rubella and BCG) should not usually be given to children who are immunodeficient (e.g. cytotoxic therapy or high dose steroids)

Paediatrics at a Glance, Fourth Edition. Lawrence Miall, Mary Rudolf and Dominic Smith. © 2016 John Wiley & Sons, Ltd. Published 2016 by John Wiley & Sons, Ltd.
Companion website: www.ataglanceseries.com/paediatrics

Diseases protected against by immunizations in childhood

Diphtheria

Diphtheria is now very rare in developed countries. It is caused by the organism *Corynebacterium diphtheriae*. Infection occurs in the throat, forming a pharyngeal exudate, which leads to membrane formation and obstruction of the upper airways. An exotoxin released by the bacterium may cause myocarditis and paralysis.

Tetanus

Tetanus is caused by an anaerobic organism, *Clostridium tetani*, found universally in the soil, which enters the body through open wounds. Progressive painful muscle spasms are caused by a neurotoxin produced by the organism. Involvement of the respiratory muscles results in asphyxia and death.

Pertussis (whooping cough)

Whooping cough is caused by the bacterium *Bordetella pertussis*. It lasts for 6–8 weeks and has three stages: catarrhal, paroxysmal and convalescent. Paroxysms of coughing are followed by a whoop (a sudden inspiratory effort against a narrowed glottis), with vomiting, dyspnoea and sometimes seizures. Complications include bronchopneumonia, convulsions, apnoea and bronchiectasis. The diagnosis is clinical and can be confirmed by nasopharyngeal culture. Erythromycin given early shortens the illness but is ineffective by the time the whoop is heard. There is high morbidity and mortality in children under the age of 2.

Polio

Polio is caused by the poliomyelitis virus, which produces a mild febrile illness, progressing to meningitis in some children. Anterior horn cell damage leads to paralysis, pain and tenderness. It may also cause respiratory failure and bulbar paralysis. Residual paralysis is common in those who survive.

Haemophilus influenzae B

Haemophilus influenzae type B (Hib) was the main cause of meningitis in young children before the vaccine was introduced. It led to severe neurological sequelae such as profound deafness, cerebral palsy and epilepsy in 10–15% of cases and death in 3%. The vaccine is only effective against type B infection.

Pneumococcal disease

Pneumococcal disease is caused by *Streptococcus pneumoniae*, which can lead to septicaemia, meningitis and pneumonia.

Meningococcal C

Meningococcus C causes purulent meningitis in young children with a purpuric rash and septicaemic shock. Mortality is as high at 10% and morbidity includes hearing loss, seizures, brain damage, organ failure and tissue necrosis.

Rotavirus

Rotavirus is highly infectious and causes diarrhoea, vomiting, abdominal pain and fever. It can cause severe dehydration and even death in small babies.

Measles

Measles is characterized by a maculopapular rash, fever, coryza, cough and conjunctivitis. Complications include encephalitis leading to neurological damage and a high mortality rate. In the United Kingdom, there has been a recent reduction in vaccine uptake due to unfounded concerns about an association with autism and inflammatory bowel disease. These have now been disproved.

Mumps

Mumps causes a febrile illness with enlargement of the parotid glands. Complications include aseptic meningitis, sensorineural deafness and orchitis in adults. It is a cause of subfertility in men.

Rubella

Rubella is a mild illness causing rash and fever. Its importance lies in the devastating effects it has on the fetus if infection occurs in the early stages of pregnancy. These include multiple congenital defects such as cataracts, deafness and congenital heart disease.

Tuberculosis (TB)

Tuberculosis remains a major problem in many countries and is re-emerging in eastern Europe. It affects the lungs, meninges, bones and joints. Most children are identified because they are contacts of infected adults. Symptoms include cough, tiredness, weight loss, night sweats, haemoptysis and lymphadenopathy. Most have a positive reaction on Mantoux skin testing. Active TB requires treatment that must be continued over many months. BCG is recommended at birth for babies born in communities where there is a high prevalence and for children whose parents or grandparents were born in countries with a high prevalence.

Hepatitis B

Hepatitis B is an important cause of acute and chronic liver disease. It can be transmitted perinatally from carrier mothers or through blood transfusion, needlestick injuries and biting insects. Children with HBV may be asymptomatic. Babies born to HBsAg +ve mothers receive vaccination at birth.

Human papillomavirus (HPV)

Infection with human papillomavirus is common, with over 50% of sexually active women infected over their lifetime. Two strains (16 and 18) are the cause of cervical cancer in >70% of cases. The vaccine is given to girls and gives some protection against genital warts too. Some countries have also started to vaccinate boys.

Chicken pox

Chickenpox is a common childhood infection, which is usually mild. It causes serious morbidity in immunosuppressed individuals and immunisation is recommended for health workers and other close contacts of individuals on chemotherapy.

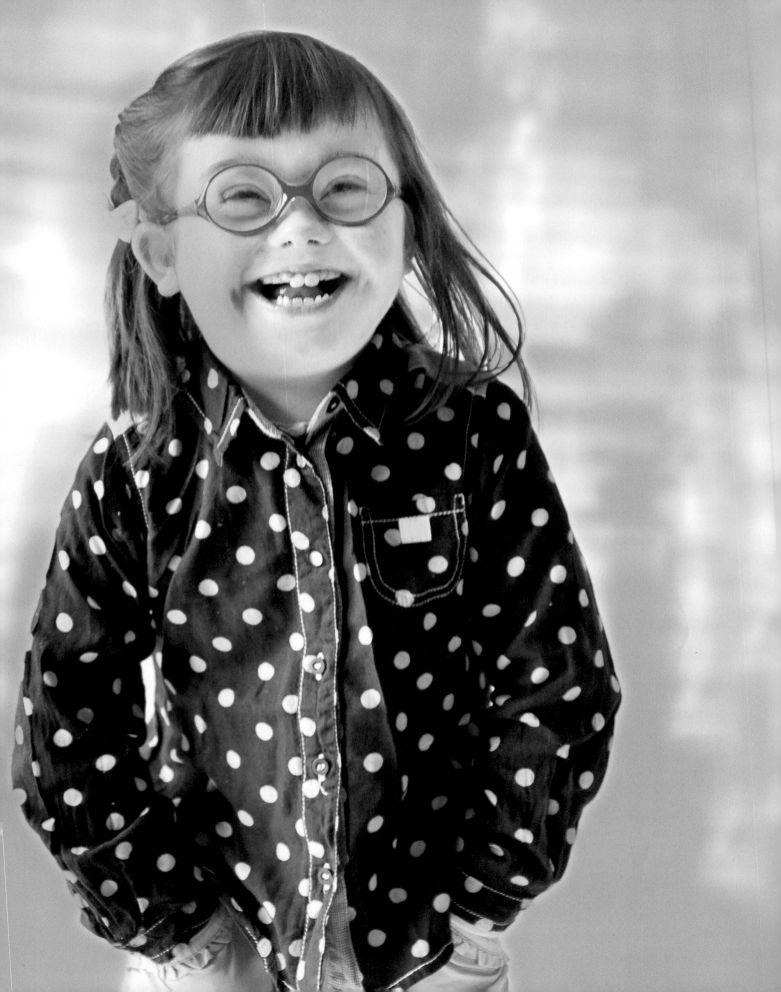

Growth, endocrine and metabolic

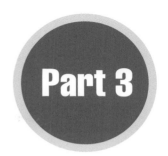

Part 3

Chapters

Weight faltering and failure to thrive

Weight faltering

Catch down growth and 'constitutional'
- Babies commonly cross centiles in first year
- Large babies cross down to reach genetically destined centile
- Important not to cause iatrogenic distress

Environmental/psychosocial (non-organic)
- Most common cause of weight faltering
- Weight is usually affected first, then height and head growth
- Eating difficulties are common
- Disturbed maternal–infant interaction may be present
- Maternal depression/psychiatric disorder may be present
- Neglect may be a factor

Cystic fibrosis
(see Chapter 30)
- Diarrhoea
- Chest infections

IUGR
- Low birthweight
- If birth length and head size were also small, catch-up is less likely
- May have features of TORCH
- May be due to a genetic syndrome

Immunodeficiency (rare)
- Recurrent infections
- HIV, SCID are causes

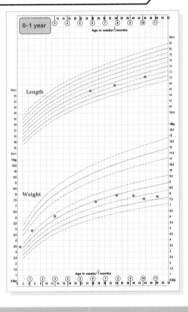

Genetic syndromes
- Low birthweight common
- Dysmorphic features

Chronic illness
- Only rarely an occult cause
- Features depend on the illness

Gastro-oesophageal reflux
(see Chapter 32)
- Pain from oesophagitis
- Apnoea
- Vomiting/possetting
- Common in babies with neuro-developmental problems

Coeliac disease (see Chapter 34)
- Weight may fall off at weaning when gluten is introduced
- Diarrhoea
- Irritability

Endocrine dysfunction
- Developmental delay in hypothyroidism
- Growth hormone deficiency very rare

What you need from your evaluation

History

- **Nutritional history.** Take a dietary history (a food diary can be helpful).
  Ask about feeding difficulties: did they start at birth, weaning or as a toddler? Consider whether they are a result or cause of weight faltering
- **Review of symptoms.** A good history identifies most organic conditions. Look for diarrhoea, colic, vomiting, irritability, fatigue or chronic cough
- **Developmental history.** Are there neurodevelopmental problems? Has weight faltering affected the baby's developmental progress?
- **Past medical history.** Low birthweight and prenatal problems may jeopardize growth potential. Recurrent or chronic illness may affect growth
- **Family history.** Is there a family history of weight faltering or genetic problems? Are there psychosocial problems?

Examination

- **General observations.** Does the child look neglected, ill or malnourished (thin, wasted buttocks, a protuberant abdomen and sparse hair)?
  How does the mother relate to the baby?
- **Growth.** Plot growth on a chart (remember to correct for prematurity!)
- **Physical examination.** Look for signs of chronic illness

Investigations

'Fishing' for a diagnosis by carrying out multiple investigations is wasteful and unhelpful. Obtaining a blood count and ferritin level is useful as iron deficiency is common and affects development and appetite. Otherwise, investigations should be based on clinical findings.

Paediatrics at a Glance, Fourth Edition. Lawrence Miall, Mary Rudolf and Dominic Smith. © 2016 John Wiley & Sons, Ltd. Published 2016 by John Wiley & Sons, Ltd.
Companion website: www.ataglanceseries.com/paediatrics

Investigations and their significance			
• Full blood count, ferritin	Iron deficiency is common in FTT and can cause anorexia	• Thyroid hormone and TSH	Congenital hypothyroidism causes poor growth and developmental delay
• Urea and electrolytes	Unsuspected renal failure	• Karyotype	Chromosomal abnormalities are often associated with short stature and dysmorphism
• Stool for fecal elastase	Low levels suggest malabsorption	• Hospitalization	Hospitalization can be a form of investigation Observation of baby and mother over time can provide clues to the aetiology
• Coeliac antibodies, jejunal biopsy, sweat test	Coeliac disease and cystic fibrosis are the most important causes of malabsorption		

Concern about growth is usually raised when:

- Weight is below the second centile
- Height is below the second centile
- *Or* when height or weight crosses down two centiles.

Growth and weight faltering are common in the first 2 years of life, and expertise is needed to diagnose a normal growth pattern from a pathological cause. There is some debate about the terms used. *Weight faltering* has replaced *failure to thrive* and tends to imply that the condition is not serious and is transient. *Failure to thrive (FTT)* implies not only growth failure but also failure of emotional and developmental progress. It usually refers to babies or toddlers who have been subject to neglect. The most common causes of weight faltering and failure to thrive are non-organic.

It can be very distressing when a young child's weight falters, and the evaluation needs to be carried out sensitively. The purpose is to differentiate the child with a problem and to identify contributing factors whether organic or non-organic (which may coexist). It is important that a normal, healthy but small baby is not wrongly labelled. Investigations need to be requested judiciously.

'Catch down' growth and 'constitutional' causes

Short parents tend to have small children and small, healthy children with short parents should not arouse concern. Usually, growth is steady along lower centiles, but large babies may cross down centiles before settling onto their destined line. It is very important that professionals do not engender unnecessary anxiety, leading to feeding difficulties and sustained weight faltering.

Weight faltering due to environmental or psychosocial causes

Psychosocial causes include eating difficulties, difficulties in the home and limited parenting skills. Fall off in weight can be initiated by poor appetite following a minor illness, which has been handled poorly creating a cycle of stress. More serious causes include disturbed attachment and maternal depression or psychiatric disorder. Uncommonly, neglect is a factor.

Most commonly the child is from a caring home, where parents are anxious and concerned. The problem is often one of eating difficulties, where meals are very stressful and parents do their utmost (often counterproductively) to persuade the child to eat. The picture is quite different from the neglected child who shows physical signs of poor care and emotional attachment. In this case, the problem is often denied and compliance with intervention poor.

Management must suit the underlying problem. An organic cause needs to be excluded and nutritional advice and help with eating problems provided. Stopping breastfeeding is rarely helpful. Practical support can ease the stress, and nursery placement can be helpful as well as helping to resolve eating difficulties. Occasionally, it is necessary to admit the baby for observation.

Failure to thrive

FTT implies not only growth failure but also failure of emotional and developmental progress. Weight gain is usually first affected, followed in some by a fall in length and head circumference. The child's development may also be delayed. Where neglect is the cause and the family is not amenable to help, social care must be involved. A few children need to be removed from their homes.

Malabsorption

Malabsorption is an important cause of poor weight gain. Diarrhoea and colic are usually present. The commonest causes of malabsorption are coeliac disease and cystic fibrosis. In the former, the growth curve characteristically shows fall-off in weight coincident with the introduction of gluten.

Chronic illness

Children and babies with any chronic illness may grow poorly. They rarely present as a diagnostic dilemma as the manifestations of the disease are usually evident. However, organic causes may be compounded by psychosocial difficulties, and these need to be addressed. Very rarely, chronic disease can be occult and present as weight faltering.

Genetic and intrauterine causes

Genetic syndromes are quite commonly associated with short stature, often with congenital abnormalities or dysmorphic features. Intrauterine growth retardation (IUGR) results from adverse uterine conditions that affect infant growth. When this occurs early in the pregnancy, length and head circumference may also be affected, and growth potential jeopardized. The cause of the IUGR should, where possible, be identified.

KEY POINTS

- Be sensitive and do not generate anxiety. It can be very distressing if a baby has weight faltering or fails to thrive.
- Differentiate significant weight faltering from the normal baby who is 'catching down' centiles.
- Identify symptoms and signs suggesting organic conditions.
- Only do investigations if there are leads in the history and examination.
- Identify psychosocial problems and provide help and support.

19 Short stature and poor growth

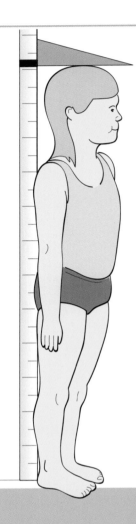

Steady growth below centiles

Constitutional (familial) short stature
- Short parents
- Normal history and examination
- No delay in bone age

Maturational delay
- Delayed onset of puberty
- Family history of delayed puberty
- Delayed bone age

Turner's syndrome
- Features of Turner's syndrome (not always present)
- XO karyotype
- No pubertal signs
- No delay in bone age

IUGR
- Low birthweight
- The underlying reason for the IUGR may be evident

Skeletal dysplasias (rare)
- Body disproportion with shortened limbs
- Achondroplasia is the most common form

Fall-off in growth across centiles

Chronic illness
- Usually identifiable on history and physical examination
- Crohn's disease and chronic renal failure may be occult
- Some delay in bone age occurs

Acquired hypothyroidism
- Clinical features of hypothyroidism
- Goitre may be present
- Low T4, high TSH and thyroid antibodies
- Delayed bone age

Cushing's disease (rare)
- Usually iatrogenic due to prescribed steroids
- Cushingoid features
- Delayed bone age

Growth hormone deficiency (rare)
- Congenital or acquired
- May occur with other hormone deficiencies
- Delayed bone age

Psychosocial
- Neglected appearance
- Behavioural problems
- Catch-up growth occurs when child is removed from home

What you need from your evaluation

History

- **Medical history and review of systems.** Identify any chronic condition, such as asthma, arthritis or diabetes, that can affect growth. Ask about symptoms of raised intracranial pressure, malabsorption and hypothyroidism. Long-term steroid administration stunts growth
- **Family history.** Compare the child's growth with parental heights. It normally lies on the centile between parents' height centiles. Late maternal menarche suggests familial maturational delay
- **Birth history.** A child born small for gestational age may have reduced growth potential. Enquire too about perinatal problems
- **Psychosocial history.** Emotional neglect and abuse can stunt growth but also ascertain whether there are social or emotional difficulties resulting from short stature

Physical examination

- **Pattern of growth.** Obtain previous growth measurements from the GP or school nurse. A fall-off in growth suggests a medical condition requiring treatment
- **Anthropometric measures.** Obtain accurate measures of length (to 24 months of age) or height, and weight. Plot on a growth chart
- **General examination.** Look for signs of hypothyroidism, body disproportion, stigmata of Turner's syndrome and dysmorphism. Each organ system should be examined for evidence of occult disease
- **Head circumference**

Investigations and their significance

If a decrease in growth velocity has occurred, investigations are always required.

- Blood count and plasma viscosity — Inflammatory bowel disease
- Urea and electrolytes — Chronic renal failure
- Coeliac antibodies — Screening test for coeliac disease
- Thyroxine and TSH — Hypothyroidism
- Karyotype (in girls) — Turner's syndrome
- Growth hormone tests — Hypopituitarism, growth hormone deficiency
- X-ray of the wrist for bone age — Delayed bone age suggests maturational delay, hypothyroidism, GH deficiency or corticosteroid excess. A prediction of adult height can be made from it

Paediatrics at a Glance, Fourth Edition. Lawrence Miall, Mary Rudolf and Dominic Smith. © 2016 John Wiley & Sons, Ltd. Published 2016 by John Wiley & Sons, Ltd.
Companion website: www.ataglanceseries.com/paediatrics

Short stature is usually physiological and is due to reduced genetic potential or maturational delay (slow physical development). Fall-off in growth is much more concerning as it suggests a pathological cause. Short stature can cause social difficulties, particularly for adolescent boys, and occasionally psychological counselling is required.

Constitutional or familial short stature

Short parents tend to have short children. In this case, the history and physical examination are normal, and the bone age is appropriate for age. Reassurance is often all that is needed. Prescribing growth hormone in children with physiological short stature is controversial and probably has little effect on children's final adult height.

Maturational delay

Children with maturational delay are often called 'late developers' or 'late bloomers'. These children are short and reach puberty late. Their final height depends on their genetic constitution and may be normal. There is often a family history of delayed puberty and menarche, and the bone age is delayed. Most families simply require reassurance that final height will not be so affected. Sometimes, teenage boys find the social pressures are so great that it is helpful to trigger puberty early using low doses of testosterone, so causing an early growth spurt. This treatment does not have an effect on final height.

Hypothyroidism

The most common causes of hypothyroidism are Hashimoto's autoimmune thyroiditis, which is more common in girls, and hypothyroidism secondary to hypopituitarism. A lack of thyroid hormone has a profound effect on growth, and short stature is often the presenting sign. Other features include a fall-off in school performance, constipation, dry skin and delayed puberty. Low thyroxine (T4) and high thyroid stimulating hormone (TSH) levels are found on investigation, along with antithyroid antibodies if the cause is autoimmune. Treatment with thyroid hormone is lifelong. Parents are often alarmed when their placid, hypothyroid child is transformed into a normal, active teenager. The prognosis is good.

Rarer hormonal problems

Cushing's syndrome and disease are extremely rare in childhood. However, growth suppression from exogenous steroids (e.g. high-dose inhaled steroids for asthma) is not uncommon. When children require long-term, high-dose oral steroid therapy, the deleterious effect on growth is reduced by giving steroids on alternate days.

Growth hormone deficiency is a rare cause of short stature. It may be idiopathic or may occur secondary to pituitary tumours or cranial irradiation. It may be accompanied by deficiency of other pituitary hormones. The diagnosis is made by growth hormone testing, and brain imaging is needed to identify any underlying pathology. Treatment involves daily subcutaneous injections of synthetic growth hormone.

Chronic illness

Any chronic illness can cause stunting of growth. However, chronic illnesses rarely present as short stature as the features of the illness are usually all too evident. Chronic conditions that present with poor growth before other clinical features become obvious include inflammatory bowel disease, coeliac disease and chronic renal failure.

Turner's syndrome

Turner's syndrome or gonadal dysgenesis is an important cause of short stature and delayed puberty in girls. It is caused by the absence of one X chromosome, although mosaicism also occurs. The gonads are merely streaks of fibrous tissue.

At birth, Turner babies often have webbing of the neck and lymphoedematous hands and feet. In childhood, short stature is marked and girls often have the classic features of webbing of the neck, shield-shaped chest, wide-spaced nipples and a wide carrying angle. Some girls are only diagnosed in adolescence when puberty fails to occur. Growth can be promoted by small doses of growth hormone and oestrogen in childhood. Puberty has to be initiated and maintained by oestrogen therapy. Despite treatment, women with Turner's syndrome are usually short. As a result of recent advances in infertility treatment, a few women have become pregnant through in vitro fertilization (IVF) with donated ova.

Late effects of cancer treatment

Slowed growth is a common problem during childhood cancer treatment. If treatment is with chemotherapy without radiation, the change in growth rate is most often short term and many children catch up after treatment. Many of the late effects of cancer on growth are due to radiation therapy. Radiation in the head and neck area can damage the pituitary gland, leading to slow growth and pubertal development. Very young children are most likely to be affected. Treatment with growth hormone may be prescribed to improve growth.

KEY POINTS

- A good history and physical examination identify most pathological causes of short stature.
- Focus on looking for signs of intracranial pathology, hormone deficiency, chronic illness and gastrointestinal symptoms.
- Relate the child's height to the parents' heights.
- Identify any emotional and social consequences of being short.

20 Obesity

Causes of obesity

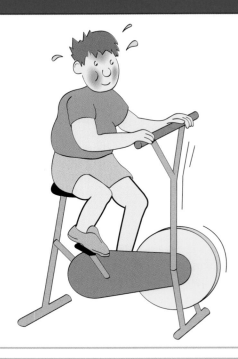

Nutritional obesity
- Family history of obesity is common
- Social/emotional difficulties
- Early puberty
- Penis may seem small (as it is buried in suprapubic fat)
- Child tends to be tall

Genetic syndromes and single gene defects (rare)
- Severe obesity from infancy
- Short stature
- Dysmorphic features
- Learning disability
- Hypogonadism
- Other congenital abnormalities

Endocrine causes (very rare)
- Hypothyroidism
- Cushing's
- Hypothalamic lesions

Consequences for obese children
- Low self-esteem
- School problems (bullied and bullies)
- Impaired glucose tolerance
- Hypertension
- Dyslipidaemia
- Abnormal liver function tests
- Orthopaedic problems
- Asthma
- Sleep apnoea
- Polycystic ovary syndrome
- Obesity in adult life

'5210' recommendations for children
- 5: at least 5 fruit or vegetables per day
- 2: no more than 2 h screen time per day (and none for children <2 years old)
- 1: 1 h physical activity most days
- 0: no sweetened drinks

What you need from your evaluation

History

- **Lifestyle and diet.** Ask about both physical activity and sedentary activities. Take a dietary history, but bear in mind this may be a sensitive issue
- **Emotional and behavioural problems.** Social and school problems are very common. Children may be depressed, bullied or be bullies
- **Complications.** Musculoskeletal symptoms occur due to increased load on the joints. Snoring, and lethargy or tiredness during the day are signs of sleep apnoea. Diabetes and cardiovascular disease are rare in childhood (but biochemical indicators are common)
- **Learning difficulties.** Children with an obesity-related genetic syndrome have special educational needs
- **Symptoms** of endocrine causes, but hypothyroidism and Cushing's are rare
- **Family history.** Ask about others who are obese, and early-onset type 2 diabetes and heart disease

Investigations

Investigate for a cause if the child is short, dysmorphic or has learning difficulties
Look for co-morbidity if child is very obese

Looking for a cause:

● T4, TSH	Low T4 / high TSH in hypothyroidism
● Urinary free cortisol	High in Cushing's disease
● Karyotype and DNA analysis	Genetic syndrome, e.g. Prader–Willi syndrome
● MRI of the brain	Hypothalamic cause

Looking for consequences of obesity:

● Urinary glucose, oral glucose tolerance test, HbA1c	Diabetes
● Fasting lipid screen	Dyslipidaemia
● Liver function tests	Fatty liver

Examination

- **Growth.** Nutritionally obese children are tall. Short stature or fall-off in height suggests a pathological cause. Calculate body mass index (BMI) and plot on a chart

- **Endocrinological signs.** If growth is poor look for signs of hypothyroidism (goitre, developmental delay, slow tendon reflexes, bradycardia) and steroid excess (moon face, buffalo hump, striae, hypertension, bruising)

- **Signs of dysmorphic syndromes.** Short stature, microcephaly, hypogonadism, hypotonia and congenital anomalies

- **Signs of complications.** Check blood pressure and look for acanthosis nigricans (a dark velvety appearance at the neck and axillae)—a sign of insulin resistance

Paediatrics at a Glance, Fourth Edition. Lawrence Miall, Mary Rudolf and Dominic Smith. © 2016 John Wiley & Sons, Ltd. Published 2016 by John Wiley & Sons, Ltd.
Companion website: www.ataglanceseries.com/paediatrics

Obesity is an increasing problem in childhood, and 1 in 10 children are already obese by the time they start primary school. Most overweight and obese children have nutritional obesity, and the diagnosis can be made clinically, as other rare causes are accompanied by poor growth and clinical findings such as learning disability and dysmorphic features. In the UK, overweight is defined as a body mass index (BMI) above the 91st centile and obesity as BMI above the 98th centile.

At one time, obesity in childhood was thought to be a cosmetic problem, but it is now clear that comorbidity can occur in children and adolescents too. The mainstay of management is lifestyle change. Lipase inhibitors to induce fat malabsorption and bariatric surgery are occasionally considered in adolescents.

Nutritional obesity

The metabolic factors that predispose some individuals to becoming obese have yet to be determined, and the correlation between nutrient intake and development of obesity is not simple. Nutritionally obese children are tall, but as they tend to develop puberty early, their final adult height is not usually excessive. Despite its prevalence, obesity remains a stigma and obese children have a high incidence of emotional and behavioural difficulties.

Lifestyle change is difficult to achieve, and it is now well recognized that traditional dietary advice that focuses on the child is not effective. Guidance needs to be holistic, family focused and delivered in a skilled way that builds motivation. It includes the following.

• **Support.** Obese children are often the victims of teasing by peers, and psychological disturbance is common. Even if weight control is not successful, their emotional difficulties can be helped.
• **Encouraging physical activity and reducing sedentary behaviour.** This may be difficult if obese children experience ridicule when trying to be active.
• **A balanced healthy diet.** Rapid decreases in weight through 'crash dieting' should not be attempted and, while the child is growing, weight maintenance is a reasonable goal.
• **Monitoring.** Identification of comorbidities and management as needed.
• Medication and surgery are generally not appropriate or licenced (although may be considered in older adolescents with comorbidity).

Most obese children can be managed in primary care or the community, although those with complex difficulties should be under the care of a paediatrician and multidisciplinary team. Group programmes providing lifestyle education and opportunities for physical activity are increasingly available.

Despite medical intervention, reduction of obesity once it is well established is difficult. Psychological difficulties may well persist into the adult years. Society deals harshly with the obese, and studies show that obesity is a handicap later in life.

In childhood, overt medical complications are few although metabolic markers for cardiovascular disease, diabetes and fatty liver are common. Obese children are more susceptible to musculoskeletal strain and slipped capital femoral epiphyses. Rarely, insulin-resistant diabetes mellitus develops in childhood.

Obesity in childhood tracks into adulthood when morbidity becomes significant; diabetes and hypertension are common, leading to early mortality from ischaemic heart disease and strokes. Gallstones and certain cancers are also more prevalent.

Infant obesity

Excessive weight gain and obesity in infancy are now recognized as being far from benign. Epidemiological studies show that this can track into childhood and on to adult life. When obesity in the early years is extreme, genetic syndromes should be considered, particularly when there is dysmorphism, developmental delay and congenital abnormalities. Health visiting teams are beginning to recognize and address excessive weight gain as a problem as concerning as weight faltering.

Public health issues
Prevention

As in most conditions, prevention is better than cure. There is some evidence that breastfeeding in infancy is protective, and promotion of good nutrition in the early years, when food habits are developing, is important. Physical activity needs to be encouraged in all children, not simply the obese. There is a need for these health issues to be addressed in baby clinics and in school, particularly during adolescence when a high intake of high-fat foods and decrease in exercise is common. If intervention is provided early in the course of obesity, weight control is likely to be more successful.

Monitoring of obesity

In the UK, the National Child Measurement Programme measures children at entry to primary school (age 4–5 years) and on leaving primary school (age 10–11 years). Parents are notified if their child is overweight or obese.

KEY POINTS

• Most obese children have nutritional obesity.
• Emotional and behavioural problems are common.
• There is a high risk of adult obesity and comorbidity.
• Lifestyle management focusing on physical activity and diet is required.
• Rare causes of obesity are associated with poor growth.

21 Diabetes

Insulin-dependent diabetes mellitus (type 1 diabetes)

Aetiology
- 1 in 500 (0–14 years)
- Destruction of beta islet cells in pancreas leads to insulin deficiency
- Onset determined by genetic predisposition plus some trigger factor (possibly viral infection related)
- Incidence is increasing, particularly in children <5years old

Initial presentation
- Polyuria, polydipsia and weight loss over a few weeks
- Diagnosis if random blood sugar >11.1 mmol/L although transient hyperglycaemia can occasionally be seen without diabetes

Poor diabetic control
- Recurrent admissions with ketoacidosis
- Recurrent severe hypoglycaemia
- Poor growth
- Hyperglycaemia, high HbA1c
- Lipodystrophy if inadequate rotation of injection sites

Hypoglycaemia
- The result of excess insulin or inadequate carbohydrate intake, especially after exercise
- Feel hungry and shaky
- Pale, sweating, tremors
- Tachycardic
- Drowsy or irritable
- Convulsions or coma
- Hypoglycaemia on testing
- May get rebound hyperglycaemia afterwards
- Urgent treatment with 20 g rapid absorbed carbohydrate (2 dextrose tablets or 100 mL high sugar drink)

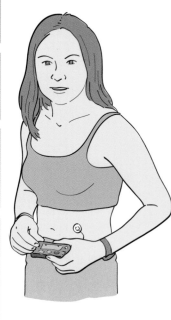

Diabetic ketoacidosis (DKA)
- May be triggered by infection or poor compliance
- Thirst and polyuria
- Vomiting
- Abdominal pain
- Acetone smell on the breath
- High blood glucose level, ketones in blood and urine
- Metabolic acidosis on blood gas
  – Severe acidosis pH<7.25 needs intravenous insulin and fluids
- Urea raised, electrolytes disturbed
- Signs of dehydration
- Kussmaul acidotic breathing
- Hypovolaemic shock, drowsiness and coma if not treated urgently
- Recurrent DKA suggests major difficulty with self-management and support—needs combined psychological support and medical intervention

Ongoing management
- Requires multidisciplinary approach
- Initial correction of metabolic state and education of family
- Treatment with insulin and specific dietary advice
- Monitoring blood sugar levels at home and HbA1c regularly in clinic
- Education about diabetic control, injection technique, diet and exercise
- Dealing with emergencies and liaison with school

Prognosis
- Retinopathy, neuropathy, renal impairment and atherosclerosis are the long-term effects of poor control of blood glucose levels

What you need from your evaluation

History
- Ask about polyuria, polydipsia, lethargy and weight loss
- Ask about bedwetting (secondary enuresis)
- Review the diabetic diary and ask about hypoglycaemic and hyperglycaemic episodes—what triggered them and were they managed appropriately?
- How is the child coping at home and at school? Also ask about siblings
- Is the child managing to eat a healthy diet and modify the diet to certain situations (e.g. snacks before heavy exercise)
- Is insulin being administered correctly with rotation of injection sites?

Examination
- Monitor height and weight as poor growth reflects poor control
- Check for signs of lipodystrophy or lipoatrophy at injection sites
- Check blood pressure annually and fundi in older children (>12 years)
- Check for signs of coexistent coeliac disease or hypothyroidism

Investigations and their significance

Blood glucose	Monitor regularly at home using finger-prick samples and handheld glucometer
HbA1c (% of glycosylated haemoglobin)	Reflects control over last 2–3 months
Urinalysis	For glycosuria, ketones, microalbuminuria
Blood gases, U&E	Need to be monitored carefully during acute diabetic ketoacidosis
Coeliac screen	Screen for coeliac disease with antitissue transglutaminase (tTG) or anti-endomysial antibodies
Thyroid function tests and antithyroid antibody screen	Screen for hypothyroidism
Glucose tolerance test (GTT)	In type 2 diabetes
Triglycerides and cholesterol	
Annual retinal screening (>12 years of age)	
Islet cell antibodies, insulin antibodies, GAD antibodies	To confirm autoimmune process at diagnosis
Insulin and C-Peptide levels	Helps distinguish type 1 from type 2 diabetes

Diabetes mellitus

Diabetes affects 1 in 400–500 children and adolescents. Diabetes is diagnosed if there are classic symptoms with fasting blood glucose >7 mmol/L or random glucose >11.1 mmol/L. The diagnosis has a major impact on the child and the family in terms of their daily life; the risk of serious illness such as diabetic ketoacidosis (DKA) and the risk of long-term complications such as retinopathy, renal failure, cardiovascular disease and neuropathy.

Type 1 diabetes mellitus

Diabetes in children is usually insulin-dependent diabetes mellitus (type 1) due to autoimmune destruction of the beta cells in the islets of Langerhans in the pancreas, resulting in lack of insulin. The lack of insulin means that glucose cannot be utilized, resulting in hyper-glycaemia. The high glucose concentration in the blood spills over into the urine, causing an osmotic diuresis with polyuria and dehy-dration. This leads to excessive thirst and weight loss. Because the cells cannot utilize glucose they switch to metabolizing fats, leading to the production of ketones, resulting in acidosis.

Type 2 diabetes mellitus

In this form of diabetes, the pancreas is able to secrete insulin, but there is peripheral insulin resistance. Until recently, type 2 diabetes was rare in childhood, but the incidence is increasing, probably related to increased calorie intake and reduced exercise. Management is dietary control of carbohydrate and oral hypoglycaemic agents (e.g. sulphonylureas). In some cases, the need to produce high levels of insulin leads the pancreas to 'burn out', such that insulin therapy becomes necessary.

Other types of diabetes mellitus

It is increasingly recognized that there are genetic forms of non-insulin-dependent diabetes mellitus that present in child-hood. They are often due to impaired secretion of insulin from the pancreatic beta cells. In other cases, the diabetes is caused by drugs (e.g. corticosteroids following transplantation) or by disease processes (e.g. cystic fibrosis or pancreatitis) or is associated with genetic syndromes.

Initial presentation of type 1 diabetes

Children usually present with a short (2–3-week) history of lethargy, weight loss, polyuria and thirst. Polyuria may cause a recurrence of bedwetting. If the symptoms are not recognized, the child may develop signs of DKA with abdominal pain, vomiting and eventually coma. Newly diagnosed children who are ketoaci-dotic will need admission to hospital to correct dehydration and commence intravenous insulin.

Intensive education of the child and family is needed under-taken by diabetic nurse specialist, paediatric diabetologist and specialist dietician. The child and the family are taught how to inject insulin, monitor blood glucose, test for ketones and recog-nize the signs of hypoglycaemia. Children are encouraged to wear a Medic-Alert bracelet, giving details of their condition in case of sudden hypoglycaemic collapse. Education should be structured so that every child has access to the full support available and their progress in building expert knowledge can be verified.

Growing up with diabetes

The education given to families at the time of diagnosis is crucial in developing the right approach to their child's diabetes. As the child gets older, they can gradually take on more of the responsibility themselves, including injecting insulin and monitoring blood glu-cose levels. Normal healthy diet should be encouraged to ease blood sugar regulation.

Managing any chronic condition places an added difficulty on emotional well-being particularly through times when it is nor-mal to show rebellious defiant behaviour such as at adolescence. Diabetes increases the risk of psychological problems (such as eating disorder) linked to poor compliance. The diabetes team need specialist skills in engaging and motivational interviewing of adolescents to help manage these problems. A psychologist should be part of the team to support emotional well-being and help patients avoid harmful behaviours associated with long-term conditions.

Insulin therapy (type 1 diabetes)

Many children go through a 'honeymoon' period soon after diag-nosis where they need very little insulin as they still produce some endogenous insulin. More insulin is often required as they go through the pubertal growth spurt. Insulin is usually delivered by an injection pen. Various insulin regimens are used.

- **Twice daily regimen**: The insulin is given as a mixture of rapid-acting insulin (peak at 2–4 h) and intermediate-acting isophane insulin (peak at 4–12 h). This is administered subcuta-neously in the arms, thighs, buttocks or abdomen, before breakfast and before the evening meal.
- **Basal bolus regimen:** This provides a long-acting insulin at night and rapid-acting insulin given before each meal, based on the cal-culated carbohydrate intake.

An alternative to these regimens is *continuous subcutaneous insulin infusion* (CSII) of rapid acting insulin via a pump, with the ability to increase the rate (bolus) during mealtimes. The insulin is infused through a cannula, which is changed every 2–3 days. This system can give better glycaemic control and fewer hypoglycaemic episodes.

Monitoring

Control is assessed by keeping a blood sugar diary and measuring HbA1c levels, which measures glycaemic control in the preced-ing few months. The family need to be warned of the symptoms of hypoglycaemia (see box) and have carbohydrate available (dex-trose tablets) at all times. Screening for complications and associ-ated conditions (thyroid disease and coeliac disease) is performed regularly.

> **KEY POINTS**
>
> - Diabetes is very common: it occurs in 1 in 500 children.
> - Presentation is with a short history of weight loss, polyuria and polydipsia.
> - DKA can be life-threatening and needs high-dependency treatment.
> - Insulin is given subcutaneously in a number of different reg-imens to best suit the child.
> - Patients must be able to recognize and treat hypoglycaemia.
> - Type 2 diabetes is becoming more common in children.

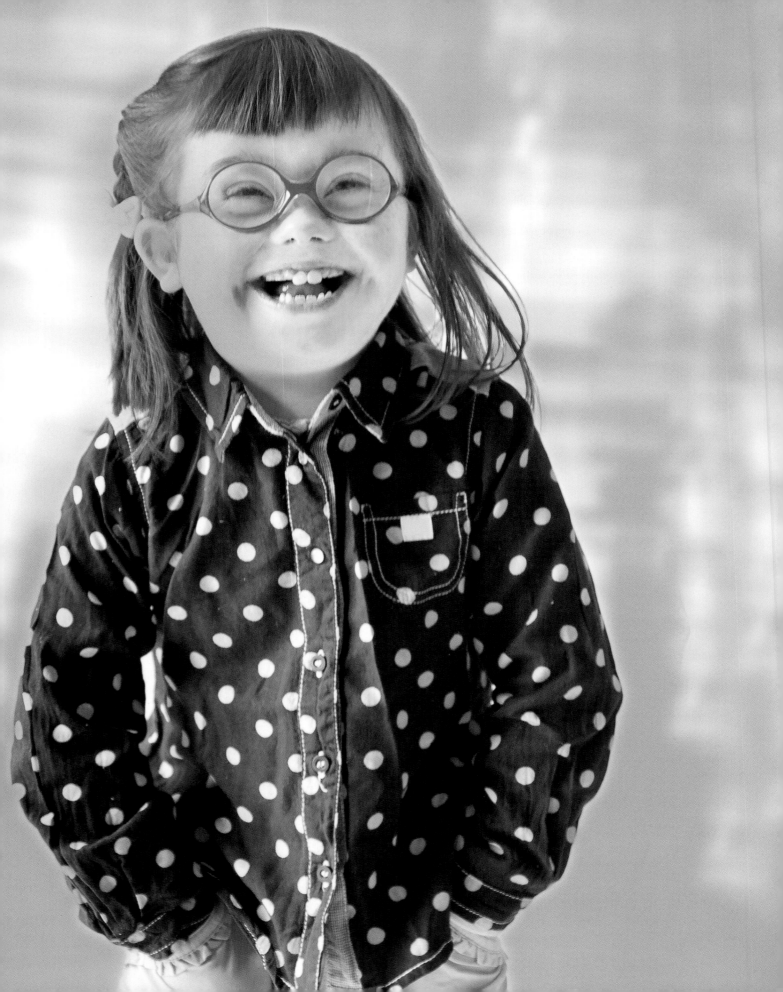

Cardiovascular disorders

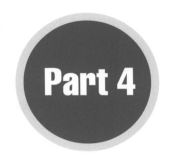

Part 4

Chapters

22 Congenital heart disease

Presentation of congenital heart disease in the neonatal period

Detected by antenatal screening
- 20 week ultrasound scan aims to identify the four chambers of the heart and the orientation of the great vessels
- Specialist fetal echo cardiography is performed if there is a strong family history, maternal diabetes, or evidence of a fetal anomaly associated with cardiac defects (e.g. Down syndrome, VACTERL)
- Antenatal detection rates vary by centre, but overall only about 45% of lesions requiring intervention in infancy are detected antenatally
- Diagnosis allows babies with duct dependent lesions (e.g. coarctation of aorta, hypoplastic left heart and transposition of the great arteries to be delivered in a cardiac centre

Presenting with cyanosis
- Obstruction to pulmonary blood flow will cause cyanosis. This is often associated with a right to left shunt across the arterial duct
- Pulmonary hypertension (PPHN) leading to right to left shunting should be excluded

Restrictive pulmonary blood flow with right to left shunting:
- Pulmonary atresia
- Severe pulmonary stenosis
- Tricuspid atresia
- Ebstein's anomaly
- Tetralogy of Fallot (pulmonary stenosis)

Abnormal connections
- Transposition of the Great Arteries (TGA) leads to separate pulmonary and systemic circulations, only connected whilst the duct is open. Causes severe cyanosis and acidosis from birth.
- Total anomalous pulmonary venous drainage (TAPVD)- the pulmonary veins do not return to the left atrium, causing cyanosis.

Common mixing
- Truncus arteriosus (single great vessel arising from the heart supplies the aorta and the pulmonary arteries)
- Massive Atrio-ventricular septal defect (AVSD)

Detected by oxygen saturation screening
- Oxygen saturations are measured in the first 24 h of life-a post ductal (foot) measurement of <95% or a pre-ductal (right hand) to post-ductal (foot) drop of >3% is a trigger for further assessment.
- If this is persistent and no other cause is found, an echocardiogram should be performed
- Can detect some duct dependent heart defects (e.g. coarctation) prior to collapse
- Generates a small number of false positives, but many of these have important disorders such as sepsis or respiratory problems

Presenting with shock
- Obstructive lesions to the left side of the heart can present with systemic shock (hypotension, acidosis and organ failure) when the duct closes, as blood can no longer reach the rest of the body.
- Coarctation of Aorta
- Interrupted aortic arch
- Hypoplastic left heart syndrome (single ventricle)
- Critical aortic stenosis

Presenting with murmur
- Valve stenosis (e.g. pulmonary stenosis)
- Ventricular septal defect (VSD)-usually after a few weeks
- Patent ductus arteriosus (PDA)-usually in pre-term babies

Presenting with breathlessness
- Left to right shunts-cause increased pulmonary blood flow and breathlessness, especially after a few weeks when the pulmonary blood pressure tends to fall
- Ventricular septal defects (VSD)
- Patent ductus arteriosus (PDA)
- Massive Arterio-venous malformations (e.g. vascular malformations and haemangiomas)

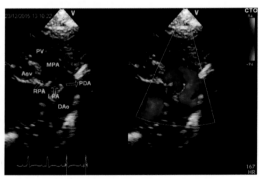

MPA = main pulmonary artery
LPA = left pulmonary artery
RPA = right pulmonary artery
DAo = descending aorta
PDA = patent ductus arterioles
PV = pulmonary valve
Aov = aortic valve

2D and colour Doppler Parasternal short axis echocardiogram view of a patent ductus arteriosus (PDA) showing left to right flow (represented as red, as flow is towards the probe) across the duct from the descending aorta to the main pulmonary artery. The flow in the pulmonary arteries is blue as it moving away from the probe.
(Figure courtesy of Dr Yogen Singh)

Cardiac investigations and their significance

Pulse oximetry	To determine degree of cyanosis or check for post ductal drop (screening for CHD)
Chest radiograph	Cardiomegaly in heart failure
	Boot-shaped heart (Fallot's tetralogy) Increased vascular markings with left to right shunts (VSD, ASD, PDA)
ECG	Varies with age (left ventricle becomes more dominant after neonatal period)
	Right ventricular hypertrophy
	Superior QRS axis (AVSD, primum ASD)
	24 h ECG can be useful in evaluating arrhythmias.
Echo	Ultrasound examination of the heart, usually performed by a paediatric cardiologist, can diagnose the vast majority of congenital heart defects
Fetal echo	Many defects can be detected antenatally
Cardiac catheter	To define complex anatomy or perform non-invasive treatment (e.g. balloon dilatation of stenosed valve)

Paediatrics at a Glance, Fourth Edition. Lawrence Miall, Mary Rudolf and Dominic Smith. © 2016 John Wiley & Sons, Ltd. Published 2016 by John Wiley & Sons, Ltd.
Companion website: www.ataglanceseries.com/paediatrics

Congenital heart disease presenting in the newborn period

Congenital heart disease (CHD) is the commonest congenital malformation (7–8 per 1000 live births). About 8% are associated with chromosomal abnormality (e.g. AVSD in Down's syndrome) or genetic abnormalities, e.g. aortic arch defects and hypocalcaemia in Di George syndrome (22q11 deletion). The risk of CHD is higher if there is a family history. CHD can be caused by teratogens (e.g. tetralogy of Fallot may be a feature of fetal alcohol syndrome and Ebstein's anomaly may occur after fetal lithium exposure). The presentation of congenital heart disease is shown opposite. Specific lesions are described below:

Presenting with shock

Coarctation of the aorta
- Narrowing of the descending aorta
- 6% of CHD
- Presents with shock as the duct closes in first days of life
- Insufficient blood to perfuse abdominal organs and lower limbs, with lactic acidosis
- Key sign is weak or absent femoral pulses
- Blood pressure may be higher in arms than legs
- Oxygen saturation in legs may be low due to right to left shunt across the duct, before it closes
- Associated with Turner's syndrome, 10% of whom have Coarctation and sometimes a bicuspid aortic valve
- Treatment: keep arterial duct open with prostaglandin E2 and then balloon dilatation or surgical repair
- Variants include hypoplastic or interrupted aortic arch

Critical aortic valve stenosis
- Narrowing of the aortic valve
- 5% of CHD
- If severe presents with shock as duct closes
- All pulses (not just femorals) are thready and difficult to feel
- Ejection systolic murmur radiating to the neck and a palpable thrill over aortic area.
- In older children may cause syncope or reduced exercise tolerance and a murmur.
- Treatment – keep the duct open with prostaglandin E2
- Requires balloon valvuloplasty or surgical valve replacement (Ross procedure involves replacing aortic valve with patient's pulmonary valve and then fitting a replacement pulmonary valve)

Presenting with heart failure

Patent ductus arteriosus (PDA)
- 12-15% of CHD
- Typically presents in preterm babies in second to third week of life
- During fetal life the arterial duct shunts blood from the pulmonary artery to the descending aorta, bypassing the unexpanded lungs.
- Normally the duct closes within hours-days of birth, first by constriction then by fibrosis, but in unstable preterm babies or hypoxic babies it can stay open
- As the aortic pressure is higher than the pulmonary artery pressure there is a left to right shunt and with increased pulmonary blood flow leading to cardiac failure and pulmonary oedema or pulmonary haemorrhage
- Presents with a systolic or continuous machinery murmur radiating to the left clavicle and very full bounding pulses
- A very large PDA is associated with intraventricular haemorrhage (IVH) and necrotising enterocolitis (NEC) in very preterm babies, as well as respiratory distress or even pulmonary haemorrhage
- Treat with ibuprofen (prostaglandin synthetase inhibitor), surgical closure with a clip, or trans-catheter closure in older children

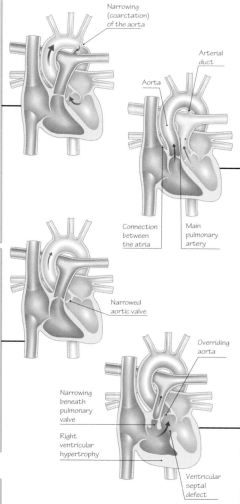
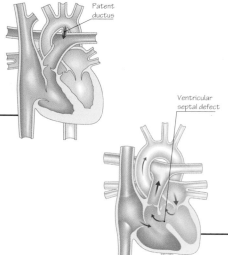

Narrowing (coarctation) of the aorta

Arterial duct

Aorta

Connection between the atria

Main pulmonary artery

Narrowed aortic valve

Overriding aorta

Narrowing beneath pulmonary valve

Right ventricular hypertrophy

Ventricular septal defect

Patent ductus

Ventricular septal defect

Presenting with cyanosis

Transposition of Great arteries (TGA)
- The aorta arises from the right ventricle and the pulmonary artery from the left ventricle (transposition)
- 6% of CHD
- Presents with severe cyanosis and acidosis after birth
- Only connection between pulmonary and systemic circulation is the duct, unless there is an associated ASD or VSD
- Emergency treatment is to keep duct open with prostaglandin E2 and perform an urgent atrial septostomy (forming a large atrial communication by inflating a catheter balloon across the foramen ovale) which allows oxygenated and deoxygenated blood to mix
- Surgical correction within 2 weeks of life involves the "switch" operation where the great vessels are switched over and the coronary arteries reconnected to the new aorta

Tetralogy of Fallot
- 'Tetralogy' refers to a large VSD, an overriding aorta that sits over the VSD defect, pulmonary infundibular stenosis and right ventricular hypertrophy
- Commonest cyanotic heart defect (6-10% of all CHD)
- The pulmonary narrowing, below the pulmonary valve, causes right to left shunting across the VSD and therefore cyanosis.
- Can present soon after birth with cyanosis or a murmur
- Classically older children develop hyper- cyanotic 'spells' which are relieved by squatting down to reverse the shunt by increasing left ventricular pressure)
- CXR may show a boot-shaped heart and oligaemic lung fields
- Treat spells with propranolol and morphine to relax the infundibulum
- Surgical correction at 2-3 months of age

Presenting with heart failure

Ventricular Septal defect (VSD)
- 25–30% of CHD (most common lesion)
- May be identified by a murmur in the newborn period or present with heart failure at 4-6 weeks as the pulmonary resistance naturally falls and the left to right shunting across the VSD increases leading to breathlessness, an enlarged liver and failure to gain weight due to feeding difficulty and work of breathing
- Defect may be in the membranous or muscular part of the septum. The latter are much more likely to close spontaneously, especially if small
- Present with a harsh, rasping pansystolic murmur at the lower left sternal edge, radiating over the whole precordium and sometimes a parasternal thrill. Loudness of the murmur is not associated with the size of the defect
- May be isolated or can commonly be found in babies with other genetic syndromes or chromosomal anomalies
- Only the largest lesions need early surgical closure, usually in the first months of life if heart failure cannot be controlled with diuretics
- If untreated the increased pulmonary flow can cause pulmonary hypertension and reversal of the shunt (Eisenmenger's syndrome)

23 Heart problems in older children

Causes of heart murmurs in older children

Innocent murmurs
- Have no clinical significance
- Are systolic and musical
- Do not radiate
- Vary with posture and position

Pathological murmurs
- Are pansystolic or diastolic
- Are harsh or long
- May radiate and have a thrill
- Often have associated cardiac symptoms or signs

Venous hum
- Blowing continuous murmur in systole and diastole
- Heard below the clavicles
- Disappears on lying down

Pulmonary flow murmur
- Brief high-pitched murmur at second left intercostal space
- Best heard with child lying down

Systolic ejection murmur
- Short systolic murmur at left sternal edge or apex
- Musical sound
- Changes with child's position
- Intensified by fever, exercise and emotion

NB: Patent ductus arteriosus and tetralogy of Fallot are discussed in Chapter 22

Aortic stenosis
- Soft systolic ejection murmur at right upper sternal border
- Radiates to neck and down left sternal border
- Causes dizziness and loss of consciousness in older children

Atrial septal defect
- Soft systolic murmur at second left intercostal space
- Wide fixed splitting of the second sound
- May not be detected until later childhood

Pulmonary stenosis
- Short systolic ejection murmur in upper left chest
- Conducted to back
- Preceded by ejection click
- Thrill in the pulmonary area

Ventricular septal defect
- Harsh pansystolic murmur at lower left sternal border
- Radiates all over chest
- Signs of heart failure may be present

Coarctation of the aorta (see Chapter 22)
- Systolic murmur on left side of chest
- Radiates to the back
- Absent or delayed femoral pulses
- Hypertension

What you need from your evaluation

History

- Fatigue is the most important symptom of cardiac failure. A baby in cardiac failure can take only small volumes of milk, becomes short of breath on sucking, and becomes sweaty. The older child tires on walking and may become breathless too
- Take a family history. The risk of heart defects is higher in siblings of children with congenital heart disease

Physical examination

- **Murmur.** The quality of the sound and the site where it is heard indicates if it is pathological. Listen for radiation over the precordium, back and neck, with the child both sitting and lying
- **Signs of heart failure:** Look for failure to thrive and poor growth, tachycardia and tachypnoea, crepitations and hepatomegaly (peripheral oedema is rare in children)
- **Pulse and blood pressure:** Remember that femoral pulses are weak, delayed or absent in coarctation of the aorta. Blood pressure will be higher in the arms than the legs
- **Sternal heave:** Indicates right ventricular hypertrophy (e.g. tetralogy of Fallot, pulmonary hypertension)
- **Cyanosis:** An unlikely finding in children presenting with a heart murmur

Investigations for heart murmurs

These are required only if the murmur is thought to be pathological.
- **Echocardiography.** Evaluates cardiac structure and performance, gradients across stenotic valves and the direction of flow across a shunt
- **Chest radiograph.** Provides information about cardiac size and shape, and pulmonary vascularity
- **ECG.** Provides information about ventricular or atrial hypertrophy
- **24h ECG.** If associated with symptoms of palpitations or syncope
- **Cardiac catheterization.** Rarely required for diagnosis. Cardiac CT or MRI scan- usually only performed as part of pre-operative assessment in complex congenital heart disease

Paediatrics at a Glance, Fourth Edition. Lawrence Miall, Mary Rudolf and Dominic Smith. © 2016 John Wiley & Sons, Ltd. Published 2016 by John Wiley & Sons, Ltd.
Companion website: www.ataglanceseries.com/paediatrics

Heart murmurs are common and most are 'functional' or 'innocent' and not associated with structural abnormalities. Once a structural lesion has been excluded, the benign nature of the murmur should be discussed with the parents. Innocent flow murmurs may be more apparent at times of illness or fever.

Left-to-right shunts

These are common. If large, a considerable volume of blood is shunted, causing congestive cardiac failure, hypertrophy, ventricular dilatation. They usually present with breathlessness.

Ventricular septal defect (VSD)

- 32% of CHD (most common)
- Membranous or muscular
- Can be asymptomatic
- Harsh pansystolic murmur at lower left sternal edge
- Parasternal thrill
- Heart failure at 4–6 weeks
- Many close spontaneously

Ventricular septal defect

Ventricular septal defect

Atrial septal defect (ASD)

- Defect of atrial septum (ostium secundum defect) or atrioventricular septum (ostium primum defect).
- Ten percent of CHD
- Soft systolic murmur due to high flow across the pulmonary valve and not due to flow across the ASD itself. Murmur may not be detected until later childhood. The second heart sound is widely split and 'fixed' (does not vary with respiration).
- May experience breathlessness, tiredness or chest infections.
- Large defects are closed surgically, but smaller defects can be closed with a catheter-inserted occlusion device.
- Untreated, cardiac arrhythmias can develop in early adulthood.

Atrial septal defect

Atrial septal defect
High flow through pulmonary valve causes a systolic murmur

Atrioventricular septal defect (AVSD)

- An atrial and ventricular communication, sometimes with a single atrioventricular valve
- Five percent of CHD
- 40% have Down's syndrome
- Superior axis on ECG
- Causes heart failure or a murmur
- May show mild cyanosis due to common mixing of the oxygenated and deoxygenated blood at atrial level
- Requires open-heart surgery to close the defects, usually in infancy.

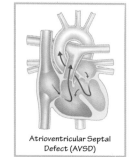

Atrioventricular Septal Defect (AVSD)

Obstructive lesions

Obstructive lesions occur at the pulmonary and aortic valves and in the aorta. The heart chamber proximal to the lesion hypertrophies, and heart failure may develop.

Aortic stenosis (see Chapter 22)

Mild forms of aortic stenosis may present in older children with a murmur (sometimes preceded by an ejection click), lethargy, syncope or dizziness on exertion. There may be left ventricular hypertrophy on ECG. Balloon valvuloplasty can stretch the valve open or a valve replacement may be required. Very strenuous sports should be discouraged.

Pulmonary stenosis

The pulmonary valve is narrowed and the right ventricle hypertrophied. A short ejection systolic murmur is heard over the upper left anterior chest and is conducted to the back. Mild stenosis is asymptomatic. In severe stenosis, a systolic thrill is palpable in the pulmonary area. On CXR, dilatation of the pulmonary artery is seen beyond the stenosis, and if severe an enlarged right atrium and ventricle. The extent of the stenosis can be measured by echocardiography and cardiac catheterization. If severe, balloon valvuloplasty is performed.

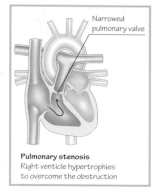

Narrowed pulmonary valve

Pulmonary stenosis
Right ventricle hypertrophies to overcome the obstruction

Cardiac arrhythmias in childhood

Arrhythmias are unusual in children compared with adults. Some children may have an irregular heart beat (sinus arrhythmia) that causes mild palpitations. Tachy-arrhythmias include supra-ventricular tachycardia (SVT) and ventricular tachycardia (VT)—the latter is much more dangerous and is often associated with long QT interval on the ECG. Certain ion-channel problems can predispose to VT or ventricular fibrillation (VF) and be genetically inherited (e.g. Brugada syndrome). Implantable defibrillators are sometimes fitted.

SVT is more common and caused by an accessory conduction pathway between the atria and ventricles. This causes episodic tachycardia (>200 bpm) with severe palpitations or dizziness. Vagal manoeuvres can be tried to convert back into sinus rhythm including carotid massage, ice on the face or the valsalva manoeuvre. Cardioversion with drugs such as adenosine or synchronized DC shock. In recurrent cases (e.g. Wolff–Parkinson–White syndrome), radio-ablation of the aberrant electrical pathway can lead to a complete cure.

Myocarditis

Some viral infections can affect the heart muscle itself leading to severe, acute cardiac failure. Whilst the viral infection may be self–limiting, the heart function may be so poor as to require intensive care and sometimes heart transplantation. Myocarditis can also occur as part of Kawasaki disease, which presents with high fever, conjunctivitis, erythematous rash and desquamation, and can also lead to coronary artery aneurysms.

Inherited cardiac disorders

Some genetic conditions are associated with cardiac symptoms in later childhood and early adulthood—for example, in Marfan's syndrome and Turner's syndrome, there is a high risk of aortic dissection. In hypertrophic cardiomyopathy (HOCM), there may be abnormal thickening of the heart muscle with the small but real risk of VT and sudden death.

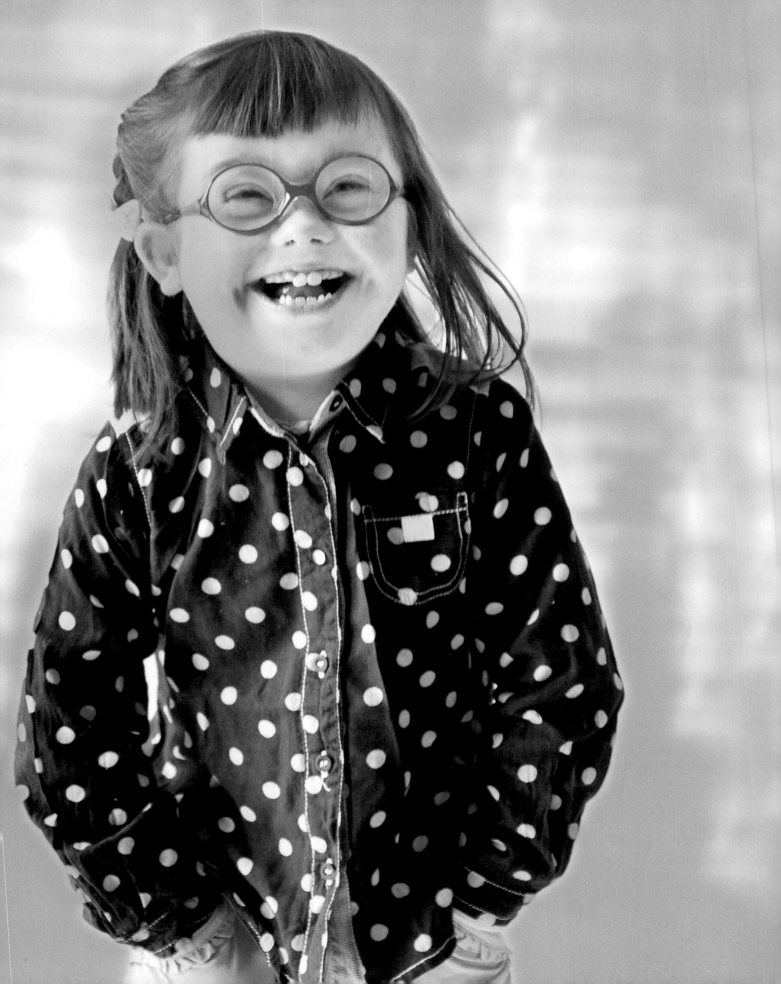

Fever

Part 5

Chapters

(24) Acute fever

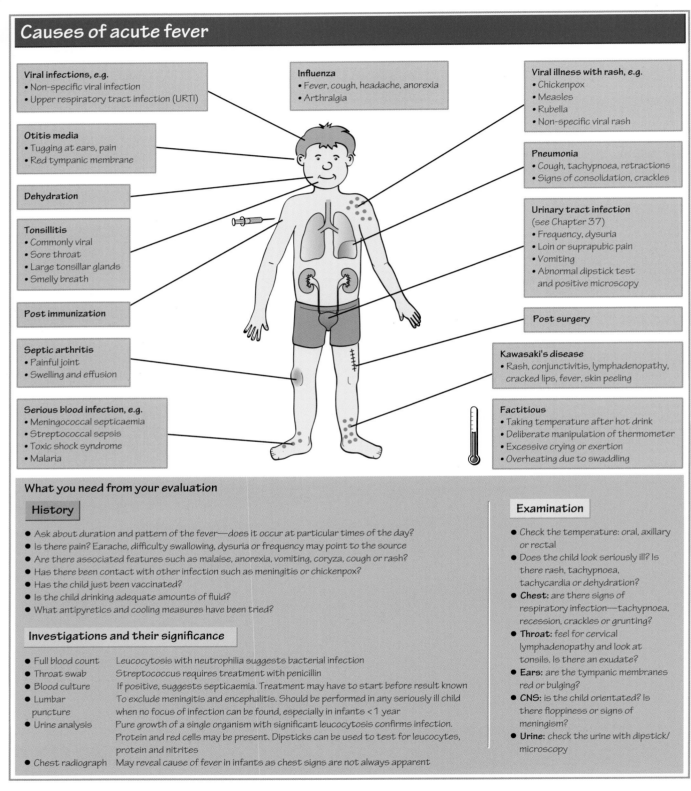

Causes of acute fever

Viral infections, e.g.
- Non-specific viral infection
- Upper respiratory tract infection (URTI)

Otitis media
- Tugging at ears, pain
- Red tympanic membrane

Dehydration

Tonsillitis
- Commonly viral
- Sore throat
- Large tonsillar glands
- Smelly breath

Post immunization

Septic arthritis
- Painful joint
- Swelling and effusion

Serious blood infection, e.g.
- Meningococcal septicaemia
- Streptococcal sepsis
- Toxic shock syndrome
- Malaria

Influenza
- Fever, cough, headache, anorexia
- Arthralgia

Viral illness with rash, e.g.
- Chickenpox
- Measles
- Rubella
- Non-specific viral rash

Pneumonia
- Cough, tachypnoea, retractions
- Signs of consolidation, crackles

Urinary tract infection
(see Chapter 37)
- Frequency, dysuria
- Loin or suprapubic pain
- Vomiting
- Abnormal dipstick test and positive microscopy

Post surgery

Kawasaki's disease
- Rash, conjunctivitis, lymphadenopathy, cracked lips, fever, skin peeling

Factitious
- Taking temperature after hot drink
- Deliberate manipulation of thermometer
- Excessive crying or exertion
- Overheating due to swaddling

What you need from your evaluation

History

- Ask about duration and pattern of the fever—does it occur at particular times of the day?
- Is there pain? Earache, difficulty swallowing, dysuria or frequency may point to the source
- Are there associated features such as malaise, anorexia, vomiting, coryza, cough or rash?
- Has there been contact with other infection such as meningitis or chickenpox?
- Has the child just been vaccinated?
- Is the child drinking adequate amounts of fluid?
- What antipyretics and cooling measures have been tried?

Investigations and their significance

- Full blood count — Leucocytosis with neutrophilia suggests bacterial infection
- Throat swab — Streptococcus requires treatment with penicillin
- Blood culture — If positive, suggests septicaemia. Treatment may have to start before result known
- Lumbar puncture — To exclude meningitis and encephalitis. Should be performed in any seriously ill child when no focus of infection can be found, especially in infants < 1 year
- Urine analysis — Pure growth of a single organism with significant leucocytosis confirms infection. Protein and red cells may be present. Dipsticks can be used to test for leucocytes, protein and nitrites
- Chest radiograph — May reveal cause of fever in infants as chest signs are not always apparent

Examination

- Check the temperature: oral, axillary or rectal
- Does the child look seriously ill? Is there rash, tachypnoea, tachycardia or dehydration?
- **Chest:** are there signs of respiratory infection—tachypnoea, recession, crackles or grunting?
- **Throat:** feel for cervical lymphadenopathy and look at tonsils. Is there an exudate?
- **Ears:** are the tympanic membranes red or bulging?
- **CNS:** is the child orientated? Is there floppiness or signs of meningism?
- **Urine:** check the urine with dipstick/microscopy

Paediatrics at a Glance, Fourth Edition. Lawrence Miall, Mary Rudolf and Dominic Smith. © 2016 John Wiley & Sons, Ltd. Published 2016 by John Wiley & Sons, Ltd.
Companion website: www.ataglanceseries.com/paediatrics

Fever is usually a response to infection or inflammation and may form part of the body's defence against infection. The height of the fever does not necessarily correlate with the severity of the illness, and fever can commonly occur in children with minor illnesses. The child often appears flushed as blood vessels in the skin vasodilate in an attempt to lose heat. Some young children experience febrile convulsions if their temperature rises very rapidly (see Chapter 43). Temperature can be measured rectally, orally or in the axilla using a thermometer, or using a thermal device in the ear canal or skin. Fever is usually defined as a temperature above 37.5 °C. Persistent or recurrent fever is discussed in Chapter 25.

Treatment of fever

Fever can be treated by undressing the child, so heat is lost through the skin. Sponging with tepid water can help. Fever can be treated with antipyretics such as paracetamol or ibuprofen when it causes discomfort—aspirin should not be used for children younger than the age of 12 years as it can lead to severe liver failure (Reye's syndrome, see Chapter 51).

Fever in young infants

Fever in infants less than 8 weeks old must be taken seriously as signs of sepsis at this age can be non-specific. Significant fever should always prompt a careful examination and investigations. If ill, infants require a full infection screen including urine culture, chest radiograph and possibly lumbar puncture.

Viral upper respiratory tract infections

Upper respiratory tract infections (URTIs) are extremely common in children, occurring on average 6–8 times a year. They are especially common when toddlers start nursery and on starting school when children become exposed to a large number of viral infections to which they have no immunity. Symptoms include coryza (runny nose), acute pharyngitis and fever. In acute pharyngitis, the tonsillar fauces and palate are inflamed, cervical lymph nodes may be enlarged and the tympanic membranes inflamed. Young infants may have difficulty breathing and feeding because they are obligate nose breathers. Treatment is symptomatic, with antipyretics such as paracetamol. Saline drops may improve nasal congestion in infants. The infection usually lasts 3–4 days. Antibiotics should not be given.

Tonsillitis

Tonsillitis is usually viral in origin and bacterial infection is rare in children under the age of 2 years. In older children, the commonest bacterial organism is group A beta-haemolytic streptococcus. Symptoms include sore throat or dysphagia and usually a fever. There is often tender cervical lymphadenopathy, which may cause neck stiffness, and associated adenitis in the mesenteric nodes may cause abdominal pain. On examination, the tonsils are enlarged and acutely inflamed. In bacterial tonsillitis, the breath may smell offensive and there may be a white exudate, although this is not always a reliable sign. Exudates can also occur with infectious mononucleosis (glandular fever) and with diphtheria (now very rare). Acute tonsillitis should be distinguished from hypertrophied but non-inflamed tonsils, which are common in preschool children.

Most children do not require antibiotics. If bacterial infection is suspected, this should ideally be confirmed by a throat swab. Streptococcal tonsillitis may be treated with phenoxymethylpenicillin for 10 days.

Complications of tonsillitis are rare and include otitis media, peritonsillar abscess (quinsy), post-streptococcal glomerulonephritis and in some parts of the world, rheumatic fever. Chronically enlarged tonsils can cause upper airway obstruction and obstructive sleep apnoea. This is an indication for tonsillectomy.

Infectious mononucleosis

Glandular fever is due to Epstein–Barr virus (EBV) infection and is usually a self-limiting infection in adolescents. It presents with low-grade fever, malaise, pharyngitis and cervical lymphadenopathy. Occasionally, hepatosplenomegaly and jaundice may occur. Peripheral leucocytosis with atypical lymphocytes is seen; EBV serology is diagnostic. The symptoms may last many weeks. Amoxicillin is contraindicated as it causes a maculopapular rash in EBV infection.

Acute otitis media

Otitis media is very common, especially in young children and can occur in babies. The commonest causes are *Streptococcus pneumoniae*, *Haemophilus influenzae* and viruses. It is especially common when there is Eustachian tube dysfunction, which occurs as a result of URTIs, obstruction from enlarged adenoids, cleft palate and in Down's syndrome. Symptoms include fever, deafness and pain in the ear. The child may be irritable and pull at the ear although infection may also be asymptomatic. Examination shows a red, inflamed and bulging tympanic membrane, with loss of the light reflex. Most cases resolve spontaneously and a trial of symptomatic treatment (paracetamol) for 72 hours is recommended before considering antibiotics. Bacterial otitis media is shortened by treatment with amoxicillin. Prognosis is generally good even if the tympanic membrane has perforated.

Complications include conductive deafness, mastoiditis and secretory otitis media (glue ear)—a thick, glue-like exudate in the middle ear. In secretory otitis media, the tympanic membrane looks thickened and retracted with an absent light reflex. If there is significant hearing loss, ventilation tubes (grommets) may be inserted through the tympanic membrane to allow the middle ear to drain. They often fall out after a period of months to years and their use is controversial; but they are indicated, if there is language delay secondary conductive deafness due to glue ear.

KEY POINTS

- Fever is very common in children and can usually be managed by simple cooling and paracetamol.
- Any ill child with high fever must be examined carefully to exclude serious infections such as meningitis, urinary tract infection or pneumonia.
- Fever in babies less than 8 weeks old must be taken seriously.
- Otitis media and tonsillitis are common causes of fever in young children.
- Most fevers are due to non-specific viral infections or URTIs.

25 Persistent fever and serious recurrent infections

Causes of persistent fever

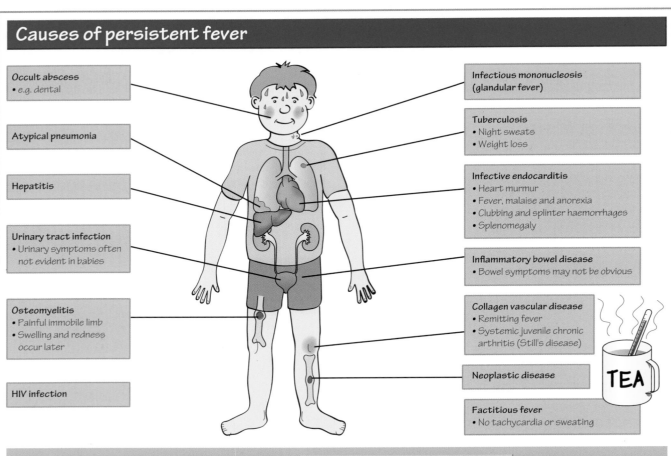

Occult abscess
- e.g. dental

Atypical pneumonia

Hepatitis

Urinary tract infection
- Urinary symptoms often not evident in babies

Osteomyelitis
- Painful immobile limb
- Swelling and redness occur later

HIV infection

Infectious mononucleosis (glandular fever)

Tuberculosis
- Night sweats
- Weight loss

Infective endocarditis
- Heart murmur
- Fever, malaise and anorexia
- Clubbing and splinter haemorrhages
- Splenomegaly

Inflammatory bowel disease
- Bowel symptoms may not be obvious

Collagen vascular disease
- Remitting fever
- Systemic juvenile chronic arthritis (Still's disease)

Neoplastic disease

Factitious fever
- No tachycardia or sweating

TEA

What you need from your evaluation?

History

- Review symptoms related to all organ systems
- Immunization history
- Contact with infectious diseases (e.g. TB)
- Travel history (including visitors)
- Exposure to animals (e.g. tick bites)

Physical examination

(Repeat physical examinations may be required.)
- **Check the temperature chart.** Repetitive chills (rigors) and temperature spikes suggest septicaemia, abscess, pyelonephritis or endocarditis. There is no tachycardia or sweating in factitious fever
- **Examine the mouth and sinuses.** Oral candida may indicate immune deficiency. A red pharynx may suggest infectious mononucleosis. Tap the sinuses and teeth for tenderness
- **Palpate muscles and bones.** Point tenderness suggests osteomyelitis or neoplastic disease. Generalized muscle tenderness occurs in collagen vascular disease. Examine joints carefully for signs of inflammation
- **Heart.** A new murmur or changed murmur may suggest infective endocarditis

Investigations and their significance

Investigation	Significance
Full blood count	High white cell count in bacterial infection. Very high in leukaemia
Urinalysis and culture	Occult urinary tract infection
Examination of blood smear	Parasitic infections, e.g. malaria
CRP	Raised in infection and inflammation. Trend may be more important than exact level
ESR or plasma viscosity	High in bacterial infection. Very high in collagen vascular disease, malignancy
Blood cultures (aerobic and anaerobic)	Bacterial infection. Repeat samples needed to diagnose endocarditis, osteomyelitis and occult abscess
Liver function tests	Hepatitis
Mantoux	TB
Radiographs—chest, bones, sinuses	Characteristic findings with bacterial infection
Bone marrow aspirate	Leukaemia, metastatic neoplasms, rare infections
Serological tests	Infectious mononucleosis, other infections, rarely helpful in collagen vascular disease
Isotope scans	Bone scans or radiolabelled white cell scans may help identify cryptogenic infection such as osteomyelitis or intra-abdominal abscess
Echocardiography	Vegetations seen on heart valves in endocarditis
Abdominal ultrasound	Identification of intra-abdominal abscess

Paediatrics at a Glance, Fourth Edition. Lawrence Miall, Mary Rudolf and Dominic Smith. © 2016 John Wiley & Sons, Ltd. Published 2016 by John Wiley & Sons, Ltd.
Companion website: www.ataglanceseries.com/paediatrics

Persistent fever and pyrexia of unknown origin

Pyrexia of unknown origin (PUO) refers to prolonged fever (more than 1 week in young children and 2–3 weeks in adolescents). Often the diagnosis becomes apparent or the fever resolves within a short period of time. The cause is usually an atypical presentation of a common illness such as urine infection or pneumonia, but more significant causes include endocarditis, collagen vascular diseases, malignancy and inflammatory bowel disease. Sometimes no diagnosis is made, but the fever abates spontaneously.

The child should be hospitalized for careful observation. Antipyretics should not be given as they obscure the pattern of fever. Blood cultures should be obtained at the time of fever peaks when the yield is higher.

Kawasaki's disease

Kawasaki's disease should be considered particularly in younger children and in infants with pyrexia beyond 5 days. Raised inflammatory markers and platelet count are sometimes seen; complications include coronary artery aneurysms.

Infective endocarditis

Infective endocarditis usually occurs as a complication of congenital heart disease. The commonest causal organism is *Streptococcus viridans*, which may be introduced during dental or other surgery. Endocarditis can also be seen in children with indwelling central venous catheters (e.g. for parenteral nutrition or chemotherapy).

The child presents with fever, malaise and anorexia. Signs include clubbing, splinter haemorrhages in the nails and splenomegaly, and the pre-existing heart murmur may change in character. Microscopic haematuria may be found. The diagnosis is made on blood culture and echocardiography, which shows vegetations on the heart valves. Intravenous antibiotics are required for 6 weeks.

Osteomyelitis

Osteomyelitis affects long bone metaphyses. Organisms are *Staphylococcus aureus*, *Haemophilus influenzae*, enterobacter species and *Streptococcus pyogenes*. Although the child may present with PUO, more usually the infected limb is obviously painful and held immobile. Swelling and redness eventually appear, and the adjacent joint may contain a sterile 'sympathetic' effusion. Repeated blood culture or direct aspiration of the bone abscess determines the causative organism. Radiographs are not helpful at presentation, as changes only become apparent after 10 days, but bone scans or MRI may be diagnostic. High-dose antibiotics are needed for up to 6 weeks, with surgical drainage if there is no immediate response. Inadequate treatment leads to bone necrosis, chronic discharge and limb deformity.

Serious recurrent infection and immunodeficiency

Most children experience recurrent trivial infections. These are commonly respiratory and peak on starting school or nursery. Despite parental concern, they do not require investigation. However, recurrent serious infections or recurrent infections in an unusual site need to be thoroughly evaluated. There may be an anatomical cause (e.g. a fistula causing recurrent urinary tract infection or splenectomy) or an inherited or acquired immunodeficiency.

Splenectomy and hyposplenism

Children who lack an effective spleen are at increased risk of sepsis, especially pneumococcal septicaemia. Hyposplenism may occur as a result of sickle cell disease (autoinfarction of the spleen) or after splenectomy for trauma, metabolic and haematological conditions (e.g. severe idiopathic thrombocytopenia purpura (ITP)). The risk of bacterial infection is especially high in children under 5 years old, and pneumococcal vaccination and prophylaxis with penicillin is recommended.

Congenital immunodeficiency

Most immunodeficiency disorders present in early childhood with recurrent infections and failure to thrive. In DiGeorge's syndrome, there is cell-mediated immunodeficiency due to thymic aplasia, cardiac abnormality and hypoparathyroidism. Severe combined immunodeficiency (SCID) affects 1 in 100 000 and presents with opportunistic infection failure to thrive.

Acquired immunodeficiency

This is often due to side effects of chemotherapy or immunosuppressants following a transplant. It is important that those treating the child (e.g. primary care doctors) are aware of the risk of infections. Care should be taken to avoid contact with chickenpox, herpes simplex and other common infections.

HIV and AIDS

By far the commonest acquired immunodeficiency worldwide is HIV-1 infection leading to AIDS. Over 3.3 million children live with HIV, either infants born to infected mothers or adolescents who acquire infection sexually or by intravenous drug abuse. Young children usually present by the age of 3 years with failure to thrive, diarrhoea, recurrent oral candidiasis, hepatosplenomegaly or severe bacterial infections.

Diagnosis is made by the detection of HIV antibody or viral load by PCR Techniques. Treatment uses combination highly active antiretroviral therapy (HAART), antibiotic prophylaxis with co-trimoxazole and appropriate viral vaccination. In developing countries, affected children often die in infancy or early childhood, but in the UK, with early diagnosis and treatment, the prognosis is good, with most children achieving viral suppression (an undetectable viral load by HIV PCR tests).

Without intervention, vertical transmission is 20–30%. Viral load should be reduced in pregnancy with HAART and with use of zidovudine in labour and for 4 weeks after birth, delivery by caesarean section and avoidance of breastfeeding, it can be reduced to <1%. In women with undetectable viral load, vaginal delivery may be considered. Breastfeeding doubles the risk of infection and is generally contraindicated in developed countries, but exclusive breastfeeding is still recommended in resource-poor settings, where the formula milk may risk severe gastroenteritis. Because maternal anti-HIV IgG antibody crosses the placenta, a standard HIV antibody test is not reliable in the first 18 months of life, and a quantitative RNA/DNA must be used.

KEY POINTS

- A thorough history and repeat physical examinations are required. This may save the child from multiple investigations.
- The characteristics of the fever may give a clue to diagnosis.
- Samples for culture should be taken at the peak of the fever.
- In severe, unusual or recurrent infections, consider immunodeficiency.

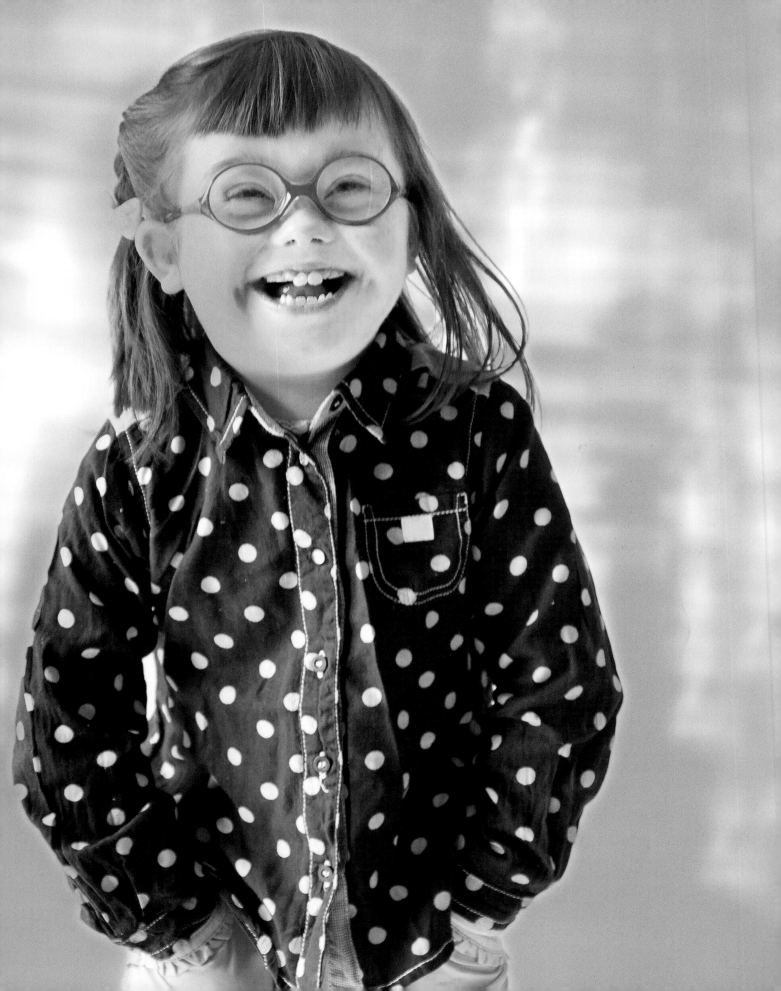

Respiratory disorders

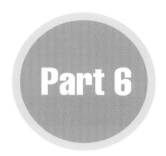

Part 6

26 Cough and wheeze

Causes of 'chestiness'

▶ Croup
- Barking cough
- Stridor

Pneumonia
- Fever, cough
- Respiratory distress
- Chest or abdominal pain
- Intercostal recession
- Crackles and signs of consolidation

Bronchiolitis
- Age: <2 years
- Coryza
- Respiratory distress
- Difficulty feeding
- Apnoea in young infants
- Wheezing and crackles

Heart failure
- Left to right shunts, e.g. ASD, VSD

Acute asthma
- Known asthmatic
- History of atopy
- Wheeze
- Cough (see Chapter 29)

Tuberculosis
- Contact with TB
- Not immunized with BCG
- Haemoptysis
- Night sweats

▶ Viral-induced wheeze
- Wheeze with URTI
- Some progress to asthma
- May respond to bronchodilators

Whooping cough (pertussis)
- Paroxysmal cough, followed by vomiting, whoop or apnoea

Inhaled foreign body
- Toddlers
- History of choking
- Unilateral wheeze
- Sudden onset

Cough without breathlessness
- Gastro-oesophogeal reflux
- Post-nasal drip
- Tracheo-oesophageal fistula
- Passive smoking
- Cystic fibrosis

What you need from your evaluation

History
- Are there features of infection such as pyrexia or poor appetite?
- Is there a history of previous episodic breathlessness suggesting recurrent asthma?
- Is the child atopic—asthma, hayfever, eczema?
- Is there a relevant family history, e.g. asthma, cystic fibrosis, TB?
- Is there an underlying condition, such as congenital heart disease or prematurity, that increases the risk of severe bronchiolitis?

Examination
- Are there signs of respiratory distress—grunting, nasal flaring, intercostal recession, tachypnoea?
- Are there any additional noises—wheeze, stridor, cough?
- Are there signs of consolidation—reduced air entry, crackles, bronchial breathing, dullness on percussion and reduced expansion? (NB: signs are often not focal in young children)
- Are there signs of a chronic respiratory condition, e.g. finger clubbing, chest deformity?
- Is there evidence of congenital heart disease?
- Is the child cyanosed?
- Is the child pyrexial?
- Can the child talk in full sentences?
- Is the peak expiratory flow rate (PEFR) normal?

Investigations and their significance
- **Chest radiograph** — Focal consolidation suggests bacterial infection; diffuse suggests viral or atypical pneumonia. Hyperinflation in asthma and bronchiolitis. May be patchy collapse in bronchiolitis
- **Full blood count** — Neutrophilia in bacterial pneumonia Lymphocytosis in pertussis
- **Sputum culture** — To isolate causative organisms. Acid-fast bacilli may be seen in TB
- **Nasopharyngeal aspirate** — Viral immunofluorescence for RSV in bronchiolitis
- **Per-nasal swab** — To isolate *Bordetella pertussis*
- **Viral titres** — In atypical pneumonia, e.g. mycoplasma
- **Blood cultures** — In suspected bacterial pneumonia may isolate *Streptococcus pneumoniae* or *Staphylococcus aureus*
- **Mantoux test** — In suspected TB
- **Bronchoscopy** — Rigid bronchoscopy to remove foreign body or flexible to perform diagnostic bronchio-alveolar lavage

The 'chesty' child

Children commonly present with coryza, breathlessness, cough, wheeze or noisy breathing. This is often due to a viral URTI (see Chapter 24) or asthma (see Chapter 29).

Pneumonia

Pneumonia (lower respiratory tract infection) can be either bacterial or viral:

- Viral causes include respiratory syncytial virus (RSV), influenza, parainfluenza, adenovirus and Coxsackie virus.
- Bacterial causes are *Streptococcus pneumoniae*, *Haemophilus influenzae*, staphylococcus, *Mycoplasma pneumoniae* and, in the newborn, group B beta-haemolytic streptococcus.
- *Pseudomonas aeruginosa* and *Staphylococcus aureus* are more common in those with underlying respiratory disease, such as cystic fibrosis (see Chapter 30).
- Predisposing factors include a congenital anomaly of the bronchi, inhaled foreign body, immunosuppression, recurrent aspiration (e.g. with a tracheo-oesophageal fistula) or cystic fibrosis.

Pneumonia usually presents with a short history of fever, cough and respiratory distress, including tachypnoea and intercostal recession. Grunting is common in infants. Signs include dullness to percussion, bronchial breathing and crackles, reflecting the underlying consolidation. Clinical signs are often not reliable in infants and the diagnosis should always be confirmed by chest radiograph. This may show a lobar pneumonia or a more widespread bronchopneumonia.

Blood and sputum cultures may reveal the organism. Amoxicillin is the first-line antibiotic for community-acquired pneumonia. Antibody titres may be useful in diagnosing mycoplasma pneumonia, which often has a more insidious onset and requires treatment with erythromycin.

Complications of pneumonia include pleural effusion, septicaemia, bronchiectasis, empyema (infected pleural effusion) or lung abscess (may follow staphylococcal pneumonia).

Bronchiolitis

Bronchiolitis is an acute cause of respiratory distress and wheezing in infants, due to obstruction of the small airways. It is usually caused by RSV and occurs in epidemics in the winter months. RSV is highly infectious and spreads rapidly in day care nurseries. Adenovirus, influenza and parainfluenza virus can also cause bronchiolitis. Coryza is followed by cough, respiratory distress and wheeze. Some infants have difficulty feeding or may have apnoea. Examination reveals widespread wheeze and fine crackles and overexpansion of the chest. Chest radiograph will show hyperinflation and patchy collapse or consolidation. A nasopharyngeal aspirate (NPA) can identify RSV using immunofluorescence.

Most children do not require any specific treatment but indications for admission to hospital include poor feeding, apnoea, increasing respiratory distress or the need for oxygen. The illness usually lasts 7–10 days, and most recover fully although there may be recurrent wheezing during infancy. A minority, particularly those with chronic lung disease or an underlying congenital heart defect, will require intensive care. There is no effective treatment other than oxygen, bronchodilators and supportive therapy. Bronchiolitis has a mortality of 1–2%. A monoclonal antibody (palivizumab) against RSV can be given prophylactically to high-risk infants throughout the winter months to provide passive immunity against infection.

Whooping cough

Bordetella pertussis pneumonia tends to occur in young infants or in those who are not fully vaccinated. Paradoxical coughing spasms during expiration are followed by a sharp intake of breath—the whoop. In infants, it can cause apnoea. Diagnosis is mainly clinical although a lymphocytosis ($>20 \times 10^9$/L) is suggestive. The organism may be cultured from a per-nasal swab. Treatment is supportive. The paroxysms of coughing can continue for months (the 100-day cough).

Croup (acute laryngotracheobronchitis)

This common condition affects children aged 6 months to 3 years and is due to a parainfluenza infection of all the upper airways. It is most common in winter and can be recurrent. Croup starts with coryzal symptoms, then proceeds to stridor (Chapter 27) and a barking cough, classically presenting at night. Children may have a hoarse voice. It is usually self-limiting but can occasionally be very severe, requiring intubation and ventilation. Signs of severe croup include increased work of breathing, cyanosis and restlessness. Milder cases can be managed by observation and reassurance. Oral or parenteral steroid can reduce the severity of symptoms and the need for hospital admission. Traditional treatments with steam and humidity have not been proven to be beneficial.

Acute epiglottitis

This life-threatening infection is caused by *Haemophilus influenzae* and is now rare thanks to immunization with the Hib vaccine. It presents in young children with signs of sepsis and an inability to swallow or talk. If epiglottitis is suspected, the child should be transferred immediately to an operating theatre for intubation by an experienced anaesthetist as examination of the throat can precipitate complete airway obstruction.

KEY POINTS

- The majority of children with 'chestiness' have a self-limiting viral URTI and do not require antibiotics.
- If a child has recurrent episodes of pneumonia, an underlying cause should be sought.
- Bronchiolitis is very common in winter, especially among infants with chest or cardiac disease.
- Whooping cough is diagnosed by the characteristic paroxysmal cough and associated colour change.
- Croup causes a barking cough and stridor, usually following a coryzal illness.

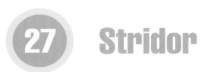

Stridor

Chronic stridor	Acute stridor

Stridor is an inspiratory noise caused by narrowing of the upper airway outside of the thorax. It is a very common symptom in young children and infants, but in a minority of cases can represent life-threatening disorders such as inhaled foreign body or epiglottitis. It may be chronic, due to a congenital abnormality, or acute, usually due to infection or obstruction.

Laryngeal anomalies
- Vocal cord palsy: may be associated with brain lesions or trauma
- Papilloma: due to vertical transmission of wart virus. Causes progressive stridor

▶ **Laryngomalacia (floppy larynx)**
- Variable sometimes biphasic stridor from birth
- Loudest when crying, disappears when settled
- Caused by prolapse of the aryepiglottic folds into upper larynx
- Usually resolves within a few months
- A well, thriving baby with characteristic mild stridor does not need investigations
- If stridor is progressive, interfering with feeding or causing respiratory distress then microlaryngo-bronchoscopy is indicated

Upper airway obstruction
- Severe micrognathia (e.g. Pierre Robin syndrome)
- Pharyngeal cysts or haemangiona

Tracheal abnormalitiy
- Subglottic stenosis—following prolonged intubation
- Tracheomalacia—abnormality of cartilage ring which may lead to recurrent lobar collapse

Vascular ring
- Congenital abnormality of great vessels (e.g. double aortic arch)
- Worsens over time, may have feeding difficulties
- Barium swallow shows indentation
- High resolution CT scan is needed to plan corrective surgery

Croup
- Infection of larynx or trachea
- Usually viral
- Coryzal illness
- Barking cough

Tonsillar abscess (quinsy)

Anaphylaxis

Epiglottitis
- Now rare due to Hib vaccine
- sudden onset
- Painful swallowing
- Septic & drooling
- Muffled voice

Inhaled foreign body
- Usually in toddlers
- Sudden onset
- History of choking
- Unilateral signs
- Requires bronchoscopy

What you need from your evaluation

History

- How long has the stridor been present? In a well baby stridor that comes and goes is usually due to laryngomalacia (floppy larynx), which usually improves with time. Persistent fixed stridor may be due to a vascular ring, vocal cord palsy, or severe micrognathia (e.g. Pierre Robin sequence)
- Does the child look acutely ill? The most common cause of stridor is croup—it is often worse at night and associated with a barking cough and preceding coryzal symptoms. Always consider epiglottitis, which presents more quickly in a very ill child who cannot swallow or speak and is a life-threatening emergency
- In any child with sudden onset of stridor, ask about choking as an inhaled foreign body must always be considered
- Is there any history of allergy that would suggest anaphylaxis?

Examination

- Assess the severity by the work of breathing, the presence of intercostal recession and the degree of oxygenation
- Unilateral wheeze or chest hyperexpansion suggests an inhaled foreign body
- An urticarial rash and angioedema suggest anaphylaxis
- If the child is sitting forwards, unable to swallow and is acutely unwell, consider epiglottitis—in this instance do not try to examine the throat until the airway has been secured. Call for senior anaesthetic help before examining the child
- In chronic stridor assess the shape and size of the jaw. Listen for murmurs which may suggest a vascular ring around the airway

Investigations and their significance

Investigations will be determined by the likely diagnosis as follows:
- Foreign body — Chest radiograph for unilateral hyperexpansion or radio-opaque objects
  Rigid bronchoscopy to find and retrieve the object
- Croup — Usually none required
- Epiglottitis — Do not perform investigations until airway secured!
  Blood culture and FBC
- Persistent stridor — Microlaryngoscopy (if infant not thriving or stridor very severe) to assess larynx and vocal cords
  Barium swallow (may show indentation of vascular ring)

> **KEY POINTS**
> - Stridor suggests upper airway obstruction.
> - Always consider an inhaled foreign body.
> - Acute epiglottitis is a life-threatening infection.
> - Croup responds to corticosteroid therapy.

Paediatrics at a Glance, Fourth Edition. Lawrence Miall, Mary Rudolf and Dominic Smith. © 2016 John Wiley & Sons, Ltd. Published 2016 by John Wiley & Sons, Ltd.
Companion website: www.ataglanceseries.com/paediatrics

28 Swellings in the neck

Causes of swellings in the neck

Mastoiditis
- Tender inflamed swelling behind ear
- Ear pushed out
- Complication of otitis media
- Medical emergency: can cause meningitis or sinus thrombosis
- Requires IV antibiotics and sometimes surgical mastoidectomy

Parotid gland: mumps
- Swelling overlies the angle of the jaw
- Ear displaced up and outwards
- Unilateral or bilateral
- Fever and malaise
- Pain on swallowing sweet or sour liquids

Thyroid gland: thyroiditis
- Anterior midline swelling
- Smooth, diffusely enlarged, non-tender
- Insidious onset
- May be clinically hypothyroid, hyperthyroid or normal
- Thyroid function tests abnormal with thyroid autoantibody present

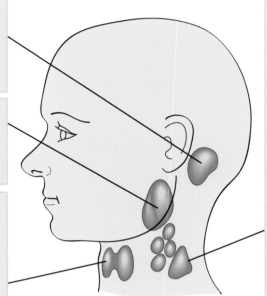

○ Lymph glands
Cervical adenitis
- Tender swollen glands, usually along anterior cervical chain
- Unilateral or bilateral
- Acutely unwell
- Fever, sore throat
- High white cell count

Infectious mononucleosis (see Chapter 24)
- Fever, sore throat
- Large purulent tonsils
- Generalized lymphadenopathy and splenomegaly
- Due to EBV
- Atypical lymphocytes on blood film

Lymphoma
- Firm, non-tender nodes
- Immobile or matted
- Malaise, night sweats, persistent fever
- Hepatosplenomegaly
- Weight loss

Atypical mycobacterium
- *Mycobacterium avium intracellulare* infection
- Cervical lymphadenitis
- Diagnosis by excision biopsy

What you need from your evaluation

History
- Ask about malaise, sore throat and fever
- What is the duration of the illness?
- In the case of thyroid swelling, ask about symptoms of hypothyroidism (tiredness, constipation, underachievement at school) or hyperthyroidism (hyperactivity, increased appetite, palpitations, heat intolerance)

Physical examination
- **Identify the site of the swelling:**
  - Lymph nodes usually lie along the anterior cervical chain
  - Parotid glands overlie the angle of the jaw, with displacement of the ear up and out
  - The thyroid is midline anteriorly, and best palpated by standing behind the child
  - The mastoid is behind the ear and pushes the ear out
- **Palpate the gland.** Infected glands are mobile and tender. Malignant glands are fixed and matted
- Look for other sites of infection, e.g. tonsillitis, otitis media
- If the child is acutely unwell, look for signs of dehydration
- If cervical lymphadenopathy is present, look for generalized lymphadenopathy and hepatosplenomegaly
- In the case of thyroid swelling, determine if the child is hypothyroid (poor growth, low pulse and BP, delayed tendon reflexes), hyperthyroid (tremor, sweating, fast pulse, high BP, eye signs) or euthyroid

Investigations and their significance

Cervical lymph nodes	FBC	High white cell count in bacterial infection; atypical lymphocytes in infectious mononucleosis
	EBV serology	Positive in infectious mononucleosis
	Throat culture	Group A haemolytic streptococcal infection needs antibiotics
	Chest X-ray	Tuberculosis; lymphoma
	Mantoux	Tuberculosis
	Interferon-Gamma release assay	Tuberculosis
	Biopsy	Lymphoma; neoplasia
Parotid glands	Serum or urine amylase	Elevated in mumps, but not usually required for diagnosis
Thyroid gland	T4 TSH Thyroid antibodies	To assess if child is hypo-, hyper- or euthyroid Often positive in thyroiditis
Mastoid process	Tympanocentesis	To identify responsible organism and drain infection

KEY POINTS
- Identify the gland involved.
- If the process is thought to be infective, assess how sick the child is and the state of hydration.
- If cervical lymphadenopathy is identified, look for generalized lymphadenopathy and hepatosplenomegaly.
- If a goitre is found, assess whether the child is hypo-, hyper- or euthyroid.
- If mastoiditis is found, admit the child as an emergency.

Paediatrics at a Glance, Fourth Edition. Lawrence Miall, Mary Rudolf and Dominic Smith. © 2016 John Wiley & Sons, Ltd. Published 2016 by John Wiley & Sons, Ltd.
Companion website: www.ataglanceseries.com/paediatrics

29 Asthma

Chronic asthma

Cough
- Recurrent dry cough
- Worse at night
- Worse with exercise

Wheeze
- Expiratory noise due to airway narrowing
- Often triggered by viral infections
- Responds to bronchodilators

Shortness of breath
- Exercise limitation
- Triggers can be exercise, cold, allergens, smoke

Uncontrolled asthma
- Poor growth
- Chronic chest deformity
- Time off school
- Frequent acute exacerbations

Pathology
- Environmental triggers cause bronchoconstriction, mucosal oedema and excess mucus production in a genetically predisposed child
- Airway narrowing causes wheeze and shortness of breath

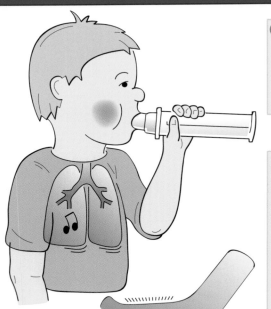

Acute asthma

▶ Acute asthma attack
- Acutely short of breath
- Cough and wheeze
- Work of breathing increased
- Child often frightened
- May be triggered by viral illness, exposure to allergens, exercise or cold air

Assessing severity

Mild
- Breathless but not distressed
- Peak expiratory flow rate (PEFR) reduced
- O_2 sat > 92%

Severe
- Too breathless to talk or feed
- Respiratory rate > 30/min (> 5 yrs) and > 40/min (2–5 yrs); pulse rate > 125/min (> 5 yrs) and > 140/min (2–5 yrs)
- PEFR < 50% of expected
- O_2 sat < 92%

Life-threatening
- PEFR < 33% of expected
- O_2 sat < 92%
- 'Silent chest' or cyanosis
- Fatigue, drowsiness, confusion
- Hypotension

What you need from your evaluation

History
- Ask about the cough and wheeze. What triggers it and at what time of day does it occur?
- How many acute exacerbations have there been? How severe was the worst attack?
- How does the asthma affect the child's life? Does it limit activities; has school been missed?
- How often has the child had to use reliever treatment? How effective was it?
- Are there other atopic symptoms such as hay fever (allergic rhinitis) or eczema or a family history of atopy?

Investigations and their significance

- PEFR — An improvement in PEFR following inhaled bronchodilator supports a diagnosis of asthma. Also useful in assessing severity of acute attacks
- Chest radiograph — To exclude pneumothorax in severe asthma. Avoid excessive radiographs
- Allergy tests — Specific IgE or skin prick testing to common inhaled allergens may identify allergens to be avoided

Examination
- In well-controlled asthmatics there may be no physical signs between acute exacerbations
- Listen for wheeze. Beware the 'silent chest' of severe asthma when there is almost no air moving
- Look for chronic chest deformity: barrel chest and Harrison's sulcus in severe uncontrolled asthma
- Measure lung function by spirometry or PEFR using handheld peak flow meter
- Check height and weight and plot on centile chart. Poorly controlled asthma stunts growth, as will overuse of oral corticosteroids
- Check inhaler technique periodically

Management
- Aim to control symptoms, prevent exacerbations and achieve best possible pulmonary function
- Make sure each child has a self-management plan
- **Medication:** 'preventers' (inhaled steroids or leukotriene receptor antagonists) and 'relievers' (bronchodilators)
- **Environmental control:** Avoid passive smoking and reduce house dust mite and other triggers if possible
- **Education:** of the child, the family and the school on good control of asthma, inhaler technique and emergency treatment of an acute exacerbation

Paediatrics at a Glance, Fourth Edition. Lawrence Miall, Mary Rudolf and Dominic Smith. © 2016 John Wiley & Sons, Ltd. Published 2016 by John Wiley & Sons, Ltd.
Companion website: www.ataglanceseries.com/paediatrics

A sthma is the most common chronic illness of childhood, occurring in up to 15% of children. The symptoms of cough, wheeze and dyspnoea are due to narrowing of the bronchi and bronchioles, mucosal inflammation and thick mucus. In a susceptible individual, this process is initiated by environmental factors such as dust mite allergens, air pollution, cigarette smoke, cold air, viral infections, stress and exercise.

Presentation

Children with asthma usually present in infancy or early childhood. The diagnosis is clinical, based on recurrent cough or wheeze that responds to bronchodilator treatment. A history of atopy (eczema or hay fever) or a family history of asthma supports the diagnosis. In infancy, it is often unclear whether recurrent wheeze is the first manifestation of asthma or merely airway obstruction due to viral respiratory tract infections. As the airways are narrow, mucosal oedema contributes more to obstruction than bronchoconstriction, and there may be poor response to bronchodilators.

In older children, recurrent episodes of wheeze and cough, especially if triggered by exercise, viral infections or allergens, suggest a diagnosis of asthma. A good response to bronchodilators, either in symptom reduction or improvement in peak expiratory flow rate (PEFR), confirms the diagnosis. In asthma, the chest radiograph may show hyperinflation (due to air trapping) and areas of collapse (due to mucous plugging). Specific IgE or skin prick testing to common inhaled allergens may identify allergens to be avoided.

Management of chronic asthma

The goal of good asthma management is to relieve the symptoms and allow normal activity, school attendance and growth. A step-wise approach is used—increasing the amount of treatment until control is obtained, then stepping back to the minimum required to maintain good control.

Medical management of asthma in children

	<5 years	5–12 years
Step 1. Mild intermittent asthma	Inhaled short-acting β₂ agonist as required	Inhaled short-acting β₂ agonist as required
Step 2. Regular preventive therapy	Add inhaled steroids *or* leukotriene antagonist if inhaled steroids cannot be used	Add inhaled steroids via MDI
Step 3. Add-on therapy (<6 months proceed to step 4)	Add leukotriene receptor antagonist if on inhaled steroids *or* if already on leukotriene receptor antagonist consider inhaled steroids	1. Add inhaled long-acting β₂ agonist (LABA) 2. Consider leukotriene receptor antagonist or oral theophylline
Step 4. Persistent poor control	Refer to respiratory paediatrician	Increase dose of inhaled steroids
Step 5. Persistent poor control	Oral steroids not used	Add oral low-dose daily steroids Refer to respiratory paediatrician

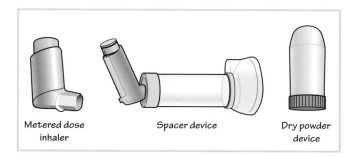

Metered dose inhaler   Spacer device   Dry powder device

Inhaler devices

Treatment is effective only if the drug is delivered in sufficient quantity to the small airways of the lungs. This is best achieved using an aerosolized drug delivery system, via a metered dose inhaler (MDI). A high degree of coordination is required to activate the MDI during inhalation, and this method is really only suitable for teenagers.

For children under 5 years, the MDI can be used in conjunction with a spacer device (e.g. AeroChamber). In infants, these should be fitted with a mask to place over the child's mouth and nose.

In children aged 5–12, the choice of device includes MDI spacer or dry powder inhaler, depending on preference for convenience and effectiveness. Nebulizers can be used for delivering high doses quickly although there is evidence that MDIs via a spacer are as effective. Nebulizers can be used in infants and for emergency treatment of acute exacerbations although there is evidence that MDIs via a spacer are as effective.

Treatment of severe exacerbation

Acute exacerbations should be treated promptly at home by using more reliever medication. If symptoms continue or worsen, then aggressive treatment with high-flow oxygen, regular β₂-agonists or ipratropium bromide via a nebulizer or spacer device (e.g. 10 puffs) and systemic corticosteroids is indicated. All children should have oxygen saturations measured and be admitted for close observation. If the oxygen saturation in air is <92% following treatment, then the child should be admitted to hospital. In life-threatening asthma, an infusion of steroids, salbutamol or aminophylline is used.

KEY POINTS

- Asthma is the most common chronic childhood illness, occurring in 10–15% of all children.
- Bronchoconstriction, viscid mucous and mucosal oedema cause airway narrowing with wheeze, cough and dyspnoea.
- Treatment is increased and decreased step by step to gain symptom control and maintain a normal lifestyle.
- It is crucial to use an inhaler device suitable for the child's age.

30 Cystic fibrosis

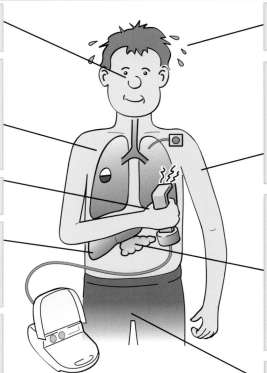

Ear, nose and throat
- Nasal polyps
- Sinusitis

Recurrent chest infections
- Cough
- Purulent sputum
- Pneumonia
- Chronic pseudomonas infection
- Bronchiectasis
- Chest deformity
- Eventual respiratory failure

Finger clubbing
- Seen with chronic lung infection

Liver disease
- Obstructive jaundice in neonatal period (rare)
- Biliary stasis may require treatment with ursodeoxycholic acid
- Eventually liver cirrhosis may develop

Airway clearance
- Regular chest physiotherapy
- Inhaled bronchodilators
- Nebulized dornase alfa can help thin viscid secretions by breaking down DNA strands within the mucus

High salt losses in sweat
- Salty taste to skin
- Risk of salt-losing crisis during very hot weather

Poor growth
- Require 40% extra energy intake compared with normal child
- Poor weight gain
- Short stature
- Normal growth is achievable with pancreatic replacement, and aggressive treatment of chest infections
- Malabsorption

Gastrointestinal effects
- Pancreatic insufficiency
- Poor fat absorption
- Steatorrhoea (fatty stools)
- Distended abdomen
- Rectal prolapse
- Distal intestinal obstruction syndrome (DIOS) – can mimic acute appendicitis
- Need to take pancreatic enzymes with food and drinks which contain fat
- May develop diabetes
- Meconium ileus (obstruction) at birth (10%)

Male infertility
- Congenital absence of the vas deferens

History

- May be a family history of cystic fibrosis, although most new diagnoses do not have a family history
- Failure to thrive with ravenous appetite
- Cough and wheeze
- Recurrent chest infections
- Recurrent sinusitis
- Bulky, pale, offensive smelling stools, often difficult to flush away
- Fall in lung function and weight loss may indicate onset of CF-related diabetes

Examination

- Finger clubbing
- Evidence of malnutrition, poor weight gain and poor growth
- Delayed puberty
- Nasal polyps
- Chest deformity (e.g. chronic hyperexpansion)
- Crackles on auscultation
- Firm enlarged liver (rare) and splenomegally
- Subcutaneous vascular access devices may be present
- Gastrostomy tube may be present

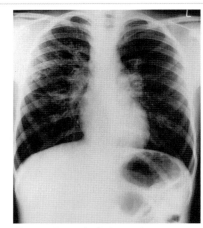

Chest radiograph of a boy with cystic fibrosis
There is gross overinflation of the lungs with hilar enlargement and ring shadows caused by bronchial wall thickening and bronchiectatic change

Paediatrics at a Glance, Fourth Edition. Lawrence Miall, Mary Rudolf and Dominic Smith. © 2016 John Wiley & Sons, Ltd. Published 2016 by John Wiley & Sons, Ltd.
Companion website: www.ataglanceseries.com/paediatrics

ystic fibrosis (CF) is the most common recessive genetic disorder in white populations of European origin (1 in 25 carriers, 1 in 2500 affected). It causes a molecular defect in a cellular membrane chloride channel, which leads to production of excessively thick mucus in many body systems. The sweat is considerably saltier than normal (>60 mmol/L). There is no cure, but effective treatment can greatly improve the quality and length of life.

Genetics

CF is caused by a gene defect in the CF transmembrane regulator (*CFTR*) gene on chromosome 7. Over 1000 different mutations have been identified, but 75% are due to a mutation known as ΔF508. The inheritance is autosomal recessive (see Chapter 8). To be affected by CF, children must inherit an abnormal *CFTR* gene from each parent. These may be two copies of the same mutation (homozygous) or two different CF-causing mutations (compound heterozygous). Carriers are unaffected. Some mutations may result in an atypical presentation and progression of the disease.

The abnormal CFTR channel in the cell membrane leads to production of excessively viscid secretions in the body. This leads to obstruction of the small and large airways and recurrent infection. Abnormal sweat gland function leads to excessive sodium and chloride in sweat, which can be measured to confirm the diagnosis. There is usually pancreatic exocrine failure and in males absence of the vas deferens leading to infertility.

Presentation

Children with CF may be diagnosed by screening soon after birth, or antenatally in affected families. One in 10 present with meconium ileus (obstruction due to viscid meconium in the newborn bowel). Others will have failure to thrive and malabsorption from infancy or may present with recurrent chest infections. Atypical cases may present much later.

Common problems and their management
Chest infections

Thick viscid mucus causes obstruction and predisposes to lung infection. Children may develop chronic respiratory infection, especially when colonized with *Pseudomonas aeruginosa* or *Burkholderia cepacia*. Infection with these bacteria can lead to a rapid deterioration in lung function, and cross-infection to other people with CF must be avoided (e.g. by avoiding mixing individuals with CF in the same clinic). Treatment may involve regular bronchodilators, antibiotics (oral, nebulized or intravenously, which can be delivered at home via an indwelling central line). Steroid therapy may be needed to suppress lung inflammation. Nebulized DNase enzymes can help break down mucus in the lung.

Preventive physiotherapy includes regular airway clearance by a variety of techniques including exercise, autogenic drainage, positive expiratory pressure, inhalation therapy and postural awareness. Prophylactic immunization against influenza and pneumococcus is recommended.

Malabsorption

Pancreatic failure means that fatty food cannot be broken down easily and causes steatorrhoea. This can lead to malnutrition and deficiency of fat-soluble vitamins (A, D, E and K). Taking pancreatic enzyme capsules with food can help with fat absorption and should be started even in babies. High-calorie diets may be required as children with CF have high metabolic demands. Fat-soluble vitamin supplements and advice from a specialist dietician are recommended.

Diabetes mellitus

25% will develop impaired glucose tolerance. Optimization of blood glucose is associated with an improvement in lung function.

Salt loss

Salt supplementation may be required to replace sweat losses. This must be carefully monitored, especially in infancy, where excessive salt intake can be dangerous.

Liver disease

Sluggish bile flow may cause biliary disease and rarely cirrhosis. Ursodeoxycholic acid can help. Children with CF may develop 'pseudo-obstruction' of the bowel, which can easily be mistaken for appendicitis but usually responds to adjustment of pancreatic enzyme replacement or osmotic laxatives and does not require surgery.

Sub-fertility

Most men with CF have absence of vas deferens, leading to infertility. Assisted conception techniques can help. Women may be sub-fertile, but most women with CF can achieve conception. Carrier testing of partners should be considered. Antenatal diagnosis of CF is possible via chorionic villus biopsy or amniocentesis.

Diagnosis

- **Newborns**: May be diagnosed by newborn bloodspot screening (see Chapter 7). Immunoreactive trypsin levels are elevated in affected babies. There is a better prognosis if CF can be diagnosed before it causes symptoms.
- **Gene testing**: Children presenting with a typical history or detected by screening should be diagnosed by mutation analysis of the *CFTR* gene. A panel of mutations are assessed, but these routinely include only 30 of over 1000 mutations. Non-white families may have unusual variants that can be missed.
- **Sweat test**: This is the diagnostic test for CF and requires measuring sodium and chloride concentration in sweat, collected by passing a small electric current across the skin.

Prognosis

There is presently no cure for CF. The prognosis has improved enormously in the last 25 years with aggressive nutritional and respiratory support, and more than half affected live beyond the age of 38 years. Children born today may be expected to live 40–50 years. Lung function tests (e.g. FEV_1) are the best measure of disease progression. Lung or heart–lung transplantation is offered to those with end-stage respiratory disease. Some individuals have survived 15 years following transplantation.

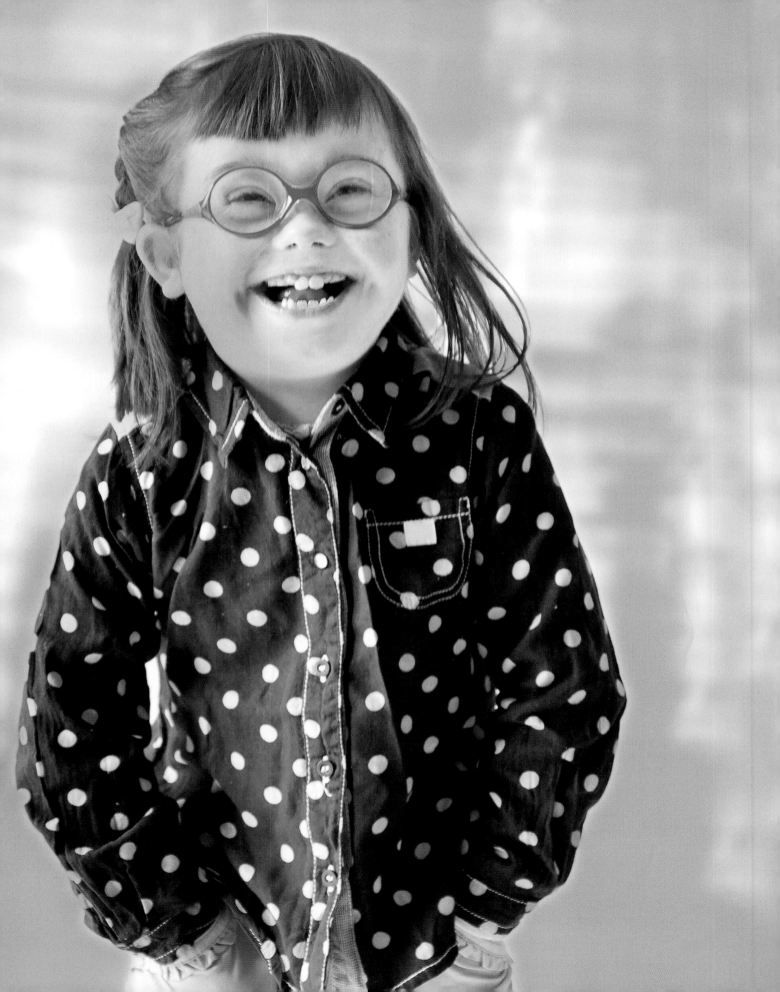

Abdominal disorders

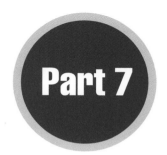

Part 7

Chapters

31 Acute abdominal pain

Causes of acute abdominal pain

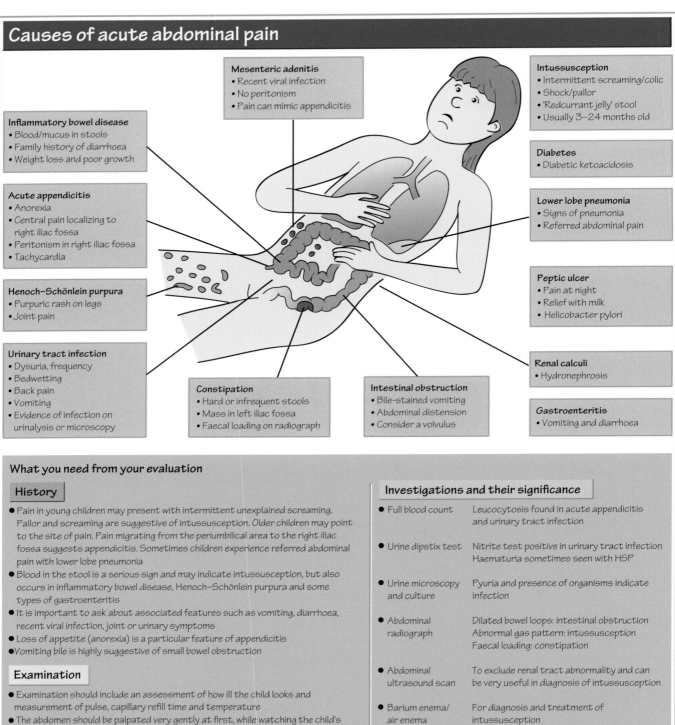

Mesenteric adenitis
- Recent viral infection
- No peritonism
- Pain can mimic appendicitis

Inflammatory bowel disease
- Blood/mucus in stools
- Family history of diarrhoea
- Weight loss and poor growth

Acute appendicitis
- Anorexia
- Central pain localizing to right iliac fossa
- Peritonism in right iliac fossa
- Tachycardia

Henoch–Schönlein purpura
- Purpuric rash on legs
- Joint pain

Urinary tract infection
- Dysuria, frequency
- Bedwetting
- Back pain
- Vomiting
- Evidence of infection on urinalysis or microscopy

Intussusception
- Intermittent screaming/colic
- Shock/pallor
- 'Redcurrant jelly' stool
- Usually 3–24 months old

Diabetes
- Diabetic ketoacidosis

Lower lobe pneumonia
- Signs of pneumonia
- Referred abdominal pain

Peptic ulcer
- Pain at night
- Relief with milk
- Helicobacter pylori

Renal calculi
- Hydronephrosis

Gastroenteritis
- Vomiting and diarrhoea

Constipation
- Hard or infrequent stools
- Mass in left iliac fossa
- Faecal loading on radiograph

Intestinal obstruction
- Bile-stained vomiting
- Abdominal distension
- Consider a volvulus

What you need from your evaluation

History

- Pain in young children may present with intermittent unexplained screaming. Pallor and screaming are suggestive of intussusception. Older children may point to the site of pain. Pain migrating from the periumbilical area to the right iliac fossa suggests appendicitis. Sometimes children experience referred abdominal pain with lower lobe pneumonia
- Blood in the stool is a serious sign and may indicate intussusception, but also occurs in inflammatory bowel disease, Henoch–Schönlein purpura and some types of gastroenteritis
- It is important to ask about associated features such as vomiting, diarrhoea, recent viral infection, joint or urinary symptoms
- Loss of appetite (anorexia) is a particular feature of appendicitis
- Vomiting bile is highly suggestive of small bowel obstruction

Examination

- Examination should include an assessment of how ill the child looks and measurement of pulse, capillary refill time and temperature
- The abdomen should be palpated very gently at first, while watching the child's face for signs of pain
- Signs of peritonism are a reluctance to move, rebound tenderness, guarding and rigidity
- In mesenteric adenitis there is often palpable lymphadenopathy elsewhere

Investigations and their significance

● Full blood count	Leucocytosis found in acute appendicitis and urinary tract infection
● Urine dipstix test	Nitrite test positive in urinary tract infection Haematuria sometimes seen with HSP
● Urine microscopy and culture	Pyuria and presence of organisms indicate infection
● Abdominal radiograph	Dilated bowel loops: intestinal obstruction Abnormal gas pattern: intussusception Faecal loading: constipation
● Abdominal ultrasound scan	To exclude renal tract abnormality and can be very useful in diagnosis of intussusception
● Barium enema/ air enema	For diagnosis and treatment of intussusception
● CRP/ESR	May be elevated in infection and in inflammatory bowel disease

Paediatrics at a Glance, Fourth Edition. Lawrence Miall, Mary Rudolf and Dominic Smith. © 2016 John Wiley & Sons, Ltd. Published 2016 by John Wiley & Sons, Ltd.
Companion website: www.ataglanceseries.com/paediatrics

Acute abdominal pain is very common. It is important to quickly assess whether surgical intervention is required as some important surgical conditions present as an acute abdomen.

Acute appendicitis

This occurs in 3–4 per 1000 children and can present at any age, especially above 5 years of age. It is difficult to diagnose in very young children. In older children, the pain is typically periumbilical and moves over a few hours to the right iliac fossa. There is loss of appetite and a reluctance to move. The most reliable signs are pain on movement and tenderness in the right iliac fossa due to peritonitis. There is often constipation, occasionally diarrhoea and vomiting and usually a low-grade fever. Investigations may show leucocytosis and neutrophilia. Urine should be checked to exclude infection. Abdominal radiograph is not helpful, but CT scan or ultrasound is performed if the diagnosis is in doubt or an appendix abscess is suspected.

The differential diagnosis of iliac fossa pain includes the following:

- Mesenteric adenitis
- Gastroenteritis
- Constipation
- Urinary tract infection
- Henoch–Schönlein purpura (HSP)
- Inflammatory bowel disease
- Ovarian pain
- Ectopic pregnancy
- Pyelonephritis.

Treatment is appendicectomy. This can be performed laparoscopically and has an excellent prognosis. Perforation is more common in children. If peritonitis has occurred, there may be severe illness and adhesions may later cause bowel obstruction.

Intussusception

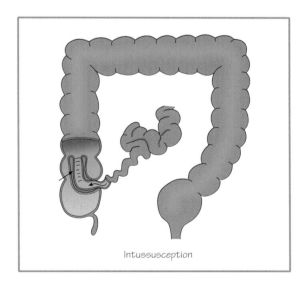

Intussusception

Intussusception is the telescoping of one part of bowel into another; usually the ileum into the caecum (75%). It is the commonest between 3 and 24 months; only 10% occur in children >3 years of age. Enlarged lymphatics may form the leading edge of the intussusception, and this often follows a viral infection (adenovirus or rotavirus). Very rarely it is due to a pathological lesion such as a polyp or lymphoma or as a complication of HSP.

A child presents with episodic screaming and pallor and between episodes may appear well. There may be shock or dehydration. Passage of blood and mucus in the stool ('redcurrant jelly' stool) occurs in 75% but is a late sign. A sausage-shaped mass may be palpable.

Abdominal radiograph may show the rounded edge of the intussusception against the gas-filled lumen of the distal bowel, with signs of proximal bowel obstruction. Ultrasound can confirm the presence of bowel within bowel—the 'doughnut sign'. The intussusception can often be reduced by an air or barium enema. If this fails or there is evidence of peritonitis, then a laparotomy is required.

Children still die of intussusception because it can present non-specifically and the diagnosis is not always considered.

Other surgical causes of acute abdominal pain
Ovarian cysts

Ovarian cysts can be present even in prepubertal children and are present in 20% of teenage girls. They are usually asymptomatic but can cause severe pain with torsion, rupture or bleeding into the cyst. Mittelschmerz pain occurs in mid-menstrual cycle due to rupture of a follicular cyst.

Volvulus

This is torsion of a malrotated intestine and presents with severe abdominal pain and bilious vomiting. Urgent surgery is required to untwist the volvulus and treat the underlying malrotation. If missed, the bowel may infarct.

Renal, ureteric and biliary stones

Stones cause severe colicky pain but are relatively rare in childhood, unless there is an underlying metabolic or haemolytic disorder.

Non-surgical causes of acute abdominal pain

- Colicky abdominal pain is a very common feature of gastroenteritis (Chapter 33) and may precede vomiting and diarrhoea by some hours.
- In sexually active girls, pelvic inflammatory disease and ectopic pregnancy should be considered. A pregnancy test and ultrasound may be indicated.
- Urinary tract infection (pyelonephritis) can cause abdominal pain more than dysuria (Chapter 37).
- Diabetic ketoacidosis may characteristically cause abdominal pain and vomiting (Chapter 1).
- Lower lobe pneumonia may cause pain referred to the abdomen.
- HSP causes abdominal pain due to widespread vasculitis (Chapter 56) and these children are at risk of intussusception.

Abdominal pain is a common symptom of anxiety and school refusal (Chapter 15).

Mesenteric adenitis

Mesenteric adenitis is caused by inflammation of intra-abdominal lymph nodes following an upper respiratory tract infection or gastroenteritis. The enlarged nodes cause acute pain, which can mimic appendicitis, but there is no peritonism or guarding and there may be evidence of infection in the throat or chest. It is a diagnosis of exclusion and treatment is with simple analgesia.

32 Vomiting

Causes of vomiting

Newborn and infants

Overfeeding
• Feeding >200 mL/kg per day

Gastro-oesophageal reflux
• Due to lax gastro-oesophageal sphincter: positional vomiting
• May lead to oesophagitis or aspiration pneumonia
• May cause apnoea and failure to thrive

Pyloric stenosis
• 4–6 weeks old
• Projectile vomiting after feed
• Hungry after vomiting
• Less frequent stools
• Palpable pyloric mass

Whooping cough
• Paroxysmal cough

Small bowel obstruction
(congenital atresia or malrotation)
• Bile-stained vomiting
• Presents soon after birth
• May have abdominal distension

Constipation

Systemic infection
• Meningitis
• UTI (pyelonephritis)

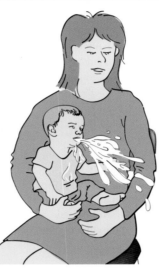

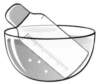

Older children and adolescents

Gastroenteritis
• Usually with diarrhoea
• History of contact with infection
• Check for dehydration
• Usually self-limiting

Migraine
• Characteristic headache

Raised intracranial pressure
• Effortless vomiting
• Usually neurological signs
• Papilloedema

Bulimia: self-induced vomiting as part of an eating disorder

Toxic ingestion or medications

Early pregnancy

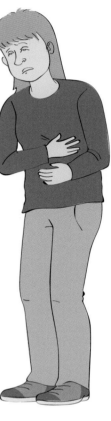

What you need from your evaluation

History

● In infants it is important to differentiate posseting from serious vomiting. With significant vomiting the child will look ill and be failing to gain weight or may even be losing weight
● Take a thorough feeding history, as overfeeding is not uncommon in a thriving baby who seems hungry but vomits the excess milk after a feed
● Always ask about projectile vomiting (pyloric stenosis) and bile-stained vomiting. The latter suggests intestinal obstruction and must be investigated urgently
● The presence of diarrhoea suggests gastroenteritis
● Fever suggests infection, and it is important to look for infection outside the gastrointestinal system; UTI, otitis media and meningitis may all present with vomiting. Vomiting with infection tends not to be projectile
● Paroxysms of coughing followed by turning red or blue and vomiting suggests whooping cough
● Gastro-oesophageal reflux should be suspected in infants and children with disability such as Down's syndrome or cerebral palsy

Examination

● Check for dehydration, especially with gastroenteritis
● Feel for a palpable pyloric mass in any young infant
● Check for abdominal distension, which suggests intestinal obstruction
● Check for papilloedema and hypertension in cases of unexplained vomiting to exclude raised ICP as a cause
● Look for signs of meningitis

Investigations and their significance

Investigations are required only in particular cases:
● Plasma urea and electrolytes — To assess electrolyte imbalance in dehydration and in pyloric stenosis
● Plasma chloride, pH and bicarbonate — To assess degree of metabolic alkalosis in pyloric stenosis
● pH monitoring and barium swallow — May show *significant gastro-oesophageal reflux*
● Upper gastrointestinal contrast study — Mandatory in bile-stained vomiting in newborn to exclude malrotation
● Ultrasound scan of pylorus- if pyloric stenosis strongly suspected

Paediatrics at a Glance, Fourth Edition. Lawrence Miall, Mary Rudolf and Dominic Smith. © 2016 John Wiley & Sons, Ltd. Published 2016 by John Wiley & Sons, Ltd.
Companion website: www.ataglanceseries.com/paediatrics

Regurgitating a small amount of milk, known as posseting, is normal in babies. Vomiting refers to more complete emptying of the stomach. Vomiting is one of the commonest symptoms in childhood and is often due to gastroenteritis. It may be associated with more serious infections such as pyelonephritis or may be the presenting symptom of life-threatening conditions such as meningitis or pyloric stenosis. In newborn infants, bile-stained vomiting suggests a congenital intestinal obstruction (e.g. duodenal or ileal atresia or volvulus). These need urgent investigation with an upper gastrointestinal (GI) contrast study.

Gastro-oesophageal reflux

Gastro-oesophageal reflux (GOR) is a common symptom in babies and in some older children with cerebral palsy or Down's syndrome. It is especially common in the preterm. It is due to weakness of the functional gastro-oesophageal sphincter, which normally prevents stomach contents refluxing into the oesophagus. GOR may present with trivial posseting or vomiting after feeds and is worse on lying flat. If there is significant oesophagitis, apnoea, aspiration or failure to thrive, it is called gastro-oesophageal reflux disease (GORD). Abnormal posturing may occur with severe acid reflux—this is known as Sandifer's syndrome and can be mistaken for seizures.

GOR is usually diagnosed clinically on the basis of a typical history. Simple reflux can be managed by nursing the infant in a more upright position and by thickening the feeds with thickening agents (carob flour or rice-flour thickeners). Formula milk is now available that thickens on contact with stomach acid, which can be helpful. Breastfed infants may be helped by taking Gaviscon before a feed. Winding the baby well after feeds is important. Most gastro-oesophageal reflux resolves over time as the infant sits more upright and is weaned on to a more solid diet.

Investigations should only be performed if the reflux is significant. These include monitoring the oesophageal pH for 24 h using a pH probe or occasionally a barium swallow. Acid in the oesophagus reflects reflux of stomach acid and the percentage of time that this occurs over 24 h is documented. Endoscopy is used to confirm oesophagitis. In GORD, drugs that affect gastric emptying and gut motility can be tried and a small number of children with recurrent aspiration require surgical fundoplication.

Pyloric stenosis

- Caused by hypertrophy of the pylorus muscle.
- Develops in the first 2–8 weeks of life and is said to be most common in first-born male infants.
- It occurs in 1 in 300 to 1 in 500 and is the commonest indication for surgery in infancy.
- Vomiting increases in intensity and is characteristically projectile, occurring immediately after a feed.
- Vomit is *not* bile-stained and the infant usually remains hungry. There may be a history of constipation.
- Weight loss and dehydration occur, and the infant is irritable due to hunger.
- Palpation after a test feed with the left hand from the left side of the body reveals a hard mobile mass to the right of the epigastric area. Prominent peristaltic waves may be visible over the stomach.
- Ultrasound shows a thickened and elongated pyloric muscle.
- Blood tests typically show a low plasma chloride, potassium and sodium, and a metabolic alkalosis secondary to protracted vomiting of stomach acid.

- The infant should be fully rehydrated with careful correction of the electrolyte imbalance before definitive surgery is performed. Rehydration may take at least 24 h.
- Surgery involves splitting the pylorus muscle without cutting through the mucosa (Ramstedt's pyloromyotomy). Laparoscopic pyloromyotomy is sometimes performed. Oral feeds can usually be commenced soon after surgery.

Vomiting due to gastroenteritis

Gastroenteritis (Chapter 33) is by far the commonest cause of vomiting in childhood and is usually associated with diarrhoea. Viral gastroenteritis may sometimes cause vomiting alone. This is typical of Norovirus infection, which causes fever, myalgia, abdominal cramps and vomiting for 24–48 h. Acute food poisoning or food allergy may also cause sudden vomiting.

Bowel obstruction

Bile-stained vomiting in the first days of life should always be investigated urgently. It may be due to duodenal or ileal atresia or malrotation of the small bowel. Duodenal atresia is more common in Down's syndrome. All newborn infants with bile-stained vomiting should have a nasogastric tube passed to aspirate the stomach and feeds should be stopped pending investigation with an upper GI contrast study. In congenital malrotation, the small bowel is rotated on its mesentery and a Doppler ultrasound scan may show malalignment of the mesenteric vessels. Once the cause of the obstruction has been identified and the child has been rehydrated, definitive surgery can take place. Bowel obstruction due to Hirschsprung's disease (colonic aganglionosis) or meconium ileus (in cystic fibrosis) causes abdominal distension before vomiting. In older infants, intussusception should be suspected (see Chapter 31). In children, bowel obstruction may be secondary to adhesions from previous abdominal surgery (e.g. appendicectomy).

Sepsis presenting with vomiting

In young infants, the signs of sepsis may be very non-specific. In an unwell infant with vomiting, urinary tract infection or early meningitis should always be considered.

Vomiting due to raised intracranial pressure

If an older child has a history of regular vomiting for more than a few days, then raised intracranial pressure (e.g. due to a brain tumour) must be excluded by careful neurological examination including examination of the optic discs. Early morning vomiting is said to be typical of raised intracranial pressure.

KEY POINTS

- Vomiting is often due to infection or gastroenteritis.
- Pyloric stenosis presents at 2–8 weeks with projectile vomiting.
- Gastro-oesophageal reflux is common and usually responds to simply thickening the feeds.
- Bile-stained vomiting in an infant is a serious symptom, which always requires investigation.

33 Acute diarrhoea and dehydration

Causes of dehydration

Inadequate intake

Inability to drink
- Herpes stomatitis
- Acute tonsillitis

Inadequate access to water

Excessive fluid loss

Excessive sweating
- High fever
- Hot climate
- Cystic fibrosis

Vomiting
- Pyloric stenosis
- Viral infections
- Gastroenteritis

Acute diarrhoea
- Viral gastroenteritis
- Bacterial gastroenteritis
    shigella
      E. coli
      salmonella
      campylobacter
- Antibiotic-induced
- Food poisoning (toxins)
- Any acute infection

Fluid loss
- Burns
- Post surgery

Polyuria
- Diabetes mellitus, especially diabetic ketoacidosis
- Diabetes insipidus

Signs of severe dehydration
- Sunken fontanelle
- Sunken eyes
- Dry lips and mouth
- Thirst++
- Tachycardia
- Delayed capillary refill time
- Reduced skin turgor
- Reduced urine output
- Weight loss

What you need from your evaluation

History

- Has there been diarrhoea and/or vomiting?
- Is the vomiting projectile (pyloric stenosis)?
- How many loose stools have there been?
- Is the child passing less urine than normal? Ask when was the last wet nappy?
- How often and for how long has the child been vomiting?
- Does the child have cystic fibrosis or diabetes?

Investigations and their significance

(Investigations are required only in moderate to severe diarrhoea or if the child is very ill)

- U&E — For electrolyte imbalance and renal function
- Blood gas — Metabolic acidosis or alkalosis
- Urinalysis — For osmolality or specific gravity
- Blood sugar — To exclude diabetic ketoacidodis
- Stool culture — In gastroenteritis and food poisoning

Examination

- Weigh the child and compare with previous weight (if known) to assess dehydration
- In young infants feel for a pyloric mass during a test feed (pyloric stenosis)
- Assess the degree of dehydration (mild, moderate or severe) as follows:

	Mild	Moderate	Severe
Mouth and lips	Dry	Dry	Dry
Urine output	Normal	Reduced	None for 12 h
Mental state	Normal	Lethargic	Irritable or coma
Pulse rate	Normal	Tachycardia	Tachycardia
Blood pressure	Normal	Normal	Low
Capillary refill time	Normal	Delayed	Very delayed
Fontanelle	Normal	Sunken	Very sunken
Skin and eye turgor	Normal	Reduced	Very reduced
Dehydration (%)	<5	5–10	>10 (shock)

Treatment

- Use oral rehydration therapy where possible
- Treat shock with boluses of IV fluids
- Rehydrate slowly to replace fluid loss over at least 24 h
- Correct any electrolyte imbalance

Paediatrics at a Glance, Fourth Edition. Lawrence Miall, Mary Rudolf and Dominic Smith. © 2016 John Wiley & Sons, Ltd. Published 2016 by John Wiley & Sons, Ltd.
Companion website: www.ataglanceseries.com/paediatrics

Dehydration

Water accounts for up to 80% of an infant's weight. Loss of more than 5% of this water represents significant dehydration. Fluid may be depleted in the intracellular or extracellular compartments. If significant fluid is lost acutely from the intravascular part of the extracellular space, then shock may ensue. Normal body fluid is a balance between intake (drinking) and output (urine output, stool volume, sweat and insensible losses such as expiration). If intake does not keep up with losses, then the child becomes dehydrated. The commonest cause of dehydration in children is diarrhoea and vomiting due to gastroenteritis.

Acute diarrhoea

Episodes of acute diarrhoea are common and are usually due to infections, although not always gastrointestinal (GI) infection. Dehydration due to gastroenteritis is sadly still a major cause of mortality in children in developing countries. Gastroenteritis is usually viral, and rotavirus is the main agent causing winter epidemics. Diarrhoea follows 1–2 days after low-grade fever, vomiting and anorexia. There may be acute abdominal pain and malaise. The diarrhoea resolves within a week and the management is adequate hydration. A rotavirus vaccine is available in the UK. Bacterial gastroenteritis has a similar presentation, and common pathogens are *Escherichia coli*, *Shigella*, *Salmonella* and *Campylobacter*. Meningism and febrile convulsions can occur with *Shigella*, whilst bloody diarrhoea occurs in *Shigella* and *Campylobacter* infection.

Any febrile illness can cause diarrhoea, especially in infants. This includes viral URTIs, chest infections, otitis media and UTI. Use of antibiotics may cause diarrhoea due to a disturbance of the normal enteric flora. Recurrence of diarrhoea on refeeding is most likely to be due to lactase deficiency and may require a lactose-free diet for a number of weeks.

Antibiotics should not be prescribed for uncomplicated gastroenteritis. Antiemetics and antimotility agents are not generally recommended. If there is evidence of septicaemia, the child should be admitted for intravenous antibiotics. There is some evidence that the use of probiotics (e.g. lactobacillus species) may reduce the duration of diarrhoea. Breastfeeding should be continued whenever possible.

Management of dehydration

- Determine the cause of diarrhoea and the degree of dehydration.
- Ask about the duration of diarrhoea, whether there has been vomiting and when the child last passed urine.
- Assess dehydration by the pulse, blood pressure, mucous membranes, urine output, skin turgor and fontanelle (see examination box).

In mild dehydration, the only physical sign may be a dry mouth. 'Red flag' warning signs that may indicate likely progression to shock include

- sunken eyes
- altered responsiveness
- tachycardia
- tachypnoea
- reduced skin turgor (pinch test).

The child should be weighed; the difference between the weight at presentation and a recent weight can be used to estimate the volume of body water that has been lost (1 kg = 1 L). If the child is significantly dehydrated, blood should be taken for urea, electrolytes and bicarbonate and interpreted as in the following table:

Finding	Interpretation
Metabolic acidosis	Bicarbonate loss in diarrhoea or shock with lactic acidosis
Metabolic alkalosis	Loss of H^+ ions from persistent vomiting in pyloric stenosis
Hyponatraemia	Dehydration where diarrhoea contains high concentration of sodium ions. When $Na^+ < 130$ mmol/L, the child is often lethargic and the skin feels dry and can be pinched into creases
Hypernatraemia	Dehydration where there is greater loss of water than sodium ions or excessive salt intake or excessively concentrated formula feeds. When $Na^+ > 150$ mmol/L, the child is very thirsty and the skin may feel doughy

Calculating fluid requirements for a 7.5 kg infant with 10% dehydration

Maintenance fluids (A) = 100 mL/kg/day (for first 10 kg body weight), 50 mL/kg/day for next 10 kg and 20 mL/kg/day thereafter. For this infant = 7.5 kg × 100 mL = 750 mL

Fluid deficit (B) = Assume 7.5 kg is all water (7.5 L = 7500 mL). 10% of 7500 mL is 750 mL.

Fluids required = A + B = 1500 mL, given over 24 h

Note: Maintenance fluid covers essential urine output and insensible losses. If there is ongoing diarrhoea or vomiting, then this volume may need to increase further.

- **Mild dehydration (<5%):** May be treated at home using oral rehydration therapy, as long as the child is not vomiting excessively. The child should be encouraged to drink a rehydration solution, which contains glucose and salt in the correct concentration to aid water absorption and restore electrolyte balance. Breastfeeding should be continued, but if the infant is formula fed, milk can be reintroduced once the diarrhoea has settled.
- **Moderate and severe dehydration:** It is usually as effective and usually safer to rehydrate using oral rehydration solution (initially 50 mL/kg) orally or via an NG tube. The volume of fluid necessary to correct the deficit of water and to provide maintenance fluids and cover ongoing losses is given over 24 h (please see the box above). If there is persistent vomiting, then intravenous rehydration may be required. If shock is present, then give a 20 mL/kg bolus of intravenous 0.9% saline. Too-rapid intravenous rehydration can lead to dangerous fluid shifts and hyponatraemia.

(34) Chronic diarrhoea

Causes of chronic or recurrent diarrhoea

Frequent stools are often normal in early childhood. Babies have one to seven loose stools per day, which become formed and adult-like in odour and colour after 12 months of age. If the child is thriving and there are no other symptoms or signs, investigations are rarely necessary. Pathological diarrhoeal illnesses can broadly be divided into malabsorption, inflammation and infections.

NON-PATHOLOGICAL

Toddler diarrhoea
• Thriving toddler
• Loose stools containing undigested food
• May have a large fluid intake
• Fast gut transit time

Non-specific diarrhoea
• Loose watery stools
• Thriving child, may follow on from acute gastroenteritis

MALABSORPTION

Cystic fibrosis (see Chapter 30)
• Starts in infancy
• Failure to thrive with chest infections
• Fatty stools
• Diagnosis by sweat test

Coeliac disease
• Failure to thrive with irritability
• Muscle wasting, abdominal distension
• Often presents after introduction of wheat into diet
• Fatty stools
• Diagnosis by jejunal biopsy

Secondary lactose intolerance
• Baby or toddler
• Follows acute gastroenteritis
• Watery stools with low pH and reducing substances

INFECTION

Parasites: *Giardia lamblia*
• Weight loss and abdominal pain
• Watery stools
• Common in nurseries

OTHER

Overflow diarrhoea in constipation
• Soiling rather than diarrhoea
• Constipated stool palpable abdominally or rectally

INFLAMMATION (rare)

Crohn's disease
• Late childhood and adolescence
• Weight loss and abdominal pain
• Anorexia and fatigue
• Exacerbations and remissions

Cow's milk protein intolerance
• Occurs in babies
• Watery stools, may be bloody
• May have urticaria, stridor or bronchospasm, eczema

Ulcerative colitis
• Late childhood and adolescence
• Bloody stools and abdominal pain
• Exacerbations and remissions

What you need from your evaluation

History

● **Bowel pattern.** Get an idea of the volume, appearance and consistency of the stools. Is there blood or mucus? A diary is helpful in assessing severity and pattern of symptoms. NB Odour and 'flushability' are usually not helpful
● **Precipitating factors.** Lactose intolerance is precipitated by acute diarrhoea. Are certain foods troublesome? Are others in the family or nursery affected?
● **Associated symptoms.** Weight loss or abdominal pain are particularly significant
● **Review of symptoms.** Non GI diseases may cause diarrhoea and failure to thrive

Investigations

● These are rarely necessary if a child is thriving and there are no accompanying symptoms or signs. Detailed investigations are listed opposite.

Physical examination

● **Growth.** Obtain height, weight, head circumference and compare with earlier measurements. Weight is useful as a baseline if symptoms persist. If growth is impaired consider chronic disease as a cause
● **Other features.** Hydration, pallor, abdominal distension, tenderness and finger clubbing are particularly relevant
● **General examination.** Does the child look ill? Look for non GI diseases which might cause diarrhoea
● **Anorectal examination.** Not routinely indicated

Paediatrics at a Glance, Fourth Edition. Lawrence Miall, Mary Rudolf and Dominic Smith. © 2016 John Wiley & Sons, Ltd. Published 2016 by John Wiley & Sons, Ltd.
Companion website: www.ataglanceseries.com/paediatrics

Investigations and their significance

Blood

● Full blood count	Anaemia indicates blood loss, malabsorption, poor diet or inflammation (as in Crohn's disease) Eosinophilia suggests parasites or atopy
● Plasma viscosity/ ESR	High in inflammatory bowel disease
● Coeliac antibodies	A tissue transglutaminase type 2 (tTGA2) antibodies positive in Coeliac disease (confirm with jejunal biopsy)

Other

● Urine culture	Urinary tract infection
● Sweat test	Cystic fibrosis
● Breath hydrogen test	High H_2 in carbohydrate maldigestion
● Jejunal biopsy	Subtotal villous atrophy with crypt hyperplasia in coeliac disease
● Barium follow through	Characteristic signs in small bowel in Crohn's disease
● Endoscopy	Characteristic lesions on histology in inflammatory bowel disease

Stool

● Occult blood	Positive in colitis e.g. inflammatory bowel disease
● Ova and parasites (three samples required)	Parasitic infection
● Reducing substances and low pH	Present in sugar intolerance (usually lactose)
● Fecal elastase	Low in pancreatic insufficiency
● Microscopy for fat globules	Globules seen in fat malabsorption/maldigestion (usually pancreatic insufficiency)
● Fecal calprotectin	Present in inflammatory bowel disease (Crohn's and Ulcerative colitis but not in irritable bowel syndrome)

Toddler diarrhoea

Toddlers often experience non-specific diarrhoea, probably due to a rapid gastrocolic reflex. Typically, they drink excessive fluids, particularly fruit juices, and pass food particles in the stool. The diagnosis should only be made if the child is thriving. Reassurance is all that is required.

Lactose intolerance

Lactose intolerance is common in babies and young children following gastroenteritis. The superficial mucosal cells containing lactase are stripped off, causing high levels of lactose in the bowel, which prolongs diarrhoea. Congenital lactose intolerance is rare. Lactose intolerance should be suspected if diarrhoea persists for weeks after a gastroenteritis illness. It is rarely necessary to perform lactose challenge or hydrogen breath tests. In bottle-fed babies, an empirical change of formula to soy milk or other lactose-free milk can be tried. The baby should revert to cow's milk once symptoms resolve. Breastfed babies should continue breastfeeding.

Coeliac disease

Coeliac disease results from intolerance to gluten, a substance found in wheat, rye and barley. Children usually present before 2 years of age with failure to thrive, irritability, anorexia, vomiting and diarrhoea. Signs include abdominal distension, wasted buttocks, irritability and pallor. The stools are pale and foul-smelling.

Investigations show iron deficiency anaemia and steatorrhoea. Coeliac antibodies (IgA anti-tissue transglutaminase type 2 (tTGA2) or anti-endomysial antibodies) are present in blood, but a definitive diagnosis is made by finding subtotal villous atrophy on endoscopic jejunal biopsy. Treatment is a gluten-free diet, eliminating all wheat and rye products. Improved mood, resolution of diarrhoea and good growth occur promptly. The diet is quite restrictive and must be continued indefinitely. Rechallenge with gluten after 2 years (to allow for full regeneration of the villi) and repeat biopsy are recommended. Coeliac disease is common—about 1 in 100 adults. It is associated with diabetes and Down's syndrome.

Inflammatory bowel disease

Inflammatory bowel disease (IBD) is a cause of chronic diarrhoea in late childhood and adolescence. Both Crohn's disease and ulcerative colitis are characterized by unpredictable exacerbations and remissions.

• **Crohn's disease** presents with recurrent abdominal pain, anorexia, growth failure, fever, diarrhoea, anaemia, oral and perianal ulcers and arthritis. Diagnosis is by endoscopic biopsy. Remission can be induced by an elemental diet, immunomodulator drugs, anti-TNF-α agents (infliximab) or steroids. Surgical resection may be indicated for localized disease.

• **Ulcerative colitis** presents with bloody diarrhoea and abdominal pain. Weight loss, arthritis and liver disturbance may also occur. Treatment is with oral or rectal mesalazine or steroid enemas. Immunosuppressive therapy, infliximab or even colectomy may be required in severe cases.

Parasites

Giardia lamblia can cause outbreaks of diarrhoea in day-care nurseries or may follow travel abroad. The child may be asymptomatic or have diarrhoea, weight loss and abdominal pain. Diagnosis is made on microscopic examination of the stool. Three separate specimens are required as excretion of the cysts can be irregular. Blood count may show eosinophilia. Treatment is with metronidazole.

Cow's milk protein intolerance

Allergy to cow's milk protein is rare and often over-diagnosed. The diarrhoea may be bloody, and urticaria, stridor, wheeze and very rarely Anaphylaxis can occur. It is less common in babies who have been breastfed. Diagnosis is clinical, and symptoms should subside within a week of withdrawing cow's milk. The child should be rechallenged after a period of time (in hospital if original symptoms were severe). Specific IgE antibodies against milk or a skin prick test are occasionally needed. A hydrolysed protein formula milk should be used. In most cases, intolerance resolves in 1–2 years.

35 Recurrent abdominal pain

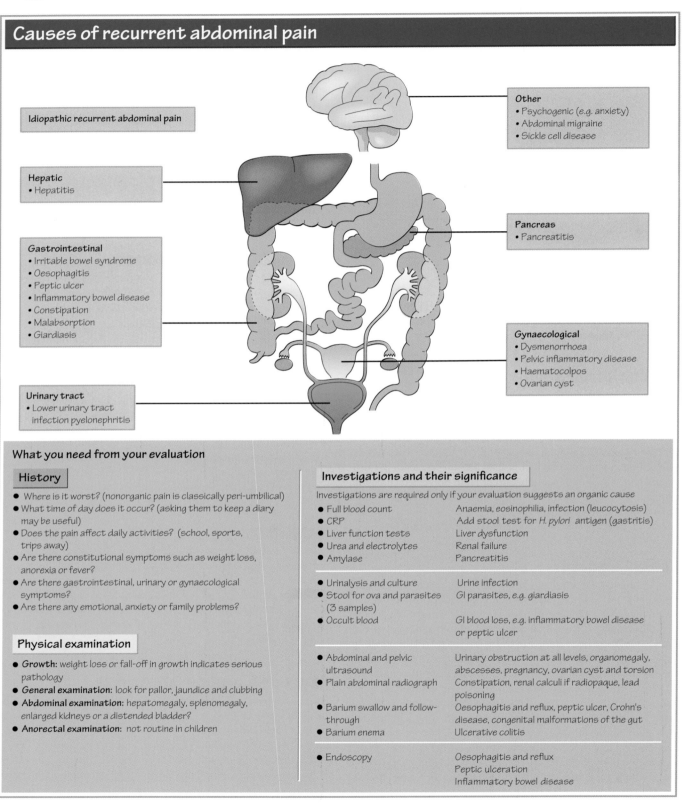

Causes of recurrent abdominal pain

Idiopathic recurrent abdominal pain

Other
- Psychogenic (e.g. anxiety)
- Abdominal migraine
- Sickle cell disease

Hepatic
- Hepatitis

Pancreas
- Pancreatitis

Gastrointestinal
- Irritable bowel syndrome
- Oesophagitis
- Peptic ulcer
- Inflammatory bowel disease
- Constipation
- Malabsorption
- Giardiasis

Gynaecological
- Dysmenorrhoea
- Pelvic inflammatory disease
- Haematocolpos
- Ovarian cyst

Urinary tract
- Lower urinary tract infection pyelonephritis

What you need from your evaluation

History

- Where is it worst? (nonorganic pain is classically peri-umbilical)
- What time of day does it occur? (asking them to keep a diary may be useful)
- Does the pain affect daily activities? (school, sports, trips away)
- Are there constitutional symptoms such as weight loss, anorexia or fever?
- Are there gastrointestinal, urinary or gynaecological symptoms?
- Are there any emotional, anxiety or family problems?

Physical examination

- **Growth:** weight loss or fall-off in growth indicates serious pathology
- **General examination:** look for pallor, jaundice and clubbing
- **Abdominal examination:** hepatomegaly, splenomegaly, enlarged kidneys or a distended bladder?
- **Anorectal examination:** not routine in children

Investigations and their significance

Investigations are required only if your evaluation suggests an organic cause

• Full blood count	Anaemia, eosinophilia, infection (leucocytosis)
• CRP	Add stool test for *H. pylori* antigen (gastritis)
• Liver function tests	Liver dysfunction
• Urea and electrolytes	Renal failure
• Amylase	Pancreatitis

• Urinalysis and culture	Urine infection
• Stool for ova and parasites (3 samples)	GI parasites, e.g. giardiasis
• Occult blood	GI blood loss, e.g. inflammatory bowel disease or peptic ulcer

• Abdominal and pelvic ultrasound	Urinary obstruction at all levels, organomegaly, abscesses, pregnancy, ovarian cyst and torsion
• Plain abdominal radiograph	Constipation, renal calculi if radiopaque, lead poisoning
• Barium swallow and follow-through	Oesophagitis and reflux, peptic ulcer, Crohn's disease, congenital malformations of the gut
• Barium enema	Ulcerative colitis

• Endoscopy	Oesophagitis and reflux Peptic ulceration Inflammatory bowel disease

Paediatrics at a Glance, Fourth Edition. Lawrence Miall, Mary Rudolf and Dominic Smith. © 2016 John Wiley & Sons, Ltd. Published 2016 by John Wiley & Sons, Ltd.
Companion website: www.ataglanceseries.com/paediatrics

Some 10–15% of school-age children experience recurrent abdominal pain at some point, but only 1 in 10 has an organic problem. A good clinical evaluation is essential as it is rare for organic problems to present with abdominal pain alone, although inflammatory bowel disease, chronic urine infections and parasites may do so.

Idiopathic recurrent abdominal pain

The majority of children presenting with recurrent abdominal pain have no identifiable organic cause. In this circumstance, the expression 'recurrent abdominal pain' is often used as a diagnostic term in itself implying that the pain is functional rather than organic. The pain can be very real and severe. The periodicity of the complaint and the intervening good health are characteristic. The children are often described as being sensitive, anxious and high-achieving individuals, although this is by no means always true. Management must be directed towards reassurance, maximizing a normal lifestyle and minimizing school absence (see following box). In the majority of children, the pain resolves over time.

Management of a child with recurrent abdominal pain

(These strategies may also be helpful for non-organic headaches and leg 'growing' pains)

• Assure the parents and child that no major illness appears to be present.
• Explain that the aetiology is not known but nonetheless the pain is very real.
• Do not communicate to the parents that the child is malingering.
• Identify those symptoms and signs that the parents should watch for and that would suggest the need for a re-evaluation.
• Develop a system of return visits to monitor the symptom. Having the family keep a diary of pain episodes and related symptoms can be helpful.
• During return visits, allow time for both the child and parent to express stresses and concerns.
• Make every effort to normalize the life of the child, encouraging attendance at school and participation in regular activities.
• Liaise with school to ensure consistent attendance.

Other causes
Psychogenic abdominal pain

In some children, the abdominal pain is truly psychosomatic and may be related to stress at home or at school. Obviously, these underlying causes must be addressed. In most cases, simply indicating the link and explaining that children tend to experience tummy aches in a similar way to how adults experience headaches is enough to reassure the parents and child. It is important to minimize absence from school.

Irritable bowel syndrome

This is a functional condition of the bowel associated with recurrent abdominal pain and minor GI symptoms such as bloating and altered bowel habit. There is sometimes alternating diarrhoea and constipation. Usually, no psychological stresses are identified.

There may be some overlap with 'recurrent abdominal pain'. It has been suggested that the discomfort results from a dysfunction of the autonomic system of the gut. The stool may be described as varying from pellets to unformed stool. Gas can also be a feature and many of these children give a history of colic as babies. Irritable bowel syndrome (IBS) is a symptom-based diagnosis (symptoms must be present for 6 months) and requires an organic cause to be excluded. It usually presents in young adults but can occur in children and teenagers. The acute symptoms resolve over time, but relapses are common. A change in symptoms (e.g. weight loss, bleeding or anaemia) should prompt further investigations and a re-evaluation of the diagnosis. Smooth muscle relaxants (e.g. mebeverine) may help abdominal spasms.

Gastritis and peptic ulcer

Gastritis and peptic ulcer are now recognized as an important cause of childhood abdominal pain. The features may be similar to adult ulcer symptoms—epigastric pain, relieved by food, and there may be a family history. If suspected, a trial of an antacid, such as ranitidine or omeprazole, may be used empirically, but if symptoms are persistent investigations for *Helicobacter pylori* are indicated. These include stool examination for helicobacter antigen, hydrogen breath test or endoscopy. Treatment consists of eradication with triple therapy (omeprazole, amoxicillin and metronidazole).

Parasitic infestations

The commonest GI parasite in the United Kingdom is *Giardia lamblia*. Inspection of the stool for presence of cysts or parasites (three separate samples are required) is merited in all children with recurrent abdominal pain. Threadworms do not cause pain, nor are they detectable on examination of the stool.

Other causes of recurrent abdominal pain

• Constipation (see Chapter 36)
• Inflammatory bowel disease (see Chapter 34)
• Urine infections (see Chapter 37)
• Sickle cell disease: Abdominal pain is a feature of sickle cell crisis (see Chapter 50).

KEY POINTS

Non-organic pain is characteristically:
• Periodic pain with intervening good health
• Periumbilical
• May be related to school hours.
    Consider organic pain if there is
• Pain occurring at night
• Weight loss, reduced appetite, lack of energy or recurrent fever
• Organ-specific symptoms, e.g. change in bowel habit, polyuria, menstrual problems, vomiting, occult or frank bleeding
• Ill appearance, growth failure or swollen joints.

36 Constipation

Causes of constipation

Acute causes

Fluid depletion
- Caused by fever or hot weather
- May require laxatives
- May lead to chronic constipation

Bowel obstruction
- Rare and usually due to congenital gut malformation or adhesions following previous surgery
- Usually presents as acute abdomen, but may present as constipation with vomiting and abdominal pain

Signs that a child may be constipated
- Infrequent stools (<3 per week)
- Pain and straining on defecation
- Abdominal pain
- Small, hard stools
- Avoiding the toilet
- Not having an urge to defecate
- Difficulty finishing defecation
- Painful bottom
- Dribbling urine
- Faecal smell
- Leaking liquid stools into underwear

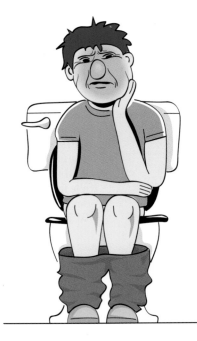

Chronic causes

Functional constipation
- Common, particularly in children with disability
- Often stems from withholding from painful defaecation
- May cause megacolon
- Management involves laxatives, bowel training and diet
- Often recurs

Hirschsprung's disease
- Onset in newborn period or infancy
- Failure to thrive and abdominal distension are features
- Diagnosis is by rectal biopsy

Secondary to other conditions
- Hypothyroidism
- Coeliac disease
- Cystic fibrosis

Behavioural
- Stool holding in toddlers and small children
- Stool gets bigger and bigger and a vicious cycle of pain and further stool holding develops

What you need from your evaluation

History
- Infrequent but normal stools are not indicators of constipation (although very long standing constipation can be painless)
- Ask about hardness of the stool, painful defecation, crampy abdominal pain and blood on the stool or toilet paper. History of an anal fissure is significant
- Onset in infancy suggests Hirschsprung's disease—functional constipation has a later onset
- Precipitating events include mismanagement of toilet training, and fluid depletion caused by hot weather, a febrile illness or vomiting
- Ask about diet as a basis for giving dietary advice on management of constipation
- Constipation can be a presenting feature of child abuse

Examination
- **Growth**
  Review the growth chart as Hirschsprung's disease is accompanied by failure to thrive
- **Abdominal examination**
  Hard indentable faeces are often palpated in the left lower quadrant
- **Anorectal examination**
  Rectal examination is not usually indicated, but will reveal hard stools. An anal fissure may be found on inspection of the anus

Investigations
- Plain abdominal radiograph is not usually required, but may show enormous quantities of faeces in the colon
- Hirschsprung's disease is diagnosed by rectal biopsy, and should be considered if constipation started in infancy and/or there is poor growth
- If there is growth faltering check for coeliac disease and hypothyroidism

Bristol stool chart

| Separate hard lumps, like nuts (hard to pass) | Sausage-shaped but lumpy | Like a sausage but with cracks on its surface | Like a sausage or snake, smooth and soft | Soft blobs with clear-cut edges (passed easily) | Fluffy pieces with ragged edges, a mushy stool | Watery, no solid pieces. Entirely liquid |

Paediatrics at a Glance, Fourth Edition. Lawrence Miall, Mary Rudolf and Dominic Smith. © 2016 John Wiley & Sons, Ltd. Published 2016 by John Wiley & Sons, Ltd.
Companion website: www.ataglanceseries.com/paediatrics

In normal children, the frequency of bowel movements ranges from more than two per day to none for several days. Infrequent bowel movements or bowel movements with every feed are common in exclusively breastfed babies.

Constipation

Constipation is the infrequent passage of hard, pellet-like stools with excessive straining or painful defecation. Using the Bristol Stool Chart can help children describe what their stool is like. Infrequent but asymptomatic bowel movements alone do not constitute constipation. Chronic constipation is commonest aged 2–4 years when they are potty training. About a third of 4 to 7 year olds are constipated at any given time. Constipation can have a sudden onset after an illness or if the child has not eaten or drunk well for a few days, or can develop insidiously.

• **Faecal impaction**: When there is no adequate bowel movement for days or weeks, a large faecal mass can become compacted in the rectum.
• **Soiling** refers to faecal staining of the underwear and results from leakage of liquid stool around impacted faeces. It can be mistaken for diarrhoea. The term is also sometimes used when a child is delayed in gaining bowel control.
• **Encopresis** is the voluntary passage of whole formed stools in inappropriate places (including underwear) by a child who is mature enough to be continent. It is indicative of severe behavioural problems.

Idiopathic constipation

This often stems from painful passage of a hard stool, which has caused an anal fissure. The child withholds further stools to avoid pain. Water is then reabsorbed from the colon making the stools harder and more painful to pass. The cycle becomes self-perpetuating and the rectum can become so stretched that colonic dilatation may occur (megacolon).

Prevention of constipation involves establishing a good toilet routine—toddlers and young children shouldn't be made to wait and shouldn't feel rushed when going to the toilet. Encourage exercise and a good diet (see following box).

Management of constipation

Stage 1: Dietary management of constipation

High-fibre foods
• Avoid excessive white bread
• Encourage whole-wheat bread or bran
• High-fibre cereals

Stool softeners
• Fruit (particularly the peel), vegetables
• Beans and nuts
• Drink 6–8 glasses of water or juice per day
• Have a bottle of water available during school time
• Fluids of any sort, especially fresh orange or prune juice
• In babies, try boiled water or fresh orange juice between milk feeds

Stage 2: Disimpaction (for 1–2 weeks or until symptoms resolve)

Laxatives:
• **Iso-osmotic agents** such as polyethylene glycol (e.g. Movicol) carry water to the stool, softening and lubricating it. Increase the dose until stools become liquid and then reduce.

• **Stimulant laxatives** such as sodium picosulfate, bisacodyl, senna or docusate sodium should be added if polyethylene glycol is ineffective.
• **Osmotic laxatives** (e.g. lactulose) draw fluid into the bowel and can be used if polyethylene glycol is not tolerated.
• **Bulking agents** absorb water and make the stool softer (e.g. Fybogel).
• **Glycerine suppositories** are useful in babies.
• **Enemas** may rarely be required in severe constipation if oral treatment has failed.
• **Manual evacuation under general anaesthetic** is occasionally required in extreme cases, usually in children with other problems such as severe learning difficulties.

Stage 3: Maintenance
• Stools should be kept soft by either diet (see box) or laxatives (polyethylene glycol ± stimulant) for 3–6 months.
• Encourage daily bowel movements by sitting the child on the toilet at a fixed time once or twice each day for 5–10 minutes. If done after eating, this makes use of the gastrocolic reflex.

Stage 4: Vigilance
• Start or escalate treatment at the first indication of recurrence of hard stools.

Management of established constipation involves checking for faecal impaction, evacuating the bowel, maintenance treatment and good diet (see boxes). Constipation often recurs but is controllable with active management.

Hirschsprung's disease

Hirschsprung's disease (congenital aganglionosis) is the absence of ganglion cells in the bowel wall nerve plexus. It usually presents in the newborn period with delayed passage of meconium (for >48 h after birth) and abdominal distension, but if only a short segment of bowel is affected, it may present later with constipation and failure to thrive. It is commoner in boys than girls. Various genes have been identified and there is an association with Down's syndrome. Diagnosis is made by barium enema and then rectal biopsy. Management is surgical with resection of the abnormal section of bowel.

Risk factors for constipation

Diet	Not drinking enough fluid or not eating enough high-fibre foods
Holding of stools	Unwillingness to use toilets (e.g. school or public toilets) or because they don't want to interrupt what they are doing
Change in routine	Going on holiday, moving house or school or even changing formula milk may upset bowel habit
Lack of exercise	Exercise can help with constipation. Lack of exercise makes it worse
Genetics	Sometimes a family history of constipation is present. Constipation is associated with various syndromes and with learning difficulties
Medication	Codeine, cough medicine, some anticonvulsants and antihistamines may cause constipation

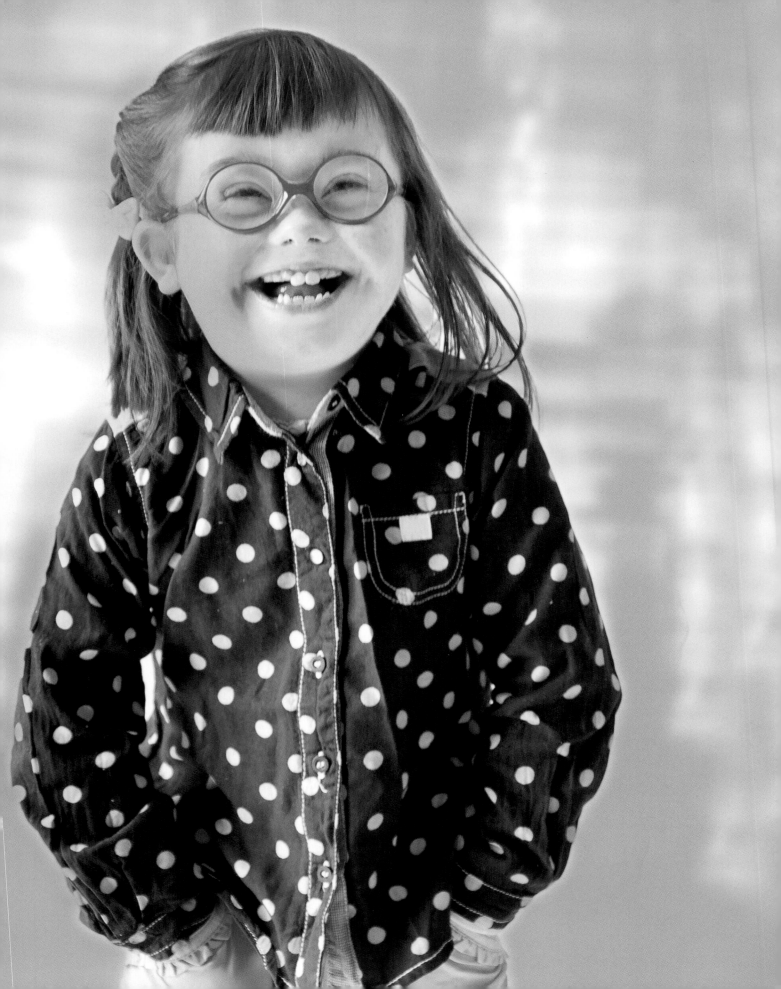

Urogenital disorders

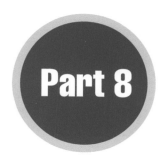

Part 8

Chapters

37 Urinary tract infections

Urinary tract infection

Urinary tract infections (UTIs) are common: they occur in 10% of girls and 3% of boys and 90% are due to infection with *Escherichia coli*. It is important to make a definite diagnosis as a UTI may indicate a congenital renal anomaly or vesicoureteric reflux, which if left untreated may lead to renal failure

Underlying causes of UTI

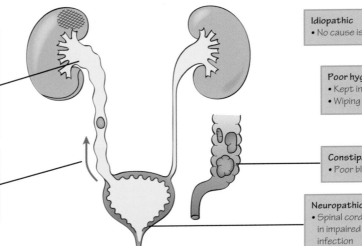

Obstructed urinary system
- Pelviureteric obstruction
- Urinary stones
- Posterior urethral valves (in boys with poor urinary stream)
- Duplex kidney with obstructed pole
- Horseshoe kidney (associated with Turner's syndrome)

Vesicoureteric reflux
- Retrograde flow of urine from the bladder up into the ureters, renal pelvis or pelvicalyceal system. Can cause hydronephrosis

Idiopathic
- No cause is found for many UTIs

Poor hygiene
- Kept in wet nappies
- Wiping 'back to front' in girls

Constipation
- Poor bladder emptying

Neuropathic bladder
- Spinal cord defect can result in impaired continence and infection

What you need from your evaluation

History
- Antenatal ultrasound (anomaly scans can detect structural urinary
- tract problems)
- In infancy UTI can present with fever, vomiting, irritability, septic shock, poor feeding, failure to thrive, jaundice
- Poor force of urinary stream can be a sign of posterior urethral valves in infant boys
- In older children UTI can present with fever, abdominal pain, dysuria, bedwetting, haematuria, offensive smelling urine
- Risk factors for UTI; constipation, dehydration, spinal disorders
- Review family history for vesico-ureteric reflux or other renal disease

Examination
- Signs of general illness — fever, perfusion, pulse rate, jaundice
- Abdominal pain, palpable kidneys or bladder
- Growth measurement and blood pressure
- Spinal abnormalities and peripheral nervous system
- Genitalia

Treatment
- Young infants <3 months are admitted and started on intravenous antibiotics such as cefotaxime or gentamicin
- Children with pyelonephritis signs are admitted and treated with intravenous antibiotic for 2–4 days followed by a course of oral antibiotics to 10 days
- Children with UTI without pyelonephritis can usually be managed in the community with oral antibiotic for 3 days (e.g trimotheprim, nitrofurantoin, cephalosporin)
- Longer term prophylactic oral antibiotic is considered for infants and children with recurrent UTI or suspected vesicoureteric reflux
- Longer term strategies are advised to ensure good hygiene, adequate fluid intake, and prompt toileting to reduce delay in voiding

Investigations
- Urine analysis is vital to confirm infection but samples can easily be contaminated by bacteria on the skin around the genitalia
- Urine collection by clean catch if possible
- Urine bag or pad sample if clean catch not possible
- Urine should reach laboratory within 4 h or be stored in fridge or boric acid container
- Presence of infection suggested by
  - MC&S - Microscopy (>50 white cells per high power field, bacteria seen)
    - Culture (>100 000 colony forming bacterial units), checks sensitivity to antibiotic
  - Urinalysis by dipstick testing for leucocyte esterase, nitrites, blood
  Note white cells can be present in urine without infection in febrile children
- Imaging

KEY POINTS
- UTIs are common, especially in girls.
- Fever may be the only symptom in infants.
- Always confirm infection by culture.
- Confirmed UTIs require investigation in all children.
- In infancy check for obstruction and reflux.

Paediatrics at a Glance, Fourth Edition. Lawrence Miall, Mary Rudolf and Dominic Smith. © 2016 John Wiley & Sons, Ltd. Published 2016 by John Wiley & Sons, Ltd.
Companion website: www.ataglanceseries.com/paediatrics

Investigating urinary tract infections

Imaging investigations	
Renal ultrasound scan (USS)	To identify anatomical abnormalities (e.g. hydronephrosis, gross vesicoureteric reflux (VUR), duplex or horseshoe kidney). May identify renal cortical damage but can miss minor scarring
DMSA isotope scan	Injection of radioisotope that is taken up by the renal tubule and measured using a gamma camera. Used to quantify differential function between the two kidneys and show areas of scarring
DTPA or MAG-3 renogram	Injection of radioisotope that is filtered through renal tubule. Shows functional clearance and can identify stasis of urine in the renal pelvis due to obstruction
Micturating cystourethrogram (MCUG)	A catheter is passed into the bladder and contrast injected to detect reflux up into the ureters with antibiotic cover

In most cases, the urinary tract infection (UTI) occurs in a child with a normal renal tract and does not cause any lasting damage. In one third of cases, there may be an anatomical congenital abnormality, which predisposes to UTI by causing stasis of urine in an obstructed or refluxing urinary system (vesicoureteric reflux). Recurrent urinary infections can cause renal parenchymal scarring, which may lead to complications of hypertension and renal impairment. This can occasionally cause end-stage renal failure. For this reason, there are recommendations regarding investigation of children with UTI:

Initial management
- **Child <3 months with signs of any sepsis**: Investigate with full septic screen including urine sample for microscopy, culture and sensitivities (MC&S) and treat with IV antibiotics.
- **Child 3 months to 3 years with signs of possible UTI**: Send urine sample MC&S and start antibiotics.
- **Child >3 years with possible UTI**:
- Use urine dipstick analysis:
  - nitrite (+) = probable UTI, send urine MC&S and start antibiotic
  - leucocyte (+) but nitrite (−) = equivocal, send urine MC&S.
- Do not start antibiotic unless good clinical evidence of UTI.
- Both leucocyte (−) and nitrite (−) = negative; do not send for culture and do not start antibiotics.

Further investigation
Further investigation for anatomical problems and scarring depends on the child's age and whether there are clinical features of more severe, recurrent or atypical infection. The aim is to screen children at a higher risk of VUR.

The level of further imaging depends on the child's age and severity of symptoms. A young baby with UTI is at high risk of reflux and should have full imaging with USS DMSA and MCUG. An older child with mild symptoms in whom infection responds quickly to antibiotics may need no further imaging.

Renal anomalies
Congenital renal anomalies are common (8/1000 live births). Less than 5% of these will have long-term renal impairment.

- **Solitary kidney**: A single kidney due to unilateral renal agenesis.
- **Ectopic kidney**: Abnormal migration during embryogenesis leads to a pelvic or horseshoe kidney.
- **Multicystic dysplastic kidney**: The kidney is non-functioning and usually involutes and disappears by school age.
- **Autosomal dominant polycystic kidney disease (ADPKD)**: Occurs in 1 in 1000 children and adults. Small cysts are present throughout the kidney. The enlarged kidneys may cause haematuria, hypertension and renal failure later in adult life.
- **Autosomal recessive polycystic kidney disease (ARPKD)**: This rare condition (1 in 20 000) is often diagnosed antenatally as the large, cystic kidneys do not produce adequate urine, leading to reduced amniotic fluid and secondary pulmonary hypoplasia. If the child survives the neonatal period, he or she will develop end-stage renal failure early in childhood.

Urological abnormalities
Obstructive uropathy may be due to an obstruction at the level of the renal pelvis, the junction of the ureter with the bladder or at the bladder outlet. Obstructive uropathy can predispose to UTI and if severe can lead to renal impairment or failure.

- **Pelviureteric obstruction** is due to abnormal tissue or external compression at the point the renal pelvis joins the ureter. 75% improve without the need for surgical intervention.
- **Posterior urethral valves** occur in 1 in 10 000 male infants. It is due to persistence of an embryological fold across the urethra, causing bladder hypertrophy, bilateral hydronephrosis and renal impairment.
- **Hypospadias**: The external urinary meatus opens on the ventral side of the penis. It may be mild, needing no treatment, or severe, requiring surgical repair. For this reason, parents should be advised not to have the child circumcised, so that the foreskin tissue can be used in reconstructive surgery.
- **Phimosis**: The foreskin is non-retractile. This is normal in infancy and requires surgery only if there is an obstruction problem.
- **Paraphimosis**: The foreskin becomes trapped behind the glans causing pain and swelling. It is usually reducible without surgery.

Circumcision is most commonly performed for persistence of these problems, or for cultural or religious reasons.

Vesicoureteric reflux
The retrograde flow of urine from the bladder into the ureters can cause hydronephrosis and predispose to UTI, pyelonephritis, hypertension or end-stage renal failure. VUR occurs because of an abnormally short and straight insertion of the ureters through the wall of the bladder, so that they are not properly occluded during bladder contraction. The severity of VUR is graded depending on the extent of reflux and degree of dilatation of ureters, renal pelvis and calyces. VUR can be managed with conservative treatment (surveillance monitoring and antibiotics for infection). Around 50% resolve, but surgery may be needed if there are breakthrough infections or deteriorating renal function.

38 Haematuria and proteinuria

Haematuria and proteinuria

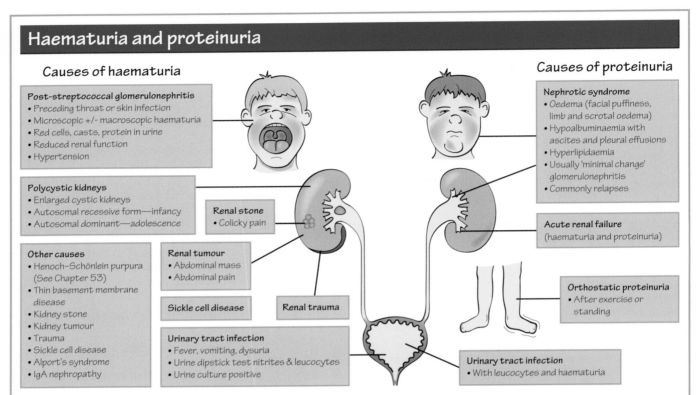

Causes of haematuria

Post-streptococcal glomerulonephritis
- Preceding throat or skin infection
- Microscopic +/- macroscopic haematuria
- Red cells, casts, protein in urine
- Reduced renal function
- Hypertension

Polycystic kidneys
- Enlarged cystic kidneys
- Autosomal recessive form—infancy
- Autosomal dominant—adolescence

Renal stone
- Colicky pain

Other causes
- Henoch–Schönlein purpura (See Chapter 53)
- Thin basement membrane disease
- Kidney stone
- Kidney tumour
- Trauma
- Sickle cell disease
- Alport's syndrome
- IgA nephropathy

Renal tumour
- Abdominal mass
- Abdominal pain

Sickle cell disease

Renal trauma

Urinary tract infection
- Fever, vomiting, dysuria
- Urine dipstick test nitrites & leucocytes
- Urine culture positive

Causes of proteinuria

Nephrotic syndrome
- Oedema (facial puffiness, limb and scrotal oedema)
- Hypoalbuminaemia with ascites and pleural effusions
- Hyperlipidaemia
- Usually 'minimal change' glomerulonephritis
- Commonly relapses

Acute renal failure (haematuria and proteinuria)

Orthostatic proteinuria
- After exercise or standing

Urinary tract infection
- With leucocytes and haematuria

What you need from your evaluation

History

Haematuria
- Make sure you are clear what is being described: is it frank blood, pink urine or a positive dipstick test. (Dipsticks are extremely sensitive to the presence of tiny quantities of blood)
- What colour is the urine? Brown suggests renal origin; fresh red blood or clots suggest bladder origin. Red urine can also be caused by eating beetroot or taking rifampicin
- Are there any other urinary symptoms? Frequency and dysuria suggest a UTI
- Is there severe pain? Renal colic or abdominal pain suggests a calculus (stone) or other obstruction
- Was there a precipitating factor? Enquire about trauma to the kidneys. Throat infections or skin infections may precede acute glomerulonephritis, or nephrotic syndrome and intense exercise may precipitate haematuria
- Is there a family history of renal disease or deafness? (Alport's syndrome causes deafness and nephritis, and is autosomal dominant)

Nephrotic syndrome
- Has oedema around the eyes been noticed in the morning? Has there been any weight gain?
- What is the urine output? Is the child fluid restricted to a certain volume per day?
- Is this the first presentation or a relapse?
- If the latter, what has the child been treated with in the past?

Investigations and their significance

- Urinalysis and culture — For presence of blood, protein, casts or white cells. Pyuria and bactiuria point to a UTI
- Full blood count — For anaemia and to exclude HUS
- ASOT/throat swab — For evidence of streptococcal infection
- U&E — To assess renal function
- Serum C3 complement level — Will be low in some types of glomerulonephritis
- Serum albumin level — Low in nephrotic syndrome
- Urinary protein/creatinine ratio — High in nephrotic syndrome
- Triglycerides and cholesterol level — High in nephrotic syndrome
- Renal ultrasound and AXR — May show renal stones
- Renal biopsy — If renal function impaired or if there is hypertension, proteinuria and haematuria

Examination

- Blood pressure measurement is mandatory. Hypertension suggests renal disease
- Palpate the abdomen for renal masses (tumour, polycystic kidneys or obstruction) and check for ascites
- Check for pitting oedema over the tibia and sacrum
- Examine for the presence of pleural effusions
- Measure weight and compare with previous values
- Look for any purpuric rash (Henoch–Schönlein purpura (p. 101) or haemolytic uraemic syndrome, HUS)

Paediatrics at a Glance, Fourth Edition. Lawrence Miall, Mary Rudolf and Dominic Smith. © 2016 John Wiley & Sons, Ltd. Published 2016 by John Wiley & Sons, Ltd.
Companion website: www.ataglanceseries.com/paediatrics

Acute post-streptococcal glomerulonephritis

Acute glomerulonephritis results from immune-mediated damage to the glomerulus. The commonest type in childhood is due to immune complex formation following group A beta-haemolytic streptococcal infection. The presenting complaint is usually haematuria, which is cola coloured and typically occurs 1–2 weeks after a throat infection or 3–6 weeks after a skin infection. The child may have malaise, oedema, loin pain and headache or be asymptomatic. Urinalysis shows gross haematuria with granular and red cell casts and often proteinuria. In most children, there is mild oliguria (reduced urine output), but in a minority there may be acute renal failure and hypertension. Useful investigations include a throat swab and antistreptolysin O (ASO) titre to look for evidence of streptococcal infection and there may be a low C3 complement level.

A 10-day course of penicillin is recommended to try to clear the nephritic strain of streptococcus, although there is no evidence that this alters the course of the disease. Acute renal failure is managed with careful monitoring of fluid balance and renal function. Salt and fluid restriction may be required and hypertension must be controlled. Rarely, acute glomerulonephritis leads to severe renal failure requiring renal dialysis.

Nephrotic syndrome

Nephrotic syndrome is characterized by proteinuria, low albumin, oedema and hyperlipidaemia. This is due to increased capillary wall permeability in the glomerulus, which allows protein to leak into the urine. The commonest cause (85%) is 'minimal change' glomerulonephritis (MCGN), where the histological changes on renal biopsy are very mild. This type usually responds to steroid therapy. The presenting feature is oedema, which is usually most noticeable in the mornings around the eyelids and as pitting oedema on the legs. There may be history of a recent viral upper respiratory tract infection (URTI). Focal segmental glomerulosclerosis (FSGS) is the second most frequent form.

With time, ascites and pleural effusions develop secondary to the hypoalbuminaemia, and there is weight gain due to oedema. Hypertension is rare, but there may be anorexia, abdominal pain, diarrhoea and oliguria. There is an increased risk of infection due to leakage of immunoglobulins and an increased risk of thrombosis.

Treatment of minimal change nephrotic syndrome involves fluid restriction, a low-salt diet and corticosteroids (prednisolone). Prednisolone is continued until there is remission of proteinuria, continued at a weaning dose over several months. Parents should be warned about the immunosuppressive effects of nephrotic syndrome and steroids and should avoid live vaccines and chickenpox at this time. Prophylactic penicillin is given until the proteinuria has cleared as pneumococcal peritonitis is a risk.

Relapses are common, occurring in up to 75% of those who initially respond. Children who are steroid resistant need a renal biopsy to confirm the pathology and may need treatment with cyclophosphamide. Long-term prognosis is good although delayed relapses may occur. Other forms of nephrotic syndrome (e.g. following Henoch–Schönlein purpura) carry a worse prognosis and may progress to chronic renal failure requiring dialysis and eventually transplantation.

Other renal conditions
Acute renal failure

Acute renal failure (acute kidney injury) is defined as a rapid onset of anuria or severe oliguria (<0.5 mL/kg per hour). Causes can be divided into pre-renal (i.e. poor perfusion), renal or post-renal (due to urinary obstruction). The commonest pre-renal cause is hypovolaemic shock. Pre-renal failure can usually be managed with fluid replacement and inotropic support of the circulation.

Intrinsic renal causes include the following:

- Acute tubular necrosis (often secondary to shock)
- Haemolytic uraemic syndrome (HUS)
- Vasculitis
- Glomerulonephritis
- Renal vein thrombosis
- Nephrotoxic drugs (e.g. gentamicin and vancomycin).

Renal failure requires careful inpatient management. Hyperkalaemia, hypertension and fluid overload can be life-threatening complications. If conservative management is failing, there is severe electrolyte imbalance, progressive acidosis or fluid overload; then renal dialysis is necessary, using peritoneal dialysis or haemodialysis.

Haemolytic uraemic syndrome

HUS is an important cause of renal failure associated with thrombocytopenia and haemolytic anaemia due to fragmentation of red blood cells. It often follows an episode of bloody diarrhoea and is associated with a verotoxin-producing *Escherichia coli* O157:H7. The disease can also affect the brain, causing encephalopathy. Intensive care treatment may be needed for renal failure, encephalopathy and associated colitis. Chronic renal failure can result.

Chronic renal failure

About 1000 children in the UK receive renal replacement therapy. The commonest cause is a congenital structural renal abnormality such as cystic–dysplastic kidneys or severe obstructive nephropathy. Rarer causes include glomerulonephritis and renal disease as part of autoimmune systemic disease. Children with untreated chronic renal failure are at risk of developing anaemia, lethargy, poor appetite, poor growth, osteodystrophy and hypertension.

Management involves a high-calorie, low-protein diet that is low in phosphate. Growth hormone and vitamin D supplements are often required, and anaemia may be treated with erythropoietin injections. When the renal disease becomes end stage, children require dialysis. Dialysis can either be haemodialysis (in hospital) or peritoneal dialysis (can be administered at home). The best long-term treatment is renal transplant from a cadaveric or living related donor.

KEY POINTS

- Careful urine analysis is essential.
- Haematuria is more likely to have serious underlying cause if associated with hypertension, proteinuria and impaired function.
- Nephrotic syndrome usually responds to steroid treatment, but relapses may occur.
- Renal transplantation is the treatment of choice for end-stage renal disease.

39 Bedwetting and daytime wetting

Bedwetting and daytime wetting

Nocturnal enuresis refers to bedwetting. It usually occurs in normal children and is due to a delay in the development of the normal sphincter control mechanisms. Day and night wetting (diurnal enuresis) may be due to poor bladder sensation or bladder muscle instability. Secondary enuresis refers to wetting in a child who had previously been dry, and is often associated with psychological stress

Primary nocturnal enuresis
- Common: 10% of 6-year-olds and 3% of 12-year-olds wet the bed once a week
- Twice as common in boys than girls

Causes
- Delayed maturation (often familial)
- May be reduced ADH production
- Reduced bladder awareness
- Emotional stress
- Urinary tract infection
- Polyuria due to diabetes or renal disease

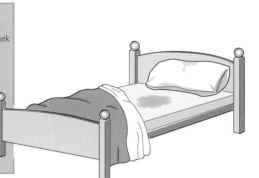

Causes of secondary enuresis
- Emotional upset
- Urinary tract infection
- Diabetes mellitus
- Threadworm infection

Causes of diurnal enuresis
- Urinary tract infection
- Neurogenic bladder
- Congenital abnormality (e.g. ectopic ureter)
- Severe constipation
- Psychogenic, due to stress
- Sexual abuse
- Physiological (urgency)

What you need from your evaluation

History

- Has the child ever been dry? If so, at what age? Was there a particular trigger that led to wetting again (e.g. birth of a sibling)?
- Is there a family history of primary nocturnal enuresis? Ask about siblings, parents and grandparents
- Is there anything to suggest stress as a cause? Is there any possibility of sexual abuse?
- Is there any dysuria, frequency or systemic upset to suggest a urinary tract infection? Is the child constipated?
- Has there been a sudden onset of polyuria, polydipsia, or weight loss to suggest diabetes mellitus or other renal disease?
- How have the parents dealt with the wetting? Have they punished or criticized the child for wetting in the past? Do they have false expectations?
- What methods have they tried, e.g. fluid restriction, lifting onto the toilet at night, star charts?
- What is the pattern of the wetting—nocturnal only, day and night, with urgency or with dribbling incontinence? Are there any features in the history to suggest a neuropathic bladder?

Examination

- Is there any evidence of a neurological or congenital abnormality? Check leg reflexes and perineal sensation
- Look for evidence of spina bifida occulta such as a lipoma or hairy patch over the sacral area
- Is there a palpable faecal mass (constipation)?
- Is there evidence of renal disease?
- Check for hypertension

Investigations and their significance

- Urine microscopy and culture — To exclude UTI
- Urine dipstick — To exclude glycosuria
- Renal ultrasound — If ectopic ureter strongly suspected. (This causes a constant connection to the vagina rather than the bladder)

KEY POINTS

- Enuresis is common—15% of 5-year-olds wet the bed
- There is rarely an organic cause
- The majority respond to behavioural management
- Psychological stress should be considered in secondary enuresis

Management of enuresis

Daytime wetting
- Encourage the child to go to the toilet to pass urine at regular intervals
- Treat any constipation or urine infections
- Consider medication with oxybutynin to give bladder muscle stability if frequent urgency and small bladder capacity

Night time wetting
- Behavioural stategies such as star charts, lifting, rewards can be helpful
- Avoid drinks in the evenings
- Enurseis alarms can be effective from around age 7 when children can be involved amd learn not to unconsciously pass uine in sleep
- Medication with desmopressin can be helpful particulalry for short periods such as holidays or sleepover nights
- Specialist enuresis nurse support is very helpful for families as it often takes a series of meetings over a few months to resolve the problem

Paediatrics at a Glance, Fourth Edition. Lawrence Miall, Mary Rudolf and Dominic Smith. © 2016 John Wiley & Sons, Ltd. Published 2016 by John Wiley & Sons, Ltd.
Companion website: www.ataglanceseries.com/paediatrics

40 Swellings in the groin and scrotum

Swellings in the groin and scrotum and impalpable testes

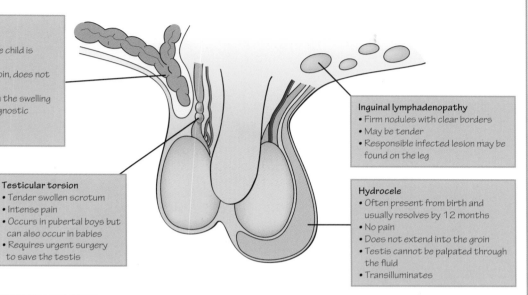

Inguinal hernia
- Common in preterm infants
- Often increases in size when the child is crying
- Swelling extends up into the groin, does not transilluminate
- Testis is palpable, distinct from the swelling
- Reduction of the swelling is diagnostic
- No pain unless incarcerated
- Requires surgery

Testicular torsion
- Tender swollen scrotum
- Intense pain
- Occurs in pubertal boys but can also occur in babies
- Requires urgent surgery to save the testis

Inguinal lymphadenopathy
- Firm nodules with clear borders
- May be tender
- Responsible infected lesion may be found on the leg

Hydrocele
- Often present from birth and usually resolves by 12 months
- No pain
- Does not extend into the groin
- Testis cannot be palpated through the fluid
- Transilluminates

Impalpable testes

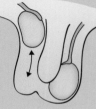

Retractile testis
- Brought down by careful palpation
- Examine the child with warm hands, and cross-legged or squatting

Undescended testis
- May be unilateral or bilateral
- More common in premature babies
- 5% undescended at term, 1% by 12 months
- May be associated with inguinal hernia
- Orchidopexy required by 1 year to avoid infertility, torsion and malignancy
- Bilateral impalpable testes need very careful evaluation (see below)

Ectopic testes
- Testes descend but along abnormal path
- May be in superficial inguinal pouch or on perineum

What you need from your evaluation

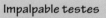

History

- **Characteristics of the swelling:** an incarcerated hernia and testicular torsion are both painful. Hernias usually cause intermittent swelling. Hydroceles are often present from birth

Physical examination

For a swelling
- **Observation:** is the boy in pain? Does the swelling extend into the groin?
- **Palpation:** in an inguinal hernia the swelling extends right up into the groin, and the testis is palpable separate from the swelling. In a hydrocele the testis cannot be palpated through the fluid. Testicular torsion is acutely tender
- Bilateral inguinal hernias in a girl should raise the possibility of the swellings being testes in an undervirilized male with ambiguous genitalia
- Bilateral impalpable testes may rarely be the manifestation of a virilized female (e.g. congenital adrenal hyperplasia or other disorders of sexual differentiation). A pelvic ultrasound should be performed urgently
- Impalpable testes can be a sign of severe anterior pituitary dysfunction, especially if associated with micro-penis
- Reduction of the swelling by manipulation or spontaneously is diagnostic of a hernia
- **Transillumination:** when a torch is held to the scrotum a hydrocele transilluminates but a hernia does not
- **General examination:** if lymphadenopathy is suspected as a cause, look for an infected lesion on the leg, lymphadenopathy elsewhere, and check for hepatosplenomegaly

KEY POINTS

- Incarcerated inguinal hernia and testicular torsion are emergencies
- Hydroceles are present from birth and usually resolve spontaneously
- Undescended testes must be referred by 1 year of age

Paediatrics at a Glance, Fourth Edition. Lawrence Miall, Mary Rudolf and Dominic Smith. © 2016 John Wiley & Sons, Ltd. Published 2016 by John Wiley & Sons, Ltd.
Companion website: www.ataglanceseries.com/paediatrics

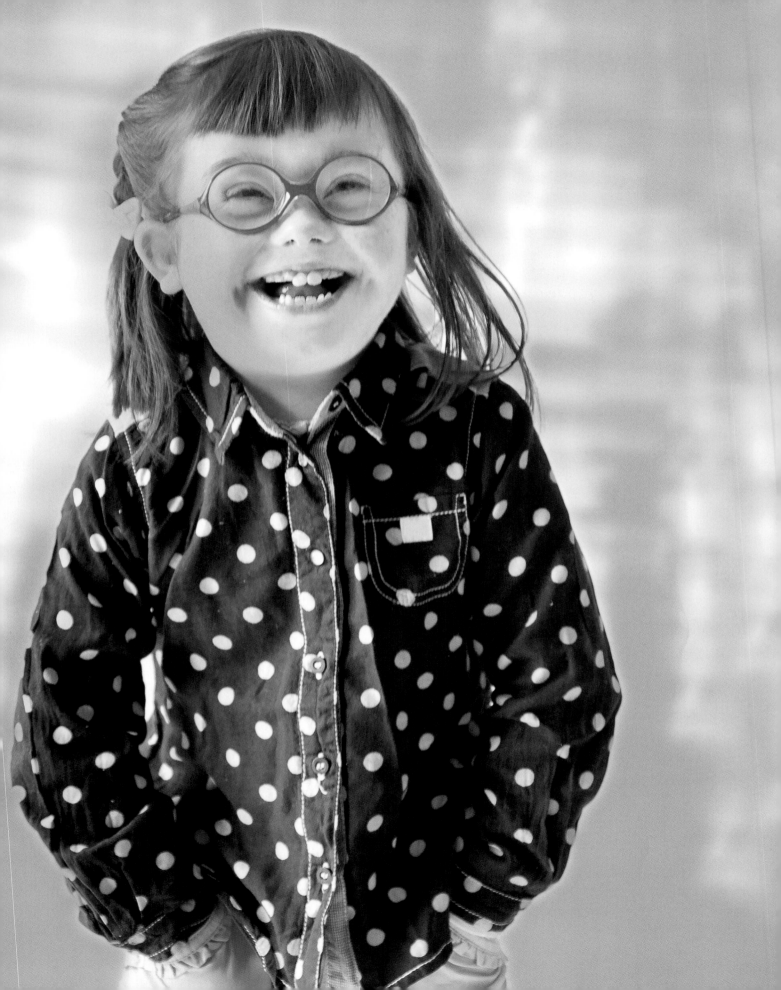

Neurological disorders

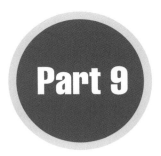

Part 9

Chapters

41 Developmental delay

Causes of developmental delay

Idiopathic
- Autism
- Various dysmorphic syndromes

Chromosomal abnormalities
- Down's syndrome
- Fragile X

Perinatal injury
- Asphyxia
- Birth trauma

Prenatal injury
- Fetal alcohol syndrome
- Intrauterine infections (TORCH)

Endocrine and metabolic defects
- Congenital hypothyroidism
- Phenylketonuria

Neurodegenerative disorders
- Leucodystrophy

Neurocutaneous syndromes
- Sturge–Weber
- Neurofibromatosis
- Tuberous sclerosis

Postnatal injury
- Meningitis
- Non-accidental injury
- Neglect

Central nervous system malformation
- Neural tube defects
- Hydrocephalus

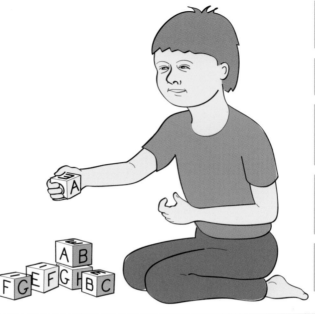

What you need from your evaluation

History

Developmental milestones
- Enquire systematically about milestones for the four developmental areas (see chapter 4)
- Ascertain the extent of delay and which areas are affected
- Remember to allow for prematurity during the first 2 years. Beyond that catch-up in development rarely occurs
- Loss in skills suggests a neurodegenerative condition
- Ask whether there are concerns about vision and hearing

Past medical history
- Enquire into alcohol consumption, medical problems and medication during pregnancy
- Enquire about prematurity and neonatal complications

Family history
- Ask about intellectual disability and consanguinity in the family

Physical examination

Children may often be uncooperative so parental report is particularly important

Developmental skills
- Assess each developmental area in turn: gross motor, fine motor/adaptive, language and social skills
- Attempt to evaluate vision and hearing
- Assess factors such as alertness, responsiveness, interest in surroundings, determination and concentration; these all have positive influences on a child's attainments

General examination
- Dysmorphic signs suggest a genetic defect, chromosome anomaly or teratogenic effect
- Microcephaly at birth suggests fetal alcohol syndrome or intrauterine infections
- Poor growth is common, but consider the possibility of hypothyroidism or non-organic failure to thrive (look for signs of neglect)
- Look for café-au-lait spots, depigmented patches and portwine stains which are indicative of neurocutaneous syndromes
- Hepatosplenomegaly suggests a metabolic disorder

Neurological examination
- Look for abnormalities in tone, strength and coordination, deep tendon reflexes, clonus, cranial nerves, primitive reflexes, and ocular abnormalities

Investigations

- Chromosome analysis, thyroid function tests and urine screen for metabolic defects are usually obtained in global developmental delay
- More sophisticated metabolic investigations and brain imaging may be indicated for some
- A hearing test is mandatory in language delay
- Comparative genomic hybridisation (CGH) analysis detects chromosomal duplications and deletions and may be useful in diagnosing the cause of severe developmental delay

Paediatrics at a Glance, Fourth Edition. Lawrence Miall, Mary Rudolf and Dominic Smith. © 2016 John Wiley & Sons, Ltd. Published 2016 by John Wiley & Sons, Ltd.
Companion website: www.ataglanceseries.com/paediatrics

The term *global* developmental delay refers to delay in all milestones (but particularly language, fine motor and social skills) and is particularly worrying as it generally indicates significant intellectual disability. Delay in a single area is much less concerning. Warning signs suggesting significant developmental problems are described in Chapter 4.

Repeat assessments may be needed to get an accurate view of a child's difficulties, and referral on to an appropriate therapist for further assessment and guidance may be required. When developmental difficulties are complex, the child should be seen by a Child Development Team (Chapter 45) for assessment and therapy. It is essential that parents' concerns are properly addressed. Ongoing parental anxiety in itself can be damaging to the child.

Severe learning/intellectual disabilities (mental retardation)

The more common causes of severe learning disability are Down's syndrome (Chapter 66), fragile X (Chapter 66) and cerebral palsy (Chapter 45). As the field of genetics advances, and genetic databases have been developed, more diagnoses are being made, particularly in children with congenital anomalies and dysmorphic features. It is therefore worth taking blood for genetic analysis. However, more than one third of children with global developmental delay still remain without a specific diagnosis.

Intrauterine infections

Primary infection with rubella, cytomegalovirus (CMV) or toxoplasmosis during early pregnancy can cause severe foetal damage, leading to multiple handicaps and microcephaly. Visual and hearing deficits are common.

Foetal alcohol syndrome

The foetal alcohol syndrome is a common cause of learning disabilities. It is caused by a moderate-to-high intake of alcohol during pregnancy. Children have a characteristic facial appearance, cardiac defects, poor growth and microcephaly. The severity of the problems relate to the quantity of alcohol consumed.

Congenital hypothyroidism

Lack of thyroid hormone in the first years of life has a devastating effect on both growth and development. However, since neonatal screening has been introduced, it is now a rare cause of developmental delay. The defect is due to abnormal development of thyroid or inborn errors of thyroxine metabolism.

The classic features of severe hypothyroidism (once called cretinism) are now very rarely seen. They include coarse facial features, hypotonia, a large tongue, an umbilical hernia, constipation, prolonged jaundice and a hoarse cry. Older babies or children have delayed development, lethargy and short stature. Thyroid function tests reveal low T4 and high TSH levels.

Congenital hypothyroidism is one of the few treatable causes of learning disabilities. Thyroid replacement is needed lifelong and must be monitored carefully as the child grows. If therapy is started in the first few weeks of life and compliance is good, normal growth and development can be achieved.

Inborn errors of metabolism

This group of disorders are caused by single-gene mutations, inherited in an autosomal recessive manner, so consanguinity is common. They present in a variety of ways, of which developmental delay is one, but neonatal seizures, hypoglycaemia, vomiting and coma may also occur. Children sometimes have coarse features, microcephaly, failure to thrive and hepatosplenomegaly. These inborn errors of metabolism are rare; phenylketonuria is the commonest and is routinely screened for in all neonates.

Neurodegenerative disorders

A neurodegenerative disease is characterized by a progressive deterioration of neurological function. The causes are heterogeneous and include biochemical defects, chronic viral infections and toxic substances although many remain without an identified cause. Children may have coarse features, fits and intellectual deterioration, and microcephaly. The course is generally one of relentless and inevitable neurological deterioration although bone marrow transplantation is now providing hope in some conditions.

Neurocutaneous syndromes

The neurocutaneous syndromes are a heterogeneous group of disorders characterized by neurological dysfunction and skin lesions. In some individuals, there may be severe learning disabilities and in others intelligence is normal. Examples include Sturge–Weber syndrome, neurofibromatosis and tuberous sclerosis. The aetiology of these problems is not known, but most are familial.

Abuse and neglect

Emotional abuse and neglect can have serious consequences for a child's developmental progress. The delay is often associated with failure to thrive. On presentation, the child may be apathetic, look physically neglected with dirty clothing, unkempt hair and nappy rash, and there may be signs of non-accidental injury. If there is any suggestion of regression of developmental skills, chronic subdural haematomas (which can occur as a result of shaking injuries) should be considered.

Intensive input and support is needed. Day nurseries can provide good stimulation, nutrition and care. If children continue to be at risk for ongoing abuse or neglect, they must be removed from the home. The prognosis depends on the degree of the damage incurred and how early the intervention is provided. Children who require removal from the home often have irreversible learning and emotional difficulties.

KEY POINTS

- All developmental areas must be accurately assessed in turn.
- Remember to correct for prematurity in the first 2 years, and carry out a full physical and neurological examination.
- Repeat evaluations may be required over time.
- Attempt to make a diagnosis or identify the aetiology for the difficulties.
- Involve the Child Development Team if difficulties are complex.

42 Headache

Causes of headache

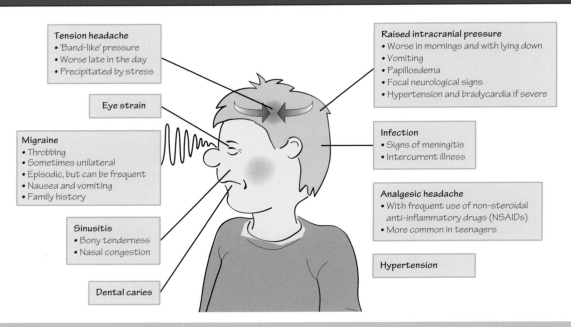

Tension headache
- 'Band-like' pressure
- Worse late in the day
- Precipitated by stress

Eye strain

Migraine
- Throbbing
- Sometimes unilateral
- Episodic, but can be frequent
- Nausea and vomiting
- Family history

Sinusitis
- Bony tenderness
- Nasal congestion

Dental caries

Raised intracranial pressure
- Worse in mornings and with lying down
- Vomiting
- Papilloedema
- Focal neurological signs
- Hypertension and bradycardia if severe

Infection
- Signs of meningitis
- Intercurrent illness

Analgesic headache
- With frequent use of non-steroidal anti-inflammatory drugs (NSAIDs)
- More common in teenagers

Hypertension

What you need from your evaluation

History

- Is there a family history of migraine? Migraine often tends to be familial
- Obtain a good description of the headaches. Are they unilateral or bilateral? Tension headaches are described as a tight band around the head. Pain in the frontal bones may suggest sinusitis. Migraine is classically throbbing
- Are there associated symptoms? Ask about vomiting and blurred vision, which may be features of raised ICP
- A headache that is worse in the morning or when lying down suggests raised ICP
- Visual auras, such as halos or zigzag lines, are suggestive of migraine
- Photophobia and neck stiffness in addition to headache suggest meningitis, although they can occur in non-specific viral infections
- Ask about nasal congestion and pain in the teeth or ears as infection around the skull can present as headache

Examination

- Measure blood pressure and the pulse Bradycardia and hypertension are signs of raised ICP
- Examine the fundi: look for signs of papilloedema
- Are there any focal neurological signs?
  - cerebellar: nystagmus, ataxia, intention tremor
  - infratentorial: cranial nerve palsies
  - cerebral: focal seizures, spasticity
  - pituitary: endocrine dysfunction, visual field defects
- Look for evidence of dental caries, sinus tenderness, audible cranial bruits (suggests arteriovenous malformation)

Investigations and their significance

- CT or MRI brain scan — Indicated if signs of raised ICP or any focal neurological signs, or if headache is persisting and not responding to normal analgesia. May show hydrocephalus or space-occupying lesion

Headaches are a common complaint in older children and are nearly always due to non-specific viral infection, local infection (e.g. sinusitis) or related to tension. Most pathological and serious headaches due to raised intracranial pressure can usually be differentiated clinically. If a headache is acute and severe, and the child is ill, then serious pathology such as intracranial infection, meningitis, haemorrhage or tumour must be considered. The following are features that should cause concern:

- Acute onset of severe pain
- Worse on lying down
- Associated vomiting
- Developmental regression or personality change
- Unilateral pain
- Hypertension
- Papilloedema
- Increasing head circumference
- Focal neurological signs
- Altered conscious level

Paediatrics at a Glance, Fourth Edition. Lawrence Miall, Mary Rudolf and Dominic Smith. © 2016 John Wiley & Sons, Ltd. Published 2016 by John Wiley & Sons, Ltd.
Companion website: www.ataglanceseries.com/paediatrics

Migraine

This is a common condition in school-age children and is slightly more common in boys than in girls. Onset is usually in late childhood or early adolescence. Classically, the attack starts with an aura such as 'zigzag' vision, followed by a throbbing unilateral headache with nausea and vomiting, although only 20% describe a preceding aura. Sleep usually ends the attack. In younger children, the headache may be bilateral with no preceding aura and no vomiting. Parents often describe the child going very pale. Migraines always cause some reduction in the child's ability to function normally during the attack. There is no diagnostic test, and physical examination is normal. The diagnosis is made clinically on the basis of the following:

- Episodic occurrence of headache (rarely every day, but can occur several times a week)
- Completely well between attacks
- Aura (often visual), though aura is less common in childhood (20%)
- Nausea, sometimes vomiting
- Throbbing headache, sometimes unilateral
- Positive family history
- Impairment of normal function during an attack
- Attack lasts between 1 and 72 h.

The first-line treatment is rest and simple analgesia (paracetamol or NSAIDs). Combination therapy containing paracetamol and anti-emetics may be useful. Sleep deprivation and stress can predispose to migraine. Avoiding cheese, chocolate, citrus fruits, nuts and caffeinated drinks may be helpful. Ask the child to keep a migraine diary so you can identify triggers. Very frequent or severe attacks may warrant prophylaxis with beta-blockers or pizotifen. Migraine often persists into adulthood, but spontaneous remission does occur. In adolescents, serotonin agonists (e.g. sumatriptan) can be given during an acute attack. Migraine can occasionally cause a post-migraine third nerve palsy or hemiparesis, though more serious cerebrovascular causes must always be excluded if this occurs.

Tension headache

Tension headaches are common in older school-age children. They may be due to contraction of neck or temporal muscles and are felt as a constricting band-like ache, which is usually worse towards the end of the day but does not interfere with sleep. The cause is often difficult to identify, but a proportion of children will be under some stress, either at home or school. Other family members may suffer similar headaches. Physical examination is normal. Management involves reassurance that there is no serious pathology, rest, sympathy and simple analgesia. Any underlying stress or anxiety in the child's life should be addressed. School absence should be minimized, and the school may need to be involved in developing a management strategy for when the headaches occur. Tension headaches usually become less frequent or resolve spontaneously as the child gets older.

Cluster headache

These may occur in older children. There is sudden onset of very severe unilateral periorbital pain. Attacks occur in clusters a few times a day for a period of weeks. The pain is non-pulsatile and can occur at night as well as during the day and is exacerbated by alcohol. There may be unilateral eye redness, orbital swelling or tears. The cause may be due to neurotransmitter activity around the superficial temporal artery. Subcutaneous or nasal triptans (serotonin agonist) can be used acutely, and calcium channel blockers may help in recurrent attacks.

Raised intracranial pressure

Brain tumours, subdural haematomas and abscesses are all rare causes of headache in children. Anxiety about brain tumours is common amongst parents though these rarely present with headache alone. If a headache is particularly persistent, then neuroimaging may be required to put everyone's mind at rest. If neurological signs (e.g. nerve palsy or weakness) are detected, then neuroimaging is mandatory.

Headaches due to raised intracranial pressure are classically worse on lying down and worse in the morning and may wake the child from sleep. There may be associated vomiting, often with surprisingly little nausea. Raised intracranial pressure may also cause blurred vision, high blood pressure, bradycardia and focal nerve palsies (e.g. sudden onset of squint). If papilloedema, hypertension, bradycardia or focal signs are present, an urgent CT or MRI brain scan is indicated. The majority of brain tumours are in the posterior fossa or brainstem, so the site of the pain is usually non-specific. They will often have cranial nerve palsies or cerebellar signs. See also Chapter 52.

Benign (idiopathic) intracranial hypertension can occur in childhood, and this should be considered in chronic headache, particularly in an older child with obesity. Brain imaging is normal but papilloedema is seen. CSF pressure is raised at lumbar puncture (which can be therapeutic). Treatment with acetazolamide is an option if headache is persistent.

Other causes of headache

Headaches are most often a feature of minor non-specific viral infections. These should be treated with simple analgesia such as paracetamol. Dental caries, sinusitis and otitis media are all treatable local infections that can cause headache.

If headaches seem particularly related to school, it is worth checking the child's visual acuity and recommend they see an optician. Always consider whether the headaches may be a manifestation of anxiety about school—is the child being bullied, or do the parents have unreasonable expectations?

KEY POINTS

- Headache is a common symptom in adolescence and is usually benign.
- Tension headaches are experienced as a constricting band.
- Migraine often has visual symptoms and nausea, and there may be a family history.
- Parents are often worried about brain tumours. Raised intracranial pressure, focal neurological signs and unusual features are indications for brain imaging.

43 Fits, faints and funny turns

Types of fits, faints and funny turns

In infants and toddlers

Apnoea and acute life-threatening events (Chapter 70)
- Found limp or twitching
- Age: <6 months old
- Usually no precipitating event, but consider reflux, sepsis, arrhythmia

Febrile convulsions
- Age: 6 months to 5 years
- Occurs on sudden rise of fever
- Lasts a few minutes

Breath holding spells (cyanotic)
- Older babies and toddlers
- Always precipitated by crying from pain or anger
- Stops breathing, becomes cyanotic and then limp
- No postictal state

Reflex anoxic spells (pallid)
- Precipitated by minor injury
- Turns pale and collapses
- Rapid recovery

Infantile spasms
- A form of myoclonic epilepsy
- Jacknife spasms occurring in clusters
- Developmental regression

Hypoglycaemia and metabolic conditions
- Rare
- Always check blood sugar in any collapsed or unconscious child

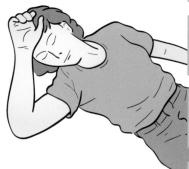

In school-age children

Epilepsy (see Chapter 44)

Simple absence
- Fleeting vacant look
- 3 per second spike and wave on EEG

Partial epilepsy
- Twitching or jerking of face, arm or leg

Complex partial epilepsy
- Altered or impaired consciousness with strange sensations or semi-purposeful movements such as chewing or sucking
- May have postictal phase

Myoclonic epilepsy
- Shock-like jerks causing sudden falls
- Usually occurs in children with known neurological disability

Syncope (vasovagal)
- Precipitated by pain, emotion or prolonged standing
- Blurred vision, light-headedness, sweating, nausea
- Resolves on lying down

Hyperventilation
- Precipitated by excitement
- Excessive deep breathing, sometimes tetany
- Resolves on breathing into a paper bag

Cardiac arrhythmias
- Palpitations may occur

What you need from your evaluation

History

- Obtain a description of the episode. Try to visualize the episode and 'replay' back to the witness. What was the child doing at the onset? Were there any precipitating factors? How long did it last? Was there loss or altered consciousness, involuntary movements, or a change in colour (pallor or cyanosis)? How did the child react to the event and was there a postictal phase?
- Home video recording—if episodes occur frequently, the parents may be able to obtain footage of an episode using a camcorder. This can provide excellent diagnostic information
- A history of developmental delay or regression is particularly important if infantile spasms or metabolic conditions are being considered
- Family history: is there anyone in the family with developmental problems, febrile seizures or a metabolic disorder? Is there a family history of cardiac arrhythmia (e.g. hypertrophic cardiomyopathy)? This is especially important if palpitations are a prominent feature of the history

Physical examination

- Rarely helpful between episodes
- Undertake a careful cardiac and neurological examination
- Dysmorphic features, micro-or macrocephaly and hepatosplenomegaly suggest a metabolic disorder

Investigations and their significance

The diagnosis is essentially clinical, but investigations must be considered if apnoea, epilepsy or a metabolic problem is suspected

- **EEG** – Hypsarrhythmia seen in infantile spasms
  – 3 per second spike and wave activity in absence seizures
  – Epileptiform activity may be seen in epilepsy (but may be present in normal children)

- **ECG** Check cardiac rhythm, PR and QT intervals on 12-lead ECG

- **24 h ECG** If arrhythmia is suspected of causing syncope

- **Blood chemistry** Hypoglycaemia, but unhelpful between episodes

- **pH monitoring** Apnoea in infants may be due to GOR

Paediatrics at a Glance, Fourth Edition. Lawrence Miall, Mary Rudolf and Dominic Smith. © 2016 John Wiley & Sons, Ltd. Published 2016 by John Wiley & Sons, Ltd.
Companion website: www.ataglanceseries.com/paediatrics

Fits, faints and funny turns refer to episodes of transient altered consciousness, which usually present to the doctor after the event is over and may occur recurrently. They may cause great anxiety although the child is often completely well in between episodes. A good description of the event should allow the different causes to be distinguished from one another, and it can be helpful to ask the family to video the episode. Most of the causes are benign and resolve with age. However, some forms of epilepsy can present in this way and need to be considered in the differential diagnosis. These include absence seizures, focal seizures such as temporal lobe seizures, and myoclonic seizures, which are covered in more detail in Chapter 44.

Breath-holding spells

Breath-holding spells (cyanotic spells) occur primarily in babies and toddlers. They normally resolve by 18 months of age. These spells are characteristically precipitated by crying due to pain or temper. The child cries once or twice, takes a deep breath, stops breathing, becomes deeply cyanotic and the limbs extend. Transient loss of consciousness may occur and even convulsive jerks. The child then becomes limp, resumes breathing and after a few seconds is fully alert again. The whole episode may last up to a minute. The key to diagnosis is the typical onset with crying and breath-holding and the absence of a postictal phase. The spells can sometimes occur several times a week, and parents are often so terrified of them that they change their behaviour to avoid upsetting the child. They need to be reassured and encouraged to treat the child normally. There is no association with behavioural disorders.

Reflex anoxic seizures

These are also known as pallid spells or 'white' breath-holding attacks. The peak age is in toddlers from 6 months to 2 years. They classically follow a bump on the head or other minor injury, which triggers an excessive vagal reflex, causing transient bradycardia and circulatory impairment. The child may or may not cry, but then turns pale and collapses. There is transient apnoea and limpness followed by a rapid recovery after 30–60 s. There may be eye-rolling and incontinence, and sometimes clonic stiffening of the limbs, but no tongue biting. After an attack, the child may be tired and emotional for a few hours. The typical history and absence of postictal drowsiness help distinguish these spells from epilepsy. Despite their appearance, the attacks are always benign and disappear before school age. Parents need to be reassured and taught to put the child in the recovery position and await recovery.

Infantile spasms

Infantile spasms (West's syndrome) are a form of generalized myoclonic epilepsy (see Chapter 44), which can sometimes cause diagnostic confusion with other causes of loss of consciousness in young children. The onset is usually in infancy, peaking between 4 and 8 months. Characteristically, there is a sudden tonic flexor spasm of the head and trunk causing the child to bend forwards ('salaam' attack). Relaxation occurs after a few seconds, and the episode may reoccur in clusters up to 10 or 20 times. Clusters are more common on awakening or just before sleep. Extensor spasms are sometimes seen. The EEG is diagnostic, showing a chaotic hypsarrhythmia pattern. In 20–30%, there is an association with tuberous sclerosis, so examination of the skin using a Wood's light is important. Infantile spasms are usually associated with severe learning disability. ACTH (corticotrophin) is the first-line treatment.

Syncope (fainting)

Syncope occurs when there is hypotension and decreased cerebral perfusion. It occurs particularly in teenage girls reacting to painful or emotional stimuli, or prolonged standing. Blurring of vision, light-headedness, sweating and nausea precede loss of consciousness, which is rapidly regained on lying flat. It is rarely a symptom of cardiac arrhythmias or poor cardiac output in childhood. Evaluation includes a cardiac examination, standing and lying blood pressure, and an ECG if there is doubt as to the cause of the faint. In unusually severe cases, diagnosis may be helped by a tilt-table test, where the patient's ECG and blood pressure are measured while being tilted from lying to standing.

Cardiac arrhythmias

These are a rare cause of syncope, but should be considered if there is a clear history of preceding palpitations or if there is a family history of cardiac tachyarrhythmias or sudden death. Hypertrophic cardiomyopathy is an autosomal dominant condition that may present with syncope often on exercise due to episodic ventricular tachycardia. Wolff–Parkinson–White syndrome causes supraventricular tachycardia due to re-entry rhythms and has a characteristic ECG with a short PR interval and a delta-wave upstroke to the R wave. A markedly increased QT interval on the ECG may be associated with ventricular tachycardia and syncope. A 24-h ECG recording may be useful in selected cases.

Hyperventilation

Excitement in some children, particularly teenage girls, may precipitate hyperventilation to the point of losing consciousness. Hyperventilation causes the carbon dioxide level to fall, triggering apnoea. The diagnosis is usually evident: breathing is excessive and deep, and tetany may also occur. Rebreathing into a paper bag allows the carbon dioxide level to rise and restores the child to normality. If episodes occur frequently, psychological therapy may be required.

Hypoglycaemia and other metabolic conditions

Metabolic disturbance, including hypoglycaemia, may cause loss of consciousness with seizures or a less dramatic alteration in consciousness. An underlying metabolic problem should be suspected if there are features such as developmental delay, dysmorphism, hepatosplenomegaly, or micro- or macrocephaly. Hypoglycaemia may be suspected if the episodes have a temporal relationship of to eating.

KEY POINTS

- Most fits, faints and funny turns are benign.
- A good history from a witness is crucial as the episodes are rarely observed by the doctor.
- The diagnosis is nearly always made on the basis of the history. Physical examination does not often contribute.
- Only carry out investigations if merited by the nature of the episode.

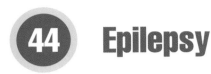

44 Epilepsy

Generalized seizures

Generalized tonic–clonic epilepsy
- Tonic phase: sudden loss of consciousness, limbs extend, back arches, teeth clench, breathing stops tongue may be bitten
- Clonic phase: intermittent jerking movements irregular breathing may urinate and salivate
- Postictal phase: child sleepy and disorientated

Absence seizures
- Fleeting (5–20 seconds) impairment of consciousness (daydreaming)
- No falling or involuntary movements
- EEG: characteristic bursts of 3/second spike and wave activity

▶ Infantile spasms (West's syndrome)
- A form of generalized myoclonic seizures
- Onset usually at 3–8 months of age
- Flexion spasms ('jacknife' or 'salaam')
- Last a few seconds, in clusters lasting up to half an hour
- Regression of developmental skills
- May have a history of perinatal asphyxia or meningitis
- EEG-characteristic hypsarrythmic pattern
- Usually occur in children with a structural neurological degenerative condition

Focal seizures

Temporal lobe seizures
- Altered or impaired consciousness associated with strange sensations, hallucinations or semi-purposeful movements
- May show chewing, sucking or swallowing movements
- Postictal phase with amnesia
- EEG may show discharges arising from the temporal lobe

Seizure types according to the International League Against Epilepsy (ILAE) classification
Generalized
- Generalized tonic–clonic seizures
- Tonic seizures
- Absence seizures
- Myoclonic seizures
- Atonic seizures

Focal
- Focal motor seizures
- Focal sensory seizures

Focal according to likely location
- Frontal lobe seizures
- Temporal lobe seizures
- Parietal lobe seizures
- Occipital lobe seizures

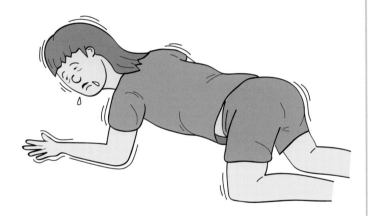

Prevalence
- Approximately 4 per 1000 school children

Pathophysiology
- Paroxysmal involuntary disturbances of brain function result in recurrent fits

How the diagnosis is made?
- The diagnosis is largely clinical, based on the description of the attacks. EEG has a limited value in the diagnostic process
- Ask yourself four key questions:
  1. Is the seizure epilepsy?
  2. What sort of seizure is it?
  3. What sort of epilepsy is it?
  4. What is the cause of the epilepsy?

Prognosis
- Generally good, with resolution of fits in >70% of children with idiopathic epilepsy. Poor prognosis for those with infantile spasms

Paediatric follow-up
Monitor:
- Frequency of fits
- Side effects of drugs
- Psychosocial and educational problems
- Anticonvulsant levels if uncontrolled

Paediatrics at a Glance, Fourth Edition. Lawrence Miall, Mary Rudolf and Dominic Smith. © 2016 John Wiley & Sons, Ltd. Published 2016 by John Wiley & Sons, Ltd.
Companion website: www.ataglanceseries.com/paediatrics

Seizures, convulsions or *fits* are non-specific terms describing any impairment of consciousness, abnormal motor activity, sensory disturbance or autonomic dysfunction. *Epilepsy* is a specific diagnosis defined as a condition where fits are recurrent, resulting from paroxysmal involuntary disturbances of brain function that are unrelated to fever or acute cerebral insult. Seizures may be *generalized* from the onset, or *focal*, when they begin in a localized or focal area of the brain. Focal fits can be motor, sensory or autonomic, or a mixture of these three, and can become generalized. Epilepsy is usually idiopathic but may result from a cerebral insult or underlying anatomical lesion when it is called secondary. In some children, a neurological problem or insult is suspected but cannot be found, and this type of epilepsy is cryptogenic.

The diagnosis of epilepsy is clinical, the key being a good detailed history. Physical examination is usually normal, but the finding of neurological signs suggests an underlying pathology. Investigations are not usually helpful as 50% of children with epilepsy have normal EEGs on first testing, and 5% of normal children have abnormal EEGs. EEG is useful in diagnosing certain syndromes, e.g. childhood absence epilepsy (formerly called petit mal) and West's syndrome (infantile spasms). Twenty-four hour and video EEG recordings are sometimes helpful. MRI is usually indicated in children with focal epilepsy, and CT scans in acute neurological insults.

Medical management of epilepsy

The goal is to achieve the greatest control of fits while producing the least degree of side effects. This is best achieved through a monotherapy approach:

• Treatment is started with the most effective drug for the type of fit.
• The dose is gradually increased to maximum recommended levels.
• A second drug is added if the first is ineffective, and the dose increased.
• The first drug, where possible, is gradually discontinued.
• Drugs should be given at intervals no longer than one half-life. Drugs with sedative effects should be given at bedtime, and, if there is a pattern, the peak level should be timed to coincide with seizures.

Most children are started on sodium valproate or carbamazepine, except for those with infantile spasms when ACTH or vigabatrin (if associated with tuberous sclerosis) is the first-line treatment. Ethosuximide is an alternative to valproate for children with absence seizures only. If medical treatment fails, surgery may rarely be tried in children with intractable fits and clinical and electrographic evidence of a discrete epileptic focus. For most children with epilepsy, restriction of physical activity is unnecessary, other than attendance by a responsible adult while bathing and swimming. As with any child, a helmet is recommended when cycling. Avoiding cycling in traffic and climbing high gymnastic equipment is prudent.

It is recommended that newly diagnosed children should receive support from an epilepsy nurse. The National Society for Epilepsy is a good source of information and support for children and families.

Management of a tonic–clonic seizure

In a tonic–clonic seizure, the child should be placed in the recovery position after the fit is over. If the fit lasts for more than 10 min, parents should be instructed to end it by giving buccal midazolam or rectal diazepam. Intravenous drugs (midazolam, valproic acid, phenytoin and phenobarbitone) should only be given in hospital, where facilities are available in the event of respiratory arrest. Children do not need to be hospitalized each time a fit occurs. Emergency treatment is not required for other forms of epileptic fits.

Monitoring a child with epilepsy

The family should be encouraged to keep a diary recording any fits along with medications received, side effects and behavioural changes. This allows you to accurately review the child's condition and the effect of drugs. Physical examination is not required at every visit but should be carried out if there is a deterioration in control. Monitoring of anticonvulsant blood levels is not routine but is helpful if fits are uncontrolled or drug toxicity is suspected. Levels below the therapeutic range can result from inadequate dosage, poor absorption, rapid drug metabolism, drug interactions and deliberate or accidental non-compliance.

Living with epilepsy

Epilepsy is a difficult condition for children to live with as it periodically and unpredictably places them in embarrassing situations. They may suffer from stigmatization and social difficulties, and their integration into school may become affected. Too often physical activities are limited for fear that a fit will place the child in danger, and a misapprehension that children will die during a fit, when in reality the mortality is extremely low.

Parents require good support and accurate information about the condition. They need to know how to safely manage an acute fit including emergency management, side effects of drugs, dangers of sudden withdrawal of medication and social and academic repercussions. There may be concern about genetic implications, and it is important that teenage girls know about the teratogenic effects of anticonvulsants.

Families may need to be encouraged to treat their child as normally as possible and not to thwart their independence. This often becomes a particular issue in adolescence when compliance too can be a problem. Career guidance is important as some occupations are closed to individuals with epilepsy. Application for a driving licence can only be made after one fit-free year whether the person is on or off medication.

Staff at school must be taught the correct management of tonic–clonic seizures. Teachers need to be aware of other types of fits such as absence seizures, as well as side effects of drugs, and report these to the parents or school nurse. When epilepsy is associated with learning difficulties, appropriate help needs to be provided.

KEY POINTS

• Ensure the diagnosis is correct.
• Only treat if fits are recurrent.
• Use monotherapy when possible.
• Check plasma levels if control is inadequate and, if low, consider non-compliance.
• For tonic–clonic epilepsy, buccal midazolam or rectal diazepam should be prescribed for home use.
• Ensure any learning difficulties are addressed.
• Help the child live a normal life with full participation at school and home.

45 Cerebral palsy

Cerebral palsy is a disorder of movement caused by a permanent, non-progressive lesion in the developing brain. Spastic cerebral palsy is the most common form where the injury is in the cerebral cortex or motor pathways. Athetoid and ataxic cerebral palsy are less common

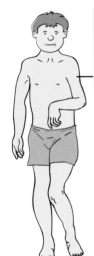

Hemiplegia
- One side of the body
- Arm often more involved than the leg
- Delayed walking
- Tiptoe gait, with arm in a dystonic posture when running

Athetoid cerebral palsy
- Due to basal ganglia damage
- Writhing movements
- Intelligence often normal
- Major physical impairment

Ataxic cerebral palsy
- Due to cerebellar damage
- Poor coordination
- Ataxic gait

Diplegia
- Both legs involved with arms less affected or unaffected
- Excessive hip adduction (hard to put on a nappy)
- Scissoring of legs
- Characteristic gait: feet in equinovarus and walking on tiptoe

Total body impairment
- Most severe form
- All extremities involved
- High association with severe learning disabilities and fits
- Swallowing difficulties and gastro-oesophageal reflux common
- Flexion contractures of the knees and elbows often present by late childhood

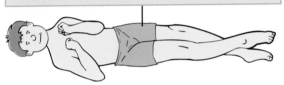

Prevalence
- 1 in 400 children

Aetiology
- Prenatal   Cerebral malformations
  Congenital infection
  Metabolic defects

- Perinatal   Complications of prematurity
  Intrapartum trauma
  Hypoxic–ischaemic insult

- Postnatal   Non-accidental injury
  (injury incurred   Head trauma
  before 2 years   Meningitis/encephalitis
  of age)   Cardiopulmonary arrest

Diagnosis
Diagnosis is clinical, based on the findings of abnormalities of tone, delays in motor development, abnormal movement patterns and persistent primitive reflexes. Diagnosis may be suspected in neonates but can only be made months later

Associated problems
Children with cerebral palsy may commonly have additional problems (especially if they have total body impairment or severe hemiplegia):
- Learning/intellectual disabilities
- Epilepsy
- Visual impairment
- Squint
- Hearing loss
- Speech disorders
- Behaviour disorders
- Undernutrition and poor growth
- Respiratory problems

Prognosis
Depends on the severity and form of cerebral palsy, level of intellectual disability and presence of other associated problems. The degree of independent living achieved relates to:
- Type and extent of cerebral palsy
- Degree of learning disability
- Presence of associated problems, e.g. visual impairment, epilepsy

Cerebral palsy is an umbrella term used to describe a disorder of movement and posture caused by a permanent and non-progressive cerebral lesion acquired early in brain development. It is often complicated by other neurological sensory and learning difficulties. Although the brain lesion itself in cerebral palsy is non-progressive, the clinical picture changes as the child grows and develops. The underlying brain lesion may result from different insults occurring at various times in the developing brain.

In the neonatal period, cerebral palsy may be suspected if a baby has difficulty sucking, irritability, convulsions, or an abnormal neurological examination. The diagnosis is usually made later in the first 18 months when the following features emerge.

- **Abnormalities of tone:** Initially, the tone may be reduced, but eventually tone alters and may be increased (spastic) or variable (dystonic).
- **Delay in motor development:** Such as marked head lag, delays in sitting and rolling over.

Paediatrics at a Glance, Fourth Edition. Lawrence Miall, Mary Rudolf and Dominic Smith. © 2016 John Wiley & Sons, Ltd. Published 2016 by John Wiley & Sons, Ltd.
Companion website: www.ataglanceseries.com/paediatrics

- **Abnormal patterns of development:** Movements are not only delayed but also abnormal in quality.
- **Persistence of primitive reflexes:** Such as the Moro, grasp and asymmetric tonic neck reflex.

The diagnosis is made on clinical grounds, with repeated examinations often being required. Once made, a multidisciplinary assessment is needed to define the extent of the difficulties. An MRI scan is useful to demonstrate cerebral injury or malformations, delineating their extent and ruling out very rare progressive or genetic causes.

Management of cerebral palsy

Most children with cerebral palsy have multiple difficulties and require a multidisciplinary input. This is provided by a Child Development Team, including a paediatrician, physiotherapist, occupational therapist, speech and language therapist, specialist nurse, dietician and psychologist. They structure a coordinated programme of treatment to meet all the child's needs and ensure good liaison between professionals and parents.

Therapy
Physiotherapy

Physiotherapists advise on handling and mobilization, and their role is crucial. The family are taught how to handle the child in daily activities such as feeding, carrying, dressing and bathing in ways that limit the effects of abnormal muscle tone. They are also taught a series of exercises to prevent the development of deforming contractures. The physiotherapist may provide a variety of aids, such as firm boots, lightweight splints and walking frames for the child when beginning to walk. Together with an occupational therapist, she provides a postural management programme, which helps prevent contractures and maximizes a child's function by appropriate seating, standing equipment and other devices.

Occupational therapy

The role of the occupational therapist overlaps with that of the physiotherapist. The occupational therapist is trained to advise on equipment such as wheelchairs and seating and on play materials and activities that best encourage the child's hand function.

Speech therapy

The speech and language therapist is involved on two accounts—feeding and language. In the early months, advice may be required for feeding and swallowing difficulties. Later, a thorough assessment of the child's developing speech and language is required and help given on all aspects of communication, including non-verbal systems when necessary.

Dietician

As feeding difficulties are common, a dietician should advise on safe nutrition either via an oral or enteral diet (e.g. gastrostomy feeds).

Paediatric management

The paediatrician's key role is supportive and involves liaison with other professionals, including school. In the long term, the child needs to be monitored for developmental progress, medical problems, including epilepsy, development of contractures or joint dislocation, behavioural difficulties and nutritional status. Drugs, other than anticonvulsants for epilepsy, have a limited role in cerebral palsy. Treatment of tone disorders is important and baclofen (for spasticity) and trihexyphenidyl (for dystonia) are first-line management. Botulinum injections for spasticity, intrathecal baclofen for spasticity and dystonia are second-line treatment.

Selective dorsal rhizotomy for spasticity and deep brain stimulation for dystonia are newer and more invasive treatments.

Cerebral visual impairment is common and all children need their vision and hearing checked. They should have yearly influenza vaccinations.

Orthopaedic problems

Even with adequate physiotherapy, orthopaedic deformities may develop as a result of long-standing muscle weakness or spasticity. Dislocation of the hip may occur as a result of spasticity in the hip adductors and children at risk require routine hip radiographs throughout the growing years to ensure this is identified. Fixed equinus deformity of the ankle may develop as a result of calf muscle spasticity. Scoliosis is often severe and follows hip dislocation and results in significant difficulties with sitting and lying and can also cause severe chest deformities and reduced respiratory capacity.

Nutrition

Undernutrition commonly occurs in children with cerebral palsy and can reduce the child's chances of achieving their physical and intellectual potential. Food must be given in a form appropriate to the child's ability to chew and swallow. Energy-rich supplements and medical treatment for reflux may be required. A child who is unable to eat adequate amounts may need a gastrostomy to meet nutritional needs. Over time, some children lose the ability to swallow safely, placing them at risk for aspiration. In this circumstance, oral feeds must be discontinued. Vitamin D is routinely prescribed and treatment for constipation is commonly needed.

Growing up with cerebral palsy

The family has to cope with all the difficulties facing any family with a disabled child. However, cerebral palsy, if severe, places particularly heavy demands in terms of time and input. Everyday tasks such as dressing and bathing take time, and feeding, in particular, may take hours each day. The child also needs regular physiotherapy at home and needs to attend appointments, both for medical follow-up and therapy. In view of this, the family needs support, often beyond what family and friends can supply. Voluntary and social service agencies can provide babysitting, respite care and financial support.

Children with milder forms of cerebral palsy can cope at mainstream school, provided minor learning difficulties and physical access are addressed. Children with more severe cerebral palsy may need special schooling in a school for the physically or severely learning/intellectually disabled, depending on the degree of their difficulties.

KEY POINTS

- Physiotherapy is needed to minimize the effects of spasticity and prevent contractures.
- Associated problems must be identified and managed.
- Any special educational needs must be met.
- The family needs adequate financial, practical and emotional support.
- The child's integration into society should be maximized.

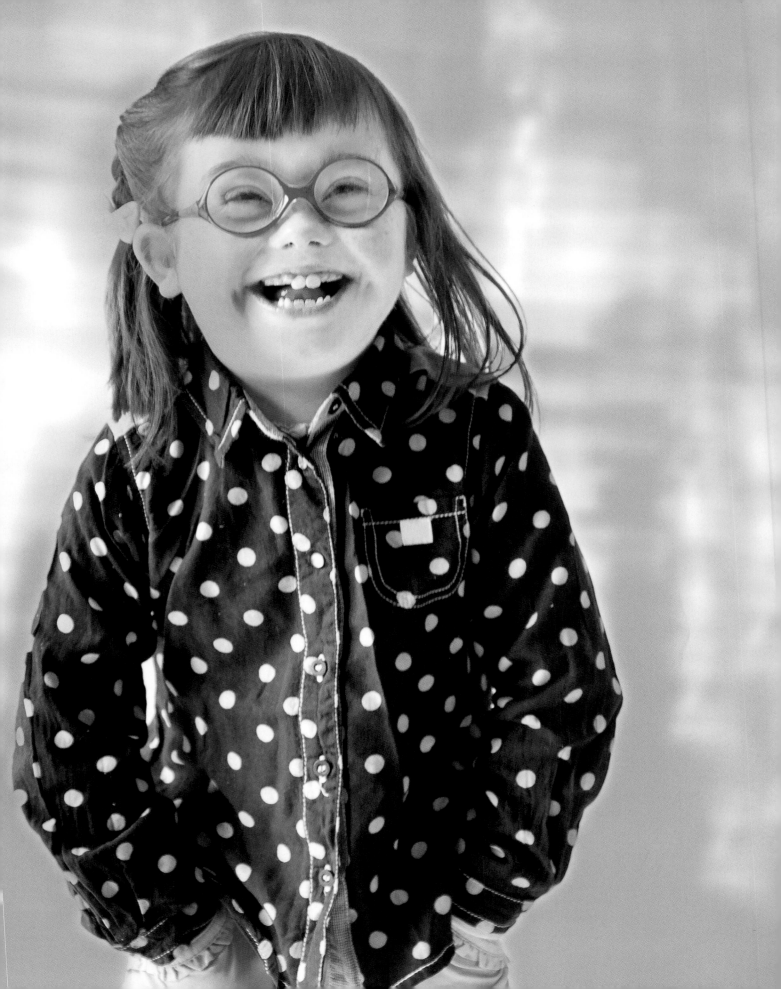

Musculoskeletal disorders

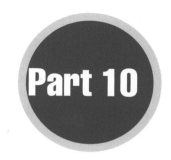

Part 10

Chapters

46 Swollen joints

Joint inflammation

Signs of joint inflammation
- Swelling
- Pain
- Heat
- Reduced range of movement

Septic arthritis
- Hot, swollen, acutely tender joint
- Fever may be present
- High white cell count, CRP
- Radiograph shows widening of the joint space
- Purulent joint fluid on aspiration

Juvenile idiopathic arthritis (see Chapter 47)
- May be systemic, polyarticular or pauciarticular
- Swelling due to oedema, effusion and synovial thickening
- Child may be irritable with morning stiffness
- Recurrent pattern
- Anaemia and high CRP
- Rheumatoid factor and ANA usually negative

Haemophilia
- Leukaemia and other malignancies
- Haemophilia
- Sickle-cell disease

Viral infection

Psoriasis

Trauma
- History of injury

Crohn's disease

Henoch–Schönlein purpura
- Painful joints +/− swelling
- Purpuric rash on buttocks and thighs

Other causes
- Trauma
- Inflammatory bowel disease
- Vasculitis (Henoch Schönlein purpura)
- Connective tissue disorder
- Psoriasis
- Haemophilia
- Leukaemia and other malignancies
- Sickle cell disease

What you need from your evaluation

History
- **Joint symptoms:** in most conditions pain is exacerbated by activity but in inflammatory arthropathies joint stiffness is alleviated by exercise
- Are there **systemic symptoms?** Fever, anorexia, weight loss, rash, weakness and fatigue suggest systemic causes
- **Past medical and family history:** important information includes previous arthritis, inflammatory bowel disease, autoimmune conditions, blood dyscrasias and psoriasis

Investigations and their significance
- Full blood count — Signs of bacterial infection, anaemia in chronic disease, haemoglobinopathies, malignancy
- CRP and plasma viscosity — Elevated in bacterial infection, collagen vascular disease and inflammatory bowel disease
- Blood culture — Positive in septic arthritis
- ASOT — High in reactive arthritis or, very rarely, rheumatic fever
- Viral titres — Viral arthritis
- Rheumatoid factor and antinuclear antibodies — Negative in most forms of juvenile chronic arthritis
- Radiography of the joint — Characteristics differ with underlying aetiology
- Joint aspiration — Microscopy and culture to exclude or confirm septic arthritis
- Ultrasound or MRI of joint — Can identify soft tissue injury (muscle, cartilage) and may show oedema and effusions

Physical examination
- **Musculoskeletal system:** examine all four limbs and the spine. Look for skin colour changes, heat, tenderness, range of motion and asymmetry
- **Observe:** the child's gait
- **General examination:** look for anaemia, hepatosplenomegaly, cardiac murmurs and rash
- **Check for focus of infection:** *Staphylococcus aureus* can cause widespread septic emboli including septic arthritis or osteomyelitis
- **Check adjoining joints:** a painful knee may be due to problems at the hip or ankle

KEY POINTS
- Trauma is by far the commonest cause
- If the joint is acutely swollen, rule out septic arthritis as the cause
- Always enquire about systemic symptoms
- Clues to the underlying diagnosis are provided by the history and distribution of the joints involved

47 Juvenile idiopathic arthritis

Juvenile idiopathic arthritis (JIA) is a group of conditions that present in childhood with joint inflammation lasting 6 weeks for which no other cause is found. Up to 1 in 1000 children may be affected during childhood. The classification depends on the presentation, but may not be reliably assigned for 6 months. Treatment is aimed at treating the pain and inflammation and maintaining good joint mobility. In the majority there is resolution during childhood. A multidisciplinary approach with psychological support is necessary for these children

Classification
- Systemic (Still's disease): 9%
- Polyarticular: 19%
- Pauciarticular (≤4 joints): 49%
- Spondyloarthropathies (HLA B27): 7%
- Juvenile psoriatic arthritis: 7%
- Other

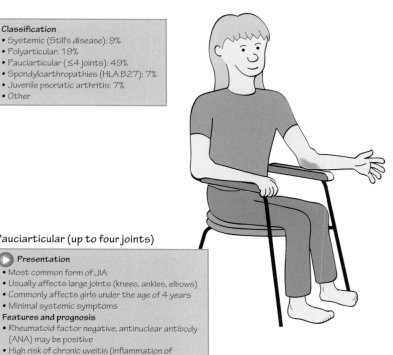

Pauciarticular (up to four joints)

Presentation
- Most common form of JIA
- Usually affects large joints (knees, ankles, elbows)
- Commonly affects girls under the age of 4 years
- Minimal systemic symptoms

Features and prognosis
- Rheumatoid factor negative, antinuclear antibody (ANA) may be positive
- High risk of chronic uveitis (inflammation of anterior eye structures), especially if ANA +ve. Needs regular slit-lamp examination to screen for this
- Arthritis resolves completely in 80%

Systemic onset (Still's disease)

Presentation
- Spiking fever, severe malaise
- Salmon-pink rash
- Anaemia, weight loss
- Hepatosplenomegaly, pericarditis
- Arthralgia and myalgia but may have minimal joint symptoms
- May resemble malignancy

Features
- Both large and small joints affected
- 25% have severe arthritis
- Rheumatoid factor negative
- Associated with HLA-DR4

Prognosis
- In 25%, arthritis persists into adulthood
- Long term prognosis improved with introduction of biological therapies

Polyarticular (more than four joints)

Presentation
- Symmetrical involvement of large and small joints
- There may be poor weight gain and mild anaemia
- Morning stiffness
- Irritability in young children

Features and prognosis
- Rheumatoid factor negative in 97%, ANA may be positive
- Low risk of eye involvement
- 12% develop severe arthritis but prognosis is generally good
- Temporomandibular joint may be involved, causing micrognathia

Management

The aims of management are to preserve joint function, to minimize complications, including complications of the treatment, and to aid the psychological adjustment to what can be a chronic disabling condition in some

The aim is to reduce joint inflammation using non-steroidal anti-inflammatory drugs (NSAIDs). Steroids may be injected into affected joints. Disease-modifying drugs are used if steroid injections need to be repeated frequently. These include methotrexate and immunosuppressants such as methotrexate and systemic steroids and systemic steroids. All have side effects. A new class of recombinant antibody drugs has been introduced that act as biological agents to reduce TNF action. These drugs are used when methotrexate is not fully controlling the inflammation (includes etanercept, infliximab, adalimumab). Non-drug therapy includes physiotherapy, hydrotherapy and wearing splints to maintain joint function and mobility. Occupational therapy can help with aids to improve function. The family needs psychological support. Children with residual disability may require help in planning a suitable career

Investigations

ESR and CRP	Raised in systemic form, may be raised in polyarticular but normal in pauciarticular arthritis
FBC	Microcytic anaemia of chronic disease
Autoantibody	(ANA) +ve in 25% (especially pauciarticular)
Rheumatoid factor	Rarely positive – marker for persistence of polyarticular arthritis into adulthood
Radiology	X-ray, Ultrasound or MRI may be useful to define inflammation
Echo	In systemic form to exclude pericarditis

Complications

Flexion contractures of the joint may develop without regular therapy and splinting. Joint destruction may require eventual joint replacement (e.g. knees, hips) in some children. Growth failure can occur due to the chronic illness, anorexia and the growth suppression effect of corticosteroid therapy. Chronic anterior uveitis (iridocyclitis) is asymptomatic but if missed can lead to visual impairment

48 Leg pain and limp

Causes of leg pain and limp in childhood

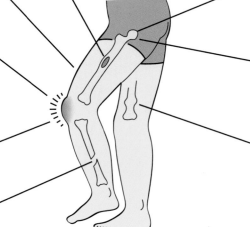

Growing pains
- Preschool children
- Pain often at night, but no limp by day
- Often bilateral and felt in shins or thighs
- Pain predominantly in muscles not bone
- Healthy child, no physical signs
- No interference with normal activities

Transient synovitis
- Benign and common in children age 2–8 years
- Limp usually resolves in 1–3 weeks
- No systemic symptoms
- Often preceded by URTI
- Normal investigations and radiographs

Septic arthritis (see Chapter 46)
- Infant and toddler
- Looks septic
- Swollen hot joint (not obvious in the hip)
- Serious condition

Trauma

Osteomyelitis
- Fever
- Swelling, erythema, tenderness, decreased movement of the limb
- High CRP, WCC
- Diagnosis by radiography, bone scan or MRI

Legg–Perthes disease
- Osteochondritis leading to avascular necrosis of femoral head
- 4:1 Male to female ratio
- Age 4–11, peak 4–7 years
- May follow transient synovitis
- Initially painless
- Pain and limp when fracture occurs
- Diagnosis by radiography or MRI

Slipped capital femoral epiphysis
- Young teenage boys (and girls)
- More common if overweight
- Gradual onset groin pain
- Diagnosis by X-ray - frog lateral pelvis

Neoplastic disease
- Benign or malignant
- Pain, tenderness and mass
- Destructive mass on radiography
- Gnawing pain in leukaemia

What you need from your evaluation

History
- Pathological pain tends to be persistent, occurring day and night, interrupts play as well as schooling, is often unilateral or located to a joint in particular
- A limp or refusal to walk is significant
- Weight loss, fever, night sweats, rash or diarrhoea point to pathological causes

Physical examination
- Examine the child lying down and walking, and fully examine the leg and groin, not only the knee
- **The limb.** Look for point tenderness, redness, swelling, muscle weakness or atrophy, and limitation of movement for each joint
- **General examination.** Look for fever, rash, pallor, lymphadenopathy or organomegaly suggesting infectious or systemic causes

Investigations and their significance
(Only if leg pain is thought to be organic)

Full blood count	High white cell count in leukaemia, infections, collagen vascular disease
CRP, ESR or plasma viscosity	High in infections, collagen vascular disease, Inflammatory bowel disease, tumours
Radiography	Bone tumours, infection, trauma, avascular necrosis, leukaemia, slipped capital femoral epiphysis
MRI, ultrasound or bone scan	Osteomyelitis

KEY POINTS
- Organic and non-organic causes can be differentiated on clinical grounds. Leg pain alone is usually non-organic
- Important features suggestive of organic disease are a child's refusal to walk, a limp, any physical signs, or constitutional symptoms
- Pain in the hip is referred to the knee, so children presenting with knee pain require a full examination of the leg and groin

Paediatrics at a Glance, Fourth Edition. Lawrence Miall, Mary Rudolf and Dominic Smith. © 2016 John Wiley & Sons, Ltd. Published 2016 by John Wiley & Sons, Ltd.
Companion website: www.ataglanceseries.com/paediatrics

Common childhood skeletal problems

Common childhood skeletal problems

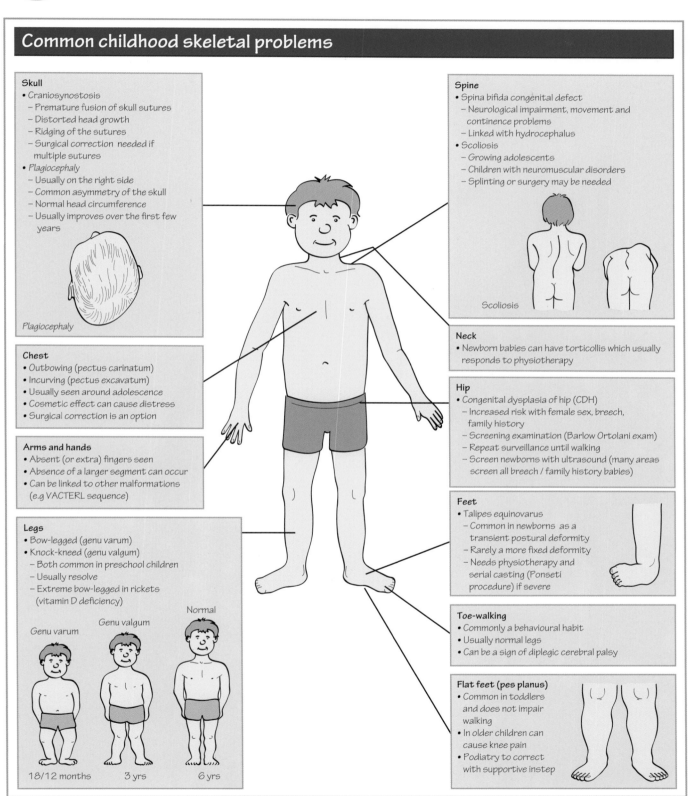

Skull
- Craniosynostosis
  - Premature fusion of skull sutures
  - Distorted head growth
  - Ridging of the sutures
  - Surgical correction needed if multiple sutures
- Plagiocephaly
  - Usually on the right side
  - Common asymmetry of the skull
  - Normal head circumference
  - Usually improves over the first few years

Plagiocephaly

Chest
- Outbowing (pectus carinatum)
- Incurving (pectus excavatum)
- Usually seen around adolescence
- Cosmetic effect can cause distress
- Surgical correction is an option

Arms and hands
- Absent (or extra) fingers seen
- Absence of a larger segment can occur
- Can be linked to other malformations (e.g VACTERL sequence)

Legs
- Bow-legged (genu varum)
- Knock-kneed (genu valgum)
  - Both common in preschool children
  - Usually resolve
  - Extreme bow-legged in rickets (vitamin D deficiency)

Genu varum — 18/12 months
Genu valgum — 3 yrs
Normal — 6 yrs

Spine
- Spina bifida congenital defect
  - Neurological impairment, movement and continence problems
  - Linked with hydrocephalus
- Scoliosis
  - Growing adolescents
  - Children with neuromuscular disorders
  - Splinting or surgery may be needed

Scoliosis

Neck
- Newborn babies can have torticollis which usually responds to physiotherapy

Hip
- Congenital dysplasia of hip (CDH)
  - Increased risk with female sex, breech, family history
  - Screening examination (Barlow Ortolani exam)
  - Repeat surveillance until walking
  - Screen newborns with ultrasound (many areas screen all breech / family history babies)

Feet
- Talipes equinovarus
  - Common in newborns as a transient postural deformity
  - Rarely a more fixed deformity
  - Needs physiotherapy and serial casting (Ponseti procedure) if severe

Toe-walking
- Commonly a behavioural habit
- Usually normal legs
- Can be a sign of diplegic cerebral palsy

Flat feet (pes planus)
- Common in toddlers and does not impair walking
- In older children can cause knee pain
- Podiatry to correct with supportive instep

Paediatrics at a Glance, Fourth Edition. Lawrence Miall, Mary Rudolf and Dominic Smith. © 2016 John Wiley & Sons, Ltd. Published 2016 by John Wiley & Sons, Ltd.
Companion website: www.ataglanceseries.com/paediatrics

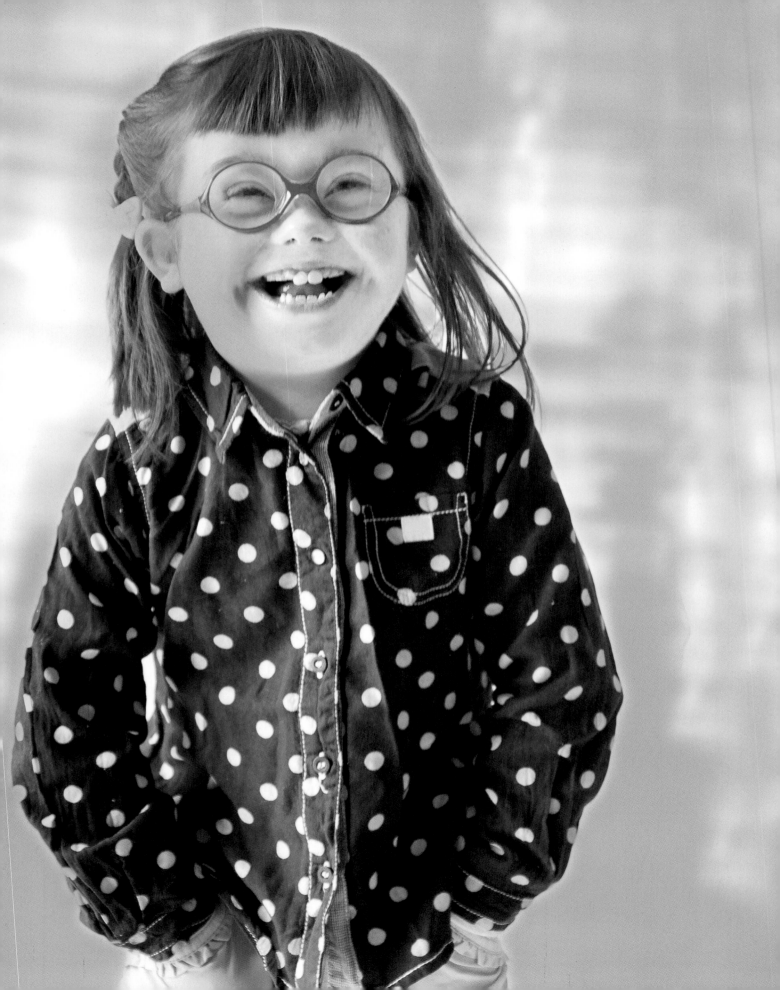

Blood disorders

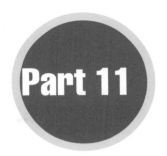

Part 11

Chapters

50 Anaemia and thrombocytopenia

Causes of anaemia and pallor

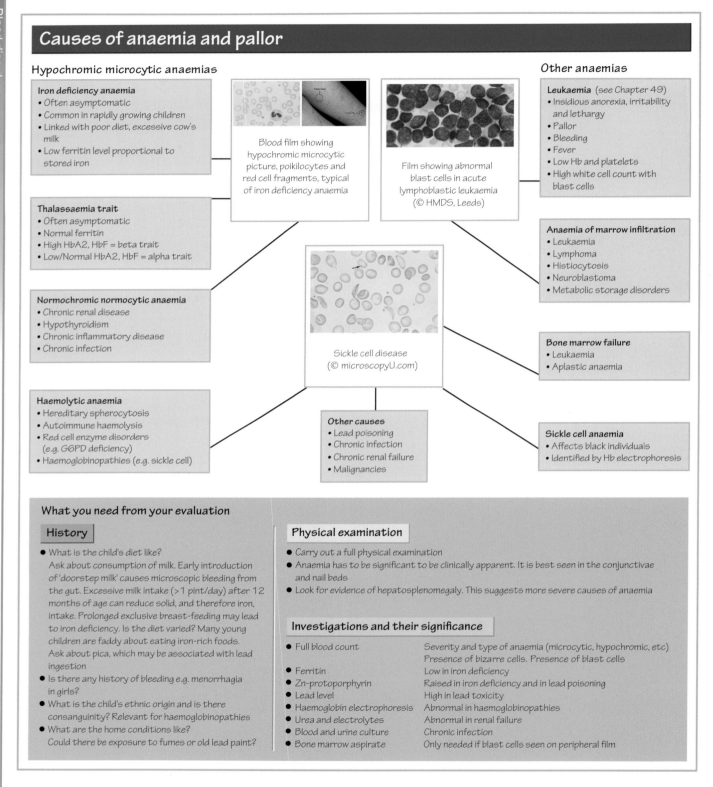

Hypochromic microcytic anaemias

Iron deficiency anaemia
- Often asymptomatic
- Common in rapidly growing children
- Linked with poor diet, excessive cow's milk
- Low ferritin level proportional to stored iron

Thalassaemia trait
- Often asymptomatic
- Normal ferritin
- High HbA2, HbF = beta trait
- Low/Normal HbA2, HbF = alpha trait

Normochromic normocytic anaemia
- Chronic renal disease
- Hypothyroidism
- Chronic inflammatory disease
- Chronic infection

Haemolytic anaemia
- Hereditary spherocytosis
- Autoimmune haemolysis
- Red cell enzyme disorders (e.g. G6PD deficiency)
- Haemoglobinopathies (e.g. sickle cell)

Blood film showing hypochromic microcytic picture, poikilocytes and red cell fragments, typical of iron deficiency anaemia

Film showing abnormal blast cells in acute lymphoblastic leukaemia (© HMDS, Leeds)

Sickle cell disease (© microscopyU.com)

Other causes
- Lead poisoning
- Chronic infection
- Chronic renal failure
- Malignancies

Other anaemias

Leukaemia (see Chapter 49)
- Insidious anorexia, irritability and lethargy
- Pallor
- Bleeding
- Fever
- Low Hb and platelets
- High white cell count with blast cells

Anaemia of marrow infiltration
- Leukaemia
- Lymphoma
- Histiocytosis
- Neuroblastoma
- Metabolic storage disorders

Bone marrow failure
- Leukaemia
- Aplastic anaemia

Sickle cell anaemia
- Affects black individuals
- Identified by Hb electrophoresis

What you need from your evaluation

History

- What is the child's diet like?
  Ask about consumption of milk. Early introduction of 'doorstep milk' causes microscopic bleeding from the gut. Excessive milk intake (>1 pint/day) after 12 months of age can reduce solid, and therefore iron, intake. Prolonged exclusive breast-feeding may lead to iron deficiency. Is the diet varied? Many young children are faddy about eating iron-rich foods. Ask about pica, which may be associated with lead ingestion
- Is there any history of bleeding e.g. menorrhagia in girls?
- What is the child's ethnic origin and is there consanguinity? Relevant for haemoglobinopathies
- What are the home conditions like?
  Could there be exposure to fumes or old lead paint?

Physical examination

- Carry out a full physical examination
- Anaemia has to be significant to be clinically apparent. It is best seen in the conjunctivae and nail beds
- Look for evidence of hepatosplenomegaly. This suggests more severe causes of anaemia

Investigations and their significance

- Full blood count — Severity and type of anaemia (microcytic, hypochromic, etc) Presence of bizarre cells. Presence of blast cells
- Ferritin — Low in iron deficiency
- Zn-protoporphyrin — Raised in iron deficiency and in lead poisoning
- Lead level — High in lead toxicity
- Haemoglobin electrophoresis — Abnormal in haemoglobinopathies
- Urea and electrolytes — Abnormal in renal failure
- Blood and urine culture — Chronic infection
- Bone marrow aspirate — Only needed if blast cells seen on peripheral film

Paediatrics at a Glance, Fourth Edition. Lawrence Miall, Mary Rudolf and Dominic Smith. © 2016 John Wiley & Sons, Ltd. Published 2016 by John Wiley & Sons, Ltd.
Companion website: www.ataglanceseries.com/paediatrics

Iron deficiency anaemia

In early childhood, the combination of a high demand for iron to keep up with rapid growth and a poor intake of iron-rich foods makes iron deficiency very common. This can be exacerbated by chronic blood loss induced by early exposure to whole cow's milk. Iron deficiency anaemia can be as high as 50% in some populations, and in many countries young children are screened routinely. Babies older than 12 months should be limited to 1 pint of milk (500 mL) daily to reduce blood loss and encourage the consumption of more iron-rich foods. Breast milk is somewhat protective as the iron is absorbed more efficiently due to the iron-binding protein, lactoferrin.

Iron deficiency anaemia is usually asymptomatic, but if the haemoglobin level falls significantly tiredness and pallor occur. Iron deficiency, even without anaemia, can affect learning. The initial finding is a low ferritin level, reflecting inadequate iron stores. As the deficiency progresses microcytosis, hypochromia and poikilocytosis develop. Zn-protoporphyrin is high as haem binds to zinc in the absence of iron. Treatment of iron deficiency is iron salts given orally for 2–3 months. Patients should be warned that iron supplements make the stool turn black and that iron is dangerous in overdose.

Thalassaemia

The thalassaemias are a group of heritable hypochromic anaemias varying in severity, caused by a defect in haemoglobin polypeptide synthesis. Beta-thalassaemia is the commonest and affects Asian and Mediterranean individuals (1 in 7 Cypriots and 1 in 20 Indians). Overall, 3% of the world's population carry thalassaemia gene mutation.

Beta-thalassaemia trait (the heterozygous form) causes a mild hypochromic, microcytic anaemia, which may be confused with iron deficiency. Diagnosis is made by haemoglobin electrophoresis, which demonstrates high levels of HbA2 and HbF. It requires no treatment. Alpha-thalassaemia trait (heterozygous) is suggested by a mild hypochromic microcytic anaemia with low or normal levels of HbA2 and HbF and no evidence of iron deficiency. It is important to recognize these conditions to avoid unnecessary iron treatment and to give patients advice that their own future children could be at risk of a more serious thalassaemia major disorder, so a future partner may need a thalassaemia screen.

Homozygous beta-thalassaemia results in a severe haemolytic anaemia, with compensatory bone marrow hyperplasia producing a characteristic bossing of the facial and skull bones and leads to dental abnormalities. There is marked hepatosplenomegaly. Blood transfusions are required on a regular basis to maintain haemoglobin levels. Haemosiderosis due to iron overload is consequence causing cardiomyopathy, diabetes and skin pigmentation but can be minimized by subcutaneous infusions of the chelating agent desferrioxamine.

Sickle-cell anaemia

Sickle-cell anaemia is the commonest haemoglobinopathy, occurring in 1 in 4 West Africans and 1 in 10 Afro-Caribbean people. One of the amino acid sequences in the beta-globin chain is substituted, causing an unstable haemoglobin (HbS). When deoxygenated, this forms highly structured polymers making brittle spiny red cells, which occlude blood vessels, causing ischaemia. Heterozygote carriers (sickle cell trait) are usually asymptomatic but can experience problems during general anaesthesia. There are over 300 haemoglobinopathies, and other forms of sickle cell disease include HbSC or Hb-beta-Thal, where the child is a compound heterozygote, inheriting HbS from one parent and HbC or beta-thalassaemia trait from the other.

In the homozygous condition, children experience recurrent acute painful crises, which can be precipitated by dehydration, hypoxia, infection or acidosis. Painful swelling of the hands and feet is a common early presentation. Repeated splenic infarctions eventually leave the child asplenic and therefore susceptible to serious infections. Pneumococcal vaccination and prophylactic penicillin is recommended. Treatment of a crisis is largely symptomatic with analgesics, antibiotics, warmth and adequate fluid hydration.

Antenatal screening is now offered to mothers and the newborn blood spot is screened for abnormal haemoglobin.

Idiopathic thrombocytopenic purpura (ITP)

ITP typically presents in young children with spontaneous onset of bruising (purpura) spots possibly with pin-prick size (petechiae) spots. The children are otherwise well. The condition can follow on after a self-limiting viral infection. Blood count shows a very low platelet count (usually <20, can be <5) but normal red cell and white cells. Most children do not need any treatment but have repeat blood counts checked to see if the problem is resolving and to check no other haematological disease is developing. Most show complete resolution over 1–2 months, but a small number can have acute bleeding problems or chronic ITP that can need treatment with steroids or immunoglobulin. A bone marrow aspirate may be needed before steroid treatment to exclude leukaemia.

KEY POINTS

- Iron deficiency is common in children as it is hard to sustain iron stores in the phase of rapid growth and a toddler's often low intake of iron-rich foods.
- If a child is ill or from an at-risk population, then consider other causes of anaemia such as sickle-cell disease.
- Haemoglobinopathies can be detected in a newborn blood spot screening test.

51 Jaundice

Causes of jaundice in the neonatal period

Unconjugated hyperbilirubinaemia

Prematurity
• Immature liver enzymes

Rhesus incompatibility
• If mother is Rh negative and baby Rh positive, then maternal IgG can cause haemolysis
• Sensitization occurs in earlier pregnancies
• If severe can cause hydrops in utero
• Coombs' test positive

ABO incompatibility
• Usually milder than rhesus

Infection
• Bacterial infection

Bruising
• Skin or scalp bruising from traumatic delivery is broken down into bilirubin

Hypothyroidism
• May be associated with pituitary disease

Breast milk jaundice
• Well baby who is breast-fed
• Jaundice develops in second week

Physiological
• Low liver enzyme activity
• Breakdown of fetal haemoglobin

Conjugated hyperbilirubinaemia

Hepatitis
• Neonatal hepatitis
• Hepatitis A,B,C
• Congenital viral infection (e.g. CMV)
• Inborn errors of metabolism (e.g. galactosaemia)
• Abnormal liver function tests

Cystic fibrosis
• Cholestasis

Choledocal cyst

Biliary atresia
• Persistent jaundice with rising conjugated fraction
• Pale, chalky stools
• Requires urgent referral for assessment, diagnostic isotope scan and surgical correction

Red blood cell breakdown

Unconjugated bilirubin (lipid soluble)

Breast milk effect

Conjugation

Conjugated bilirubin (water soluble)

Urobilinogen

Enterohepatic circulation

Stercobilinogen

What you need from your evaluation?

History

• At what age did the jaundice develop? (within 24 h of birth always requires investigation)
• Are there any risk factors for infection?
• Is there a family history (cystic fibrosis, spherocytosis)?
• Is the baby active, alert and feeding well or lethargic and having to be woken for feeds (significant jaundice)

Examination

• What is the extent of the jaundice? (it tends to spread from the head down as it becomes more significant)
• Are there other features of congenital viral infection, such as petechiae, anaemia or hepatosplenomegaly?
• Is the baby dehydrated? Failure to establish breast-feeding may present with severe jaundice and hypernatraemia in the first week of life
• Is the baby well or are there signs of infection?
• Examine the stool—pale stools may indicate obstructive jaundice

Management

• Identify the cause and severity of the jaundice
• Use phototherapy to bring down the bilirubin level
• In severe haemolytic disease, multiple exchange transfusions may be required to prevent kernicterus
• Management of conjugated jaundice depends on cause but refer early to hepatologist if biliary atresia is suspected
• Prolonged jaundice can increase the chance of bleeding disorders associated with vitamin K deficiency. Check coagulation screen and give further vitamin K supplements

Investigations and their significance

• Split bilirubin	Total bilirubin and conjugated fraction (should be <20%)
• FBC	Thrombocytopenia suggests viral infection or IUGR Anaemia in haemolytic disease Neutropenia or neutrophilia in infection
• Group and Coombs'	ABO and rhesus incompatibility
• Thyroid function	Hypothyroidism
• TORCH screen	Hepatitis B, cytomegalovirus infection
• LFTs	A high alanine transaminase (ALT) suggests hepatitis
• Urine metabolic screen	Inborn errors of metabolism
• Liver ultrasound	To visualize biliary tree
• Infection screen	Urine, blood and cerebrospinal fluid
• Liver isotope scan	To rule out biliary atresia in persistent conjugated hyperbilirubinaemia
• Coagulation	Clotting factors are not synthesized well in liver disease, and obstructive jaundice may cause vitamin K deficiency

Jaundice and liver disease in the newborn

Jaundice is the yellow pigmentation of the skin that arises due to hyperbilirubinaemia. Excessive haemolysis or impaired conjugation leads to a build-up of unconjugated bilirubin, and obstruction to drainage of bile leads to conjugated hyperbilirubinaemia. Unconjugated and unbound bilirubin is lipid soluble and can cross the blood–brain barrier.

Treatment

Phototherapy (blue light at 450 nm wavelength) helps convert unconjugated bilirubin into biliverdin, an isomer that can be excreted by the kidneys. In rhesus or ABO incompatibility, if bilirubin levels rise significantly despite phototherapy, then an exchange transfusion is sometimes required.

Haemolytic disease of the newborn

Haemolysis occurs when maternal IgG antibody crosses the placenta and reacts with fetal red blood cell antigens. The commonest causes are ABO or rhesus incompatibility. In rhesus disease, the fetus is rhesus positive and the mother rhesus negative. The mother will have been sensitized by the passage of fetal red blood cells into her circulation at a previous delivery or during a threatened miscarriage. Rhesus-negative women are now routinely immunized with anti-D antibody at 28 weeks. Fetal anaemia can lead to hydrops (severe oedema). In-utero blood transfusions can be given in severe cases. After birth, untreated babies are anaemic and rapidly develop severe jaundice. The management is to deliver the baby before severe haemolysis has occurred and then to wash out the maternal antibodies (and the bilirubin) by performing exchange transfusions, and by phototherapy. Intravenous Immunoglobulin can also be given to block antibody sites. Maternal IgG can persist in the baby's circulation for many weeks, causing ongoing haemolysis and anaemia even after the jaundice is under control.

Kernicterus

If free bilirubin crosses the blood–brain barrier in high concentrations, it is deposited in the basal ganglia, where it causes *kernicterus*. This causes an acute encephalopathy with irritability, high-pitched cry or coma. The neurotoxic damage to the basal ganglia can lead to deafness and athetoid cerebral palsy.

Physiological jaundice

Physiological jaundice is very common, especially in preterm babies and due to liver immaturity. It occasionally needs phototherapy.

Breast milk jaundice

Persistent jaundice in an otherwise well breastfed infant with normal-coloured stools and urine is probably due to inhibition of liver conjugation enzymes by substances in breast milk. It is a diagnosis of exclusion, and a split bilirubin should be measured to exclude conjugated hyperbilirubinaemia. Breast milk jaundice normally manifests itself by day 4–7 and can persist for 3 weeks to 3 months.

Biliary atresia

Biliary atresia is a rare (1 in 10 000) condition caused by the absence of intra- or extrahepatic bile ducts. A conjugated hyperbilirubinaemia develops over weeks and the stools become clay coloured. If undiagnosed, the baby will develop liver failure and may die without a transplant. If detected within the first 6 weeks, then a hepatoportoenterostomy (Kasai procedure) can usually achieve adequate biliary drainage. It is recommended that any baby still jaundiced after 2 weeks has conjugated and unconjugated bilirubin levels checked. Those with >20% conjugated fraction should be referred urgently to a paediatric hepatology service.

Liver disease in older children
Acute liver failure

Children can present with acute liver disease, which can progress to liver failure. This is seen in a number of conditions including the following:

- Infection such as hepatitis A
- Poisoning—deliberate self-harm (paracetamol overdose is a common cause)
- Reye syndrome—the combination of liver failure following aspirin use in febrile illness in young children (hence the restriction on aspirin in children <12)
- Autoimmune hepatitis
- Acute metabolic decompensation in children with metabolic disorders.

Patients with liver failure are critically ill with jaundice, encephalopathy and coagulopathy. There are limited treatment options, and emergency liver transplantation may be needed for severe cases.

Chronic liver disease

A small number of children suffer from chronic liver disease, which can also progress to liver failure requiring transplantation. Presentations include the following:

- Metabolic disorders such as Wilson's disease, galactosaemia
- Chronic infection such as hepatitis A and B
- Liver disease secondary to cystic fibrosis
- Biliary atresia can progress to chronic liver disease
- Prolonged parenteral nutrition in children with intestinal failure
- Autoimmune liver disease
- Fatty liver disease (steatohepatosis) secondary to obesity.

Children with chronic liver disease can develop clinical features of jaundice, pruritus, ascites, telangiectasia, hepatosplenomegaly with portal hypertension and varices. Growth is often impaired and nutrition may need support.

Liver transplantation requires a multidisciplinary team approach with long-term immunosuppression and monitoring for complications of infection, rejection and underlying disease management.

KEY POINTS

- Mild jaundice is extremely common in newborn infants, especially preterm babies.
- Jaundice within the first 24 h or lasting beyond 2 weeks needs investigation.
- Phototherapy and exchange transfusion are used to treat jaundice in the newborn.
- Biliary atresia causes an obstructive persistent jaundice with pale stools. Early treatment is essential.

52 # Leukaemia and childhood cancer

Types of childhood cancer

Leukaemia
- Most common childhood malignancy (35%)
- 80% acute lymphoblastic leukaemia
- Presents with
  −malaise
  −anaemia
  −bruising
  −bone pain
  −lymphadenopathy
- Chemotherapy used to induce remission and prevent relapse
- Overall prognosis good (85% survival for acute lymphoblastic leukaemia and 60–70% for acute myeloid leukaemia)

Lymphoma (10%)
- Hodgkin's disease and non-Hodgkin's lymphoma (NHL)
- Usually present with lymphadenopathy
- Mediastinal lymph node involvement is common
- Diagnostic excision biopsy followed by chemotherapy

Wilms' tumour (nephroblastoma) (5%)
- Arises in mesenchymal tissue, presents as a mass
- Occasionally causes haematuria or hypertension
- Metastasize via IVC to the lungs
- 10% associated with genetic syndromes (trisomy 8, Beckwith–Wiederman syndrome or aniridia (absent iris, coded for on chromosome 11)
- 2% have abnormalities of genitourinary tract

Rhabdomyosarcoma
- Arises in mesenchymal tissue, presents as a mass
- Head and neck and genitourinary tract are the most common sites
- 15% present with metastases
- 5-year survival 70% with optimal treatment

Retinoblastoma (3%)
- Rare but important cause of blindness
- Presents within the early years
- White pupillary reflex or squint
- Most common tumour in infancy
- Cure rate 98%

Germ cell tumours
- Sacrococcygeal tumour
- Gonadal tumours
- 90% 5 year survival

Brain tumours
- Second most common presentation of childhood cancer (25%)
- Usually primary brain tumour
- Present with raised intracranial pressure or neurological signs:
  −headache
  −nausea and vomiting
  −blurred vision
  −squint (VI nerve palsy)
  −ataxia, clumsiness
  −head tilt
  −endocrine dysfunction
- Most tumours occur in the brainstem or cerebellum
- Treatment involves neurosurgical resection, chemotherapy and/or radiotherapy
- Long-term sequelae include endocrine and growth problems

Neuroblastoma (7%)
- Usually in children under 5 years
- Arises in neural crest tissue (adrenal medulla and sympathetic nervous system)
- Presents with abdominal mass, skin nodules, periorbital bruising or an unwell child depending on site of disease
- Increase in urinary catecholamine metabolites

Bone tumours
- Usually occur in older children
- Present with bone pain or mass, usually in the long bones
- Ewing's sarcoma—a primitive neuroectodermal tumour (PNET). Associated with translocations at chromosome 11 and 22; 65% 5-year survival
- Osteosarcoma— most common primary bone tumour in childhood; 65% 5 year survival
- Treatment involves chemotherapy and surgery with bone prostheses

Management of childhood cancer

- **Diagnosis**
  The diagnosis needs to be considered in a wide range of illness presentations. Children should be referred to specialized paediatric oncology centres.
  Treatment
- The aim of treatment is eradication of the cancer, whilst minimizing damage to the normal tissues. Cancer therapy is toxic and the child requires intensive support treatment including prophylactic antibiotics and good nutritional support
  - **Surgery** is often required for diagnostic biopsy and excision of solid tumours, and for inserting indwelling central venous catheters necessary for chemotherapy and supportive care
  - **Radiotherapy** is used to treat local disease and for total body irradiation in conjunction with bone marrow transplantation. Adjacent tissues are often damaged and there may be long-term effects on growth if the spine or hypothalamo-pituitary axis is irradiated
  - **Chemotherapy** acts by killing cells during cell division. The aim is to kill the rapidly dividing malignant cells without killing normal cells. The drugs are usually given in combination at regular intervals. Side effects include hair loss, nausea, immunosuppression and bone marrow suppression. There is a particular risk of sepsis if the child becomes neutropenic, and any febrile episodes while the child is neutropenic should betreated aggressively with broad-spectrum antibiotics pending the results of blood and other cultures
  - **Bone marrow transplantation** involves either harvesting bone marrow or using compatible donated bone marrow to replace the patient's suppressed marrow; this allows more intensive chemotherapy to be used. Side effects include severe immunosuppression and graft-versus-host disease

Paediatrics at a Glance, Fourth Edition. Lawrence Miall, Mary Rudolf and Dominic Smith. © 2016 John Wiley & Sons, Ltd. Published 2016 by John Wiley & Sons, Ltd.
Companion website: www.ataglanceseries.com/paediatrics

Malignant disease affects about 1 in 600 people during childhood (1 per 10 000 children per year). The commonest malignancies are acute leukaemia and central nervous system (CNS) tumours. Overall, there has been a significant improvement in prognosis over recent years due to the use of well-researched and standardized chemotherapy regimes delivered in specialized paediatric oncology centres. The prognosis still depends largely on the particular type of malignancy and on the progression of the disease at the time of diagnosis.

Acute leukaemia

Leukaemia is the most common malignancy in childhood (30%) with an annual incidence of 3 per 100 000 children. It is due to the malignant proliferation of white cell precursors within the bone marrow. These 'blast' cells escape into the circulation and may be deposited in lymphoid or other tissue. The commonest type of leukaemia in childhood is acute lymphoblastic leukaemia (ALL), where the blast cells are precursors of lymphocytes. Chronic leukaemias are very rare in childhood.

ALL can occur at any age, but the peak is between 2 and 5 years. The prognosis is worse for those presenting under the age of 2 or over 10 years. The onset may be insidious with malaise, anorexia and then pallor, bruising or bleeding. Lymphadenopathy and splenomegaly may be present, and bone pain may occur. Peripheral blood usually, but not always, shows anaemia, thrombocytopenia and a raised white cell count. Those with an extremely high white cell count ($>50 \times 10^9$/L) carry a worse prognosis. Blast cells may be seen on the peripheral blood film. The diagnosis is confirmed by a bone marrow aspirate, which shows the marrow infiltrated with blast cells. Cells are examined by immunophenotyping and cytogenetic analysis as these give important prognostic information. In more than 90% of cases, specific genetic abnormalities can be seen in the leukaemic cell line. There may be increased numbers of chromosomes or translocations; for example, the t12:21 translocation creates a *TEL-AML1* fusion gene in 20% of children with ALL. Acute lymphoblastic leukaemia can be subdivided into common (75%), T-cell (15%), null (10%) and B-cell (1%).

Treatment of ALL involves chemotherapy to *induce* remission (i.e. remove all blast cells from the circulation and restoration of normal marrow function). Complete remission is induced in 95% of children. *Intensification* chemotherapy maintains remission, and methotrexate or cranial irradiation protects the CNS from involvement. Monthly cycles of *maintenance* chemotherapy are then required. Children who relapse are often offered high-dose chemotherapy and bone marrow transplantation. The overall prognosis for ALL is good, with up to 85% 5-year survival. AML survival is around 60–70% depending on sub-type.

Short-term side effects of treatment
Tumour lysis syndrome

The breakdown of large number of malignant cells either before or during treatment can lead to very high serum urate, phosphate and potassium levels. Urate crystals can precipitate in the kidneys causing renal failure. Tumour lysis syndrome can be prevented by good hydration and the use of allopurinol (a xanthine oxidase inhibitor) or uric acid oxidase.

Bone marrow suppression and febrile neutropenia

Bone marrow suppression may be due to invasion by tumour cells or the effect of chemotherapy. Anaemia and thrombocytopenia can be treated with infusions of red cells and platelets. Neutropenia (neutrophil count $< 1.0 \times 10^9$) is difficult to treat and means the patient is at risk of serious infection. Consequently, any significant fever or signs and symptoms of infection while neutropenic should be investigated and treated aggressively with broad-spectrum antibiotics until culture results are known.

Immunosuppression

Severe immunosuppression may result from treatment. This leaves the child at risk from normally trivial infections. Patients should not be given live vaccines, and if exposed to varicella (chickenpox), they should be given specific immunoglobulin. If the patient goes on to develop chickenpox, they should be treated with aciclovir and immunoglobulin.

Nutrition

Inflammation and disruption of gut mucosa and mouth ulcers as well as anorexia can lead to poor calorie intake. Nutritional support with food supplements may be necessary.

Late sequelae of treatment

Short stature or asymmetrical growth may be caused by radiotherapy to the spine or hypothalamo-pituitary axis. The latter may also cause delayed puberty and other endocrine dysfunction including growth hormone deficiency, hypothyroidism, cortisol deficiency and gonadal failure. Cranial irradiation, especially in very young children, can lead to neurocognitive effects such as memory loss and poor attention, and for this reason intensive chemotherapy and intrathecal treatment is used in some centres as an alternative. Chemotherapy can lead to sub-fertility, nephrotoxicity, deafness, pulmonary fibrosis and cardiomyopathy. There is a significant risk (about 12%) of second cancers due to the carcinogenic effect of chemo- and radiotherapy and an increased genetic tendency. Chronic ill health and poor school attendance may have long-term effects on educational achievement although this may be minimized by good liaison with school and specialist staff.

KEY POINTS

- ALL is the commonest childhood malignancy, but with effective treatment the 5-year survival is in excess of 80%.
- Immunosuppression and neutropenia secondary to chemotherapy increase the risk of infection. Suspected infection must be treated aggressively.
- Survivors of childhood cancer may suffer long-term effects including poor growth and endocrine dysfunction.

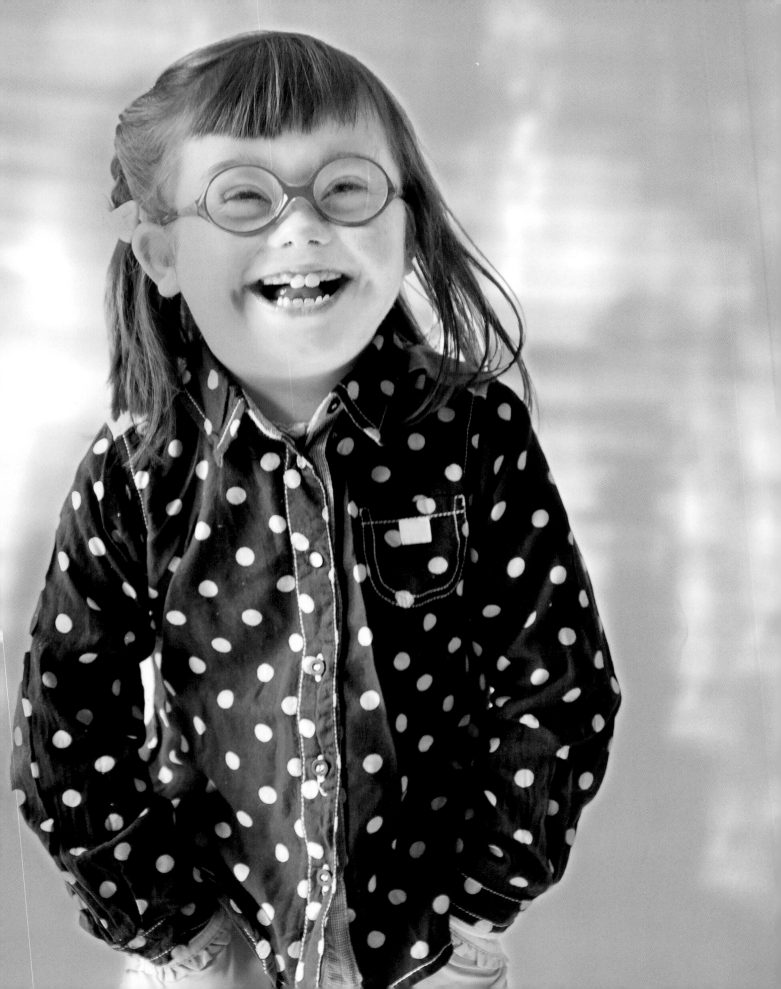

Skin disorders

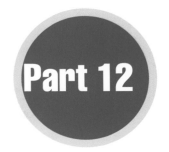

Part 12

Chapters

53 Rashes—types of skin lesions

Desquamation
- Loss of epidermal cells producing scaly eruption
- Examples: post scarlet fever, Kawasaki's disease

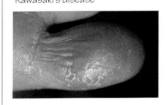

Maculopapular
- Mixture of macules and papules
- Tend to be confluent
- Examples: measles, drug rash

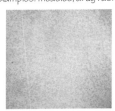

Vesicles
- Raised fluid-filled lesions <0.5 cm in diameter
- Bullae are large vesicles
- Example: chickenpox

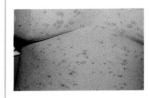

Wheals
- Raised lesions with a flat top and pale centre
- Example: urticaria

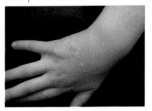

Source: Courtesy of Mollie Miall.

Papules
- Solid palpable projections above skin surface
- Example: insect bite

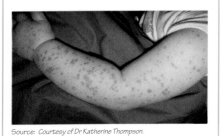

Source: Courtesy of Dr Katherine Thompson.

Purpura and petechiae
- Purple lesions caused by small haemorrhages in the skin
- Do not fade on pressure
- Petechiae are tiny (pinpoint) purpura
- Examples: meningococcaemia, ITP, HSP, leukaemia

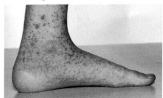

Macules
- Flat pink lesions
- Examples: rubella, roseola, café-au-lait spot

Source: Courtesy of Mollie Miall.

What you need from your evaluation?

History

- Is the child ill or febrile?
- How long has the rash or skin lesion been present?
- Could it be an insect bite or allergic reaction?
- Is it a recurrent problem?
- Is it itchy?
- Has there been contact with anyone else with a rash?

Physical examination

Describe the rash in the following terms:
- Raised or flat (papular or macular)
- Crusty or scaly
- Colour
- Blanching on application of pressure (the glass test)
- Size of the lesions
- Distribution (discrete or generalized, or limited to certain sites on the body)

It is not uncommon for children to present with an unusual rash or for parents to be concerned about skin lesions or birthmarks on a child's skin. In some cases, the rash will be acute, due to infection, allergy or skin irritation. In other children, the skin changes may be part of a chronic condition or even a marker for a neurocutaneous syndrome such as neurofibromatosis or tuberous sclerosis. In babies, skin lesions may be due to congenital naevi.

While the diagnosis of skin lesions often depends on pattern recognition and having seen similar lesions before, it is important to approach this problem with a systematic, logical approach. It is also important to be able to describe the lesions appropriately, either when seeking second opinions (e.g. from a dermatologist) or consulting databases and textbooks to establish the diagnosis. Following a systematic approach is likely to reveal the diagnosis and prevent the need for requesting further investigations or causing unnecessary anxiety.

Paediatrics at a Glance, Fourth Edition. Lawrence Miall, Mary Rudolf and Dominic Smith. © 2016 John Wiley & Sons, Ltd. Published 2016 by John Wiley & Sons, Ltd.
Companion website: www.ataglanceseries.com/paediatrics

54 Rashes—infancy and congenital

Common transient neonatal rashes

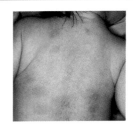

Source: Harper, J., Oranje, A. & Prose, N. S. (2006)
Figure 1.4.7, p. 60. Textbook of Pediatric
Dermatology, 2nd edition, Blackwell Publishing,
Ltd., Oxford.

Erythema toxicum neonatorum
• Commonest rash in newborns
• Small erythematous macules
• +/− Central small pustules
• Resolves over a few days

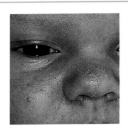

Milia
• Very common
• Tiny epidermal cysts
• 1–2 mm white/yellow popular spots
• Usually on nose, cheeks, chin, forehead
• Resolve

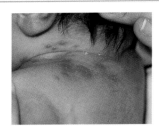

Miliaria*
• Occlusion of sweat ducts
• More common in hot humid environment
• Miliaria rubra usually at 10–15 days of age
• Resolves with reduced temperature

Nappy rash

Ammoniacal dermatitis
• Erythematous or papulovesicular
  lesions, fissures and erosions
• Skin folds spared
• Caused by irritation from excretions
  and chemicals
• Rare with modern disposable nappies
• Secondary bacterial and candidal
  infection common, and limited use of
  hydrocortisone and nystatin cream
  Treat by regular washing and changing,
  exposure to air and use of protective
  barrier creams

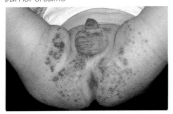

Candidal nappy rash
• Bright red rash with clearly
  demarcated edge
• Satellite lesions beyond border
• Inguinal folds usually involved
• May have oral thrush
  (white plaques in mouth)
• Treatment with nystatin
  cream, and orally if
  necessary

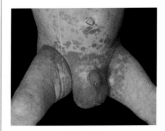

Seborrhoeic nappy rash
• Pink, greasy lesions with yellow scale
• Often in skin folds
• Cradle cap may be present
• Treat with mild topical
  corticosteroids

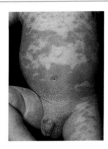

Psoriatic nappy rash
• Appearance similar to seborrhoeic
  dermatitis
• Family history of psoriasis

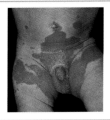

Vascular birthmarks

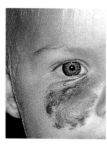

Capillary haemangioma
- Very common, especially in preterm infants
- Bright red lumpy lesion due to proliferation of blood vessels
- Enlarges until age 2–4 years then regresses
- Usually resolves spontaneously with no treatment
- If near important structures (airway, eyes)
- Oral or topical propranalol treatment can shrink down the lesions

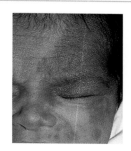

Capillary malformation
- Sharply circumscribed, pink to purple lesion
- Present from birth (3 in 1000 births)
- Abnormal dilatation of normal dermal capillaries
- May be a sign of Sturge–Weber syndrome with an underlying meningeal haemangioma, intracranial calcification and fits
- Do not resolve but some lesions may be improved with laser therapy

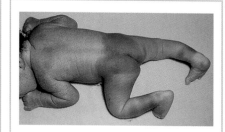

Mongolian blue spot
- Blue/grey lesions in the sacral area
- More common in racial groups with pigmented skin
- Fade during the early years
- Can be confused with bruises

Pigmentation disorders

Pigmented naevus
- Can be present from birth (congenital naevus) or appear during childhood (moles)
- Contains melanocytes
- May require surgical excision if large
- If large, at risk of malignant change

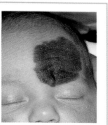

Café au lait*
- May develop increasing size and number through childhood
- Seen in genetic conditions
- Neurofibromatosis
- McCune–Albright syndrome
- Links with neurological and skeletal problems

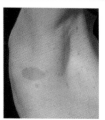

Source: Harper, J., Oranje, A. & Prose, N. S. (2006) Figure 19.13.2, p.1471. *Textbook of Pediatric Dermatology*, 2nd edition, Blackwell Publishing, Ltd., Oxford.

Depigmentation
- Depigmented skin patches seen in genetic disorder tuberous sclerosis
- May develop brain abnormalities, epilepsy, learning difficulties

Source: Harper, J., Oranje, A. & Prose, N. S. (2006) Figure 19.14.10, p.1496. *Textbook of Pediatric Dermatology*, 2nd edition, Blackwell Publishing, Ltd., Oxford.

55 Rashes—infections and infestations

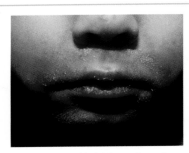

Staphylococcal scalded skin syndrome*
- Usually triggered by staphylococcal infection
- Can cause systemic illness of shock symptoms
- Swab skin to confirm infection and sensitivity
- Treat with intravenous antibiotics and systemic support measures

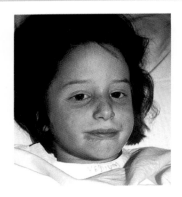

Scarlet fever
- Group A streptococcus tonsillitis
- Erythematous rash, sandpaper-like skin
- Pale around lips
- Inflamed tongue, strawberry appearance
- Risk of sequelae of glomerulonephritis and rheumatic fever
- Treat with penicillin

Meningococcal septicaemia
- Rapid onset septicaemia +/– meningitis
- Commonly due to meningococcus B, or C (other forms also seen)
- Evolves with purple (purpuric) rash that does not blanch with pressure
- Severe septicaemic shock, coma and death within hours
- Vaccination for meningococcus C has reduced rate of
- Immediate treament with antibiotic and fluid resuscitation
- A new meningococcus B vaccine has been developed and should be introduced in a new immunisation schedule in the UK

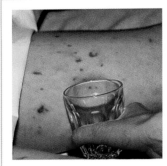

Chickenpox
- Very common childhood infection
- Onset 14–17 days after exposure
- Fever then rash (macule, vesicle, crusting)
- Sometimes see mucosal involvement (mouth, genitalia)
- Complications of pneumonia, secondary infection, encephalitis
- Treat symptomatically in healthy children without complications
- Immunosuppressed children at risk of severe complications
- Treat with zoster immune globulin after exposure, and aciclovir if signs of infection develop

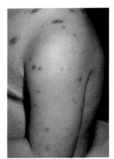

Source: Harper, J., Oranje, A. & Prose, N. S. (2006) Figure 5.3.6, p. 404. *Textbook of Pediatric Dermatology*, 2nd edition, Blackwell Publishing, Ltd., Oxford.

Measles
- Rare in immunized population (MMR vaccine protects)
- Onset 10–14 days post exposure
- Morbilliform rash
- Cough, fever, conjunctivitis and irritability
- Koplik's spots (white spots in mouth)
- Rare complication of encephalitis

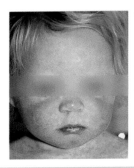

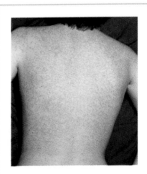

Rubella
- Rare in immunized population (MMR vaccine protects)
- Onset 14–21 days after exposure
- Pale morbilliform rash moves down body
- Severe fetal anomalies if mother develops rubella in first trimester

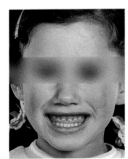

Fifth disease
- Mild illness with low-grade fever
- Slapped cheek appearance
- Lace-like rash on body
- Lasts up to 6 weeks
- Parvovirus B19 infection

Paediatrics at a Glance, Fourth Edition. Lawrence Miall, Mary Rudolf and Dominic Smith. © 2016 John Wiley & Sons, Ltd. Published 2016 by John Wiley & Sons, Ltd.
Companion website: www.ataglanceseries.com/paediatrics

Molluscum contagiosum
- Pearly dome-shaped papules with central umbilicus
- Particularly on face, axillae, neck and thighs
- Self-limited disease
- Due to molluscipox virus infection
- 'Kissing lesions' occur on opposing skin surfaces, e.g. under arms and on chest

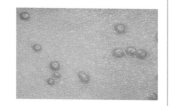

Tinea corporis (ringworm)
- Dry, scaly papule which spreads centrifugally with central clearing
- Diagnosis confirmed microscopically by scrapings in a potassium hydroxide wet mount
- Treat with topical antifungal agents for 2–4 weeks

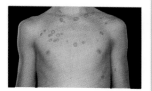

Impetigo
- Sticky, heaped-up, honey-coloured crusts
- Group A haemolytic streptococci or staphylococci
- Highly infectious
- Treat with antibiotics (flucloxacillin or erythromycin orally, or antibiotic cream if <5 lesions)

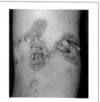

Cold sore
- Single or grouped vesicles or pustules sited periorally
- Recurrent herpes simplex infection
- Recur with colds and stress
- May be treated with aciclovir

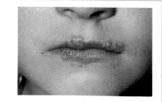

Scabies
- Wheals, papules and vesicles with superimposed eczema
- Intensely itchy
- Characteristic lesion is the mite burrow between the fingers
- Head, neck, palms and soles are spared in children but not babies
- Mites can be seen on scrapings
- Treat all the household with scabicides and launder bedding

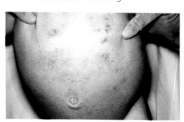

Common warts
- Roughened keratotic lesions with an irregular surface
- Occur on hands, face, knees and elbows
- Called verrucas if present on feet
- Transferred by direct contact
- Disappear spontaneously, but can be treated with salicylic acid or liquid nitrogen

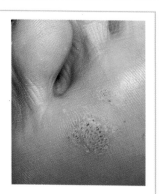

Head lice (pediculosis capitis)
- Very common in schools—affects clean hair as well as dirty
- Itchy scalp
- Nits (the eggs) are visible as white specks on hair shafts
- Transmitted on clothing, combs or by direct contact
- Treated by regularly combing out the eggs using an extra fine comb or the use of anti-pediculosis shampoos. Resistance to these agents is increasing

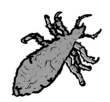
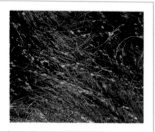

* Courtesy of Prof John Harper. Textbook of Paediatric Dermatology, 2nd Ed, 2005. Blackwell Publishing Ltd.

56 Rashes—common inflammatory disorders

Atopic dermatitis (eczema)
- Erythema, wet 'weeping' areas, dry scaly, thickened skin
- Intensely itchy
- Risk of secondary bacterial (staphylococcal) and viral (herpes zoster) infection
- Often linked with other atopic problems, e.g. asthma and hay fever
- Some cases linked with food and environmental allergens
- Breastfeeding may reduce risk of eczema
- Treat with moisturizing creams to prevent skin drying
- Cream (water based) to wet areas
- Ointment (oil based) to dry areas
- Wet wraps to prevent drying and reduce scratching
- Topical steroids to persistent inflamed areas
- Topical (tacrolimus) and oral (ciclosporin) immunomodulators if severe
- Family support and follow-up important for chronic condition

Seborrhoeic dermatitis
- Dry, scaly and erythematous
- Cradle cap in infancy
- Affects face, neck, axillae and nappy area
- Treat with olive oil and brushing or antifungal shampoo
- May look like psoriasis

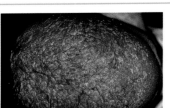

Contact dermatitis
- Erythema and weeping
- Itching
- Caused by irritants such as saliva, detergents and synthetic shoes
- Looks like atopic dermatitis

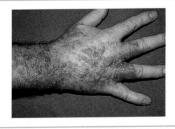

Psoriasis
- Erythematous plaques
- Silver/white scales
- Extensor surfaces—scalp, knees, elbows
- Guttate psoriasis—linked to streptococcal tonsillitis (antibiotic may improve skin)
- Pitting of nail bed
- Guttate psoriasis—multiple tiny psoriatic plaques over large area of body
- Treat with topical vitamin D analogues (calcipotriol), coal tar

Henoch–Schönlein purpura
- Vasculitic illness of uncertain aetiology, often follows viral illness
- Purpuric rash to buttocks and legs
- +/– Arthritis
- +/– Abdominal pain with gastrointestinal vasculitis, risk of intussusception
- +/– Nephritis (haematuria, proteinuria, hypertension) rarely renal failure
- Some evidence steroid helpful if abdominal pain severe

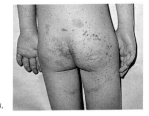

Acne*
- Very common at puberty
- Linked to androgen hormones
- Pustular erythema to face, scalp and trunk
- Treat with antibiotic erythromycin or tetracyclines (over age 12)
- Hormonal treatment with antiandrogen sometimes used
- Isotretinoin for severe cases under dermatology

Kawasaki disease*
- Acute inflammatory systemic disorder
- Many features of infectious illness
- Fever > 5 days
- Macular erythematous rash
- Peeling skin typically at fingers and toes
- Lymphadenopathy
- Mucosal changes (cracked lips, strawberry tongue)
- Conjunctivitis
- Risk of coronary artery aneurysms
- Treat with immunoglobulin and aspirin

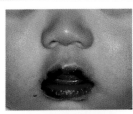

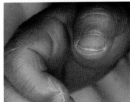

Urticaria (see Chapter 57)

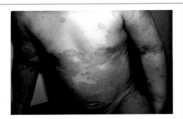

* Courtesy of Prof John Harper. Textbook of Paediatric Dermatology, 2nd Ed, 2005. Blackwell Publishing Ltd.

Paediatrics at a Glance, Fourth Edition. Lawrence Miall, Mary Rudolf and Dominic Smith. © 2016 John Wiley & Sons, Ltd. Published 2016 by John Wiley & Sons, Ltd.
Companion website: www.ataglanceseries.com/paediatrics

57 Allergy

The allergic child

Atopy
- Presents at different ages:
  - Eczema—infants and preschool
  - Food allergy—toddlers and preschool
  - Asthma—young children
  - Hay fever—teenagers
- Affects up to 1/3rd of people at some point
- Small proportion develop anaphylaxis
- Usually type I IgE mediated reaction to common allergens
- Often family history of atopy
- Breast-feeding may be protective
- Parental education and environmental adjustments may be needed

Asthma (see Chapter 29)
- Increasing prevalence—up to 11% children
- Recurrent bronchospasm
- Cough and wheeze
- Can be life threatening—status asthmaticus
- Environmental triggers—triggers, e.g. house dust mite
- Requires bronchodilators

Food intolerance
- Non-allergic aetiology
- May be due to enzyme deficiency (e.g. lactase deficiency leading to lactose intolerance)
- Sensitivity to food additives, e.g. monosodium glutamate
- Presents with colicky abdominal pain and diarrhoea
- Treat by food avoidance

Allergic conjunctivitis
- Itchy, inflamed conjunctivae with tears
- Environmental triggers similar to allergic rhinitis
- Treat with topical anti-inflammatory agents such as sodium cromoglicate drops or topical antihistamines

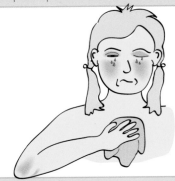

Hay fever (allergic rhinitis)
- 10–15% of population
- Commonly presents in adolescence
- Due to environmental triggers such as grass and tree pollens (most common in the summer months) or house dust mite (all year round)
- Sneezing, rhinitis, nasal congestion and sinusitis
- May develop nasal polyps
- Treat with antihistamines and topical corticosteroid

Anaphylaxis
- Rapid onset of severe systemic reaction to various allergens
- Specific IgE triggers histamine release from mast cells
- Angioedema and bronchospasm can compromise breathing causing hypoxia
- Capillary leak can lead to shock
- Triggers:
  - Foods, e.g. peanuts, tree nuts, fish, eggs and milk
  - Insects, e.g. bees, wasps
  - Drugs, e.g. antibiotics
  - Environment, e.g. severe latex allergy
- Treatment with antihistamine, steroid and intramuscular adrenaline

Eczema (see Chapter 56)
- Atopic dermatitis
- Common in infancy—extensor surfaces
- Localizes to flexoral creases in older children
- May be triggered by diet (e.g. cow's milk protein allergy) or environmental exposure (e.g. detergents)
- Treat with emollients and topical steroids

Contact dermatitis
- Type IV reaction
- Contact with nickel in cheap jewellery
- Photosensitivity rashes may be triggered by contact with certain plants
- Skin patch testing may be helpful in identifying cause

What you need from your evaluation?

History
- Is there a family history of atopy (hay fever, eczema or asthma)?
- Did the child have eczema during infancy?
- Is there an obvious environmental trigger?
- Take a full dietary history—keeping an allergy diary may help identify the cause
- What allergen avoidance has been tried so far?
- Ask about drugs—is there a history of drug allergy?
- What treatments have been needed in the past?—previous need for adrenaline shows the allergy may be life threatening
- How much is the child's daily life affected by their allergies?

Examination
- **Airway:** is there any evidence of stridor or significant angioedema of the lips or tongue? Is there nasal congestion or polyps?
- **Breathing:** observe for signs of respiratory distress and check for wheeze. Beware the 'silent chest' of severe status asthmaticus
- **Circulation:** check capillary refill for evidence of shock. Blood pressure should be measured, but hypotension is a very late sign
- **Skin:** check for urticaria (wheals), excoriation and vesicles of eczema. Lichenification suggests chronic severe eczema

Investigations
- Check for specific IgE antibodies to suspected allergens, e.g. tree pollen, peanut, milk, egg, house dust mite
- Skin prick testing may be helpful in contact dermatitis but has poor specificity—a positive test may indicate sensitization but does not necessarily correlate with symptoms
- PEFR and lung function tests in asthma, including reversibility test after bronchodilator treatment
- Controlled allergen challenge—a carefully controlled exposure to increasing quantities of allergen to test whether allergy has persisted after a period of exclusion. Must be undertaken with care, and with facilities for emergency treatment of anaphylaxis if there has been a previous severe reaction

Treatment
- Avoidance of allergens
- Antihistamines
- Steroids (topical or systemic)
- Adrenaline (for anaphylaxis)

Paediatrics at a Glance, Fourth Edition. Lawrence Miall, Mary Rudolf and Dominic Smith. © 2016 John Wiley & Sons, Ltd. Published 2016 by John Wiley & Sons, Ltd.
Companion website: www.ataglanceseries.com/paediatrics

Atopic disease

Allergy is one of the most common childhood diseases, affecting more than 1 in 4 children at some point. The incidence seems to be increasing in many countries worldwide, and the reason is not clear. Exposure to pollutants may be one factor; over-cleanliness and lack of exposure to infections and allergens in early life may be another.

Allergy is caused when an individual develops IgE antibody against specific environmental allergens. Once sensitized, an atopic individual will trigger a type I (immediate) hypersensitivity response on exposure to the same allergen, leading to local, or systemic inflammation. This inflammation is mediated by release of histamine and other cytokines from mast cells and leads to the following:

- Acute inflammation (urticaria)
- Bronchospasm (asthma)
- Chronic inflammation (e.g. eczema).

Life-threatening airway obstruction (angioedema) or shock may occur if there is a massive systemic response to allergen exposure (anaphylaxis).

The age of onset is variable, but most atopic children develop symptoms by 5 or 6 years of age. Infants are likely to show eczema and milk or egg allergy. Preschool children tend to get asthma, initially triggered by viral infection and later by environmental allergens such as house dust mite. Allergic rhinitis and conjunctivitis are commoner in older children and young adults. A family history of atopy is often present. There is good evidence that prolonged exclusive breastfeeding reduces later allergy.

Eczema

Eczema is discussed in detail in Chapter 56.

Asthma

Acute asthma is discussed in Chapter 29. Chronic asthma management is discussed in Chapter 26.

Allergic rhinitis

Allergic rhinitis (hay fever) reaches a peak in adolescence. Sneezing, rhinorrhoea, nasal congestion and itching are triggered by an IgE response to airborne allergens. Tree and grass pollens, mould spores and pet dander are common triggers. Pollens are particularly prevalent in early summer on dry, hot days. Children may exhibit the 'allergic salute' of rubbing their nose constantly with their hand. Nasal polyps can develop with chronic inflammation. Treatment involves antihistamines and nasal topical steroid.

Allergic conjunctivitis

Many children with allergic rhinitis will also have recurrent non-infective conjunctivitis; the eyes are red, feel gritty and itchy and tearful. Treatment involves topical antihistamines or topical mast cell stabilizers such as sodium cromoglycate.

Food allergy

Food allergy is IgE mediated and appears to be increasing, affecting 3–6% of preschoolers and 2–3% of school-age children. In young infants, the symptoms are often cutaneous, with eczema, urticaria, and angioedema. Wheeze, diarrhoea or vomiting may be present. Colic occurs in babies. In infants and toddlers, the commonest food allergens are cow's milk protein, egg and peanuts. There is cross-reactivity (30%) between cow's milk protein allergy and soya milk allergy. In older children, reactions to citrus fruits, tree nuts or peanuts, fish or shellfish are more common. Symptoms may be immediate or delayed by days or even weeks.

The diagnosis is made on the basis of a clear history of exposure, the presence of significant specific IgE antibody or a positive skin prick test, and preferably confirmed by a standardized controlled food challenge. Treatment involves excluding the allergen from the diet, usually for a period of 2 years, and then a controlled food challenge. A dietician should advise on maintaining a balanced diet (e.g. calcium supplements if milk is excluded). Severe anaphylaxis is relatively rare, and there is a danger of over-diagnosis, leading to a very restricted diet and lifestyle. Children with concurrent asthma are at most risk and may need to carry adrenaline and wear a MedicAlert bracelet. Very rarely there may be cross-reactivity between airborne allergens and food allergens (e.g. birch pollen and apples), leading to seasonal mucosal inflammation in response to certain foods (oral allergy syndrome).

Food *sensitivity* is not IgE mediated and causes predominantly gastrointestinal symptoms, such as abdominal pain, vomiting, diarrhoea and colitis.

Urticaria, angioedema and anaphylaxis

A variety of allergens including foods, insect stings and drugs may cause a severe acute allergic reaction. At its most extreme and life-threatening, this is known as anaphylaxis. Many allergic reactions will start with an urticarial rash—raised, well-demarcated itchy wheals with an erythematous border and a pale centre (see Chapter 56). In a few cases, urticaria may be non-allergic and triggered by mast cells releasing histamine in response to cold, pressure (the Koebner phenomenon) or other physical causes. Contact dermatitis (a delayed or type IV IgE-mediated reaction) also causes urticaria. Angioedema is acute tissue swelling around the eyes, lips or airway in response to an immediate type I IgE reaction. This may cause stridor and airway obstruction.

Anaphylaxis involves massive release of inflammatory mediators causing systemic inflammation and shock due to vasodilatation and capillary leak. Airway obstruction due to oedema and bronchospasm may occur. There is a very rapid onset of symptoms, often associated with flushing, tachycardia and a feeling of 'impending doom'. Common triggers include drugs (e.g. penicillins and anaesthetic agents), foods (peanuts and shellfish), latex (in rubber gloves) and insect stings (wasps and bees). Treatment includes removal of the allergen, intramuscular adrenaline, oral antihistamines and intravenous hydrocortisone.

Patients with a history of anaphylaxis should be referred to an allergy clinic for specialist management. It may be appropriate to provide the child with an adrenaline auto-injector (e.g. EpiPen), which can be used to administer a fixed dose of adrenaline intramuscularly at the onset of symptoms. Preventative advice to the child, their parents and school or nursery is critical, though should not over-restrict lifestyle.

KEY POINTS

- The incidence of atopy is increasing in industrialized countries.
- Eczema and milk allergy are common in infancy but normally resolve.
- Seasonal allergic rhinitis and conjunctivitis are common (up to 40% of teenagers).
- Testing for allergy is controversial as skin prick tests and IgE assays may be equivocal.
- Prevention by education and allergen avoidance is crucial for all atopic conditions.
- Severe anaphylaxis to foods is rare but does cause a few preventable deaths each year.

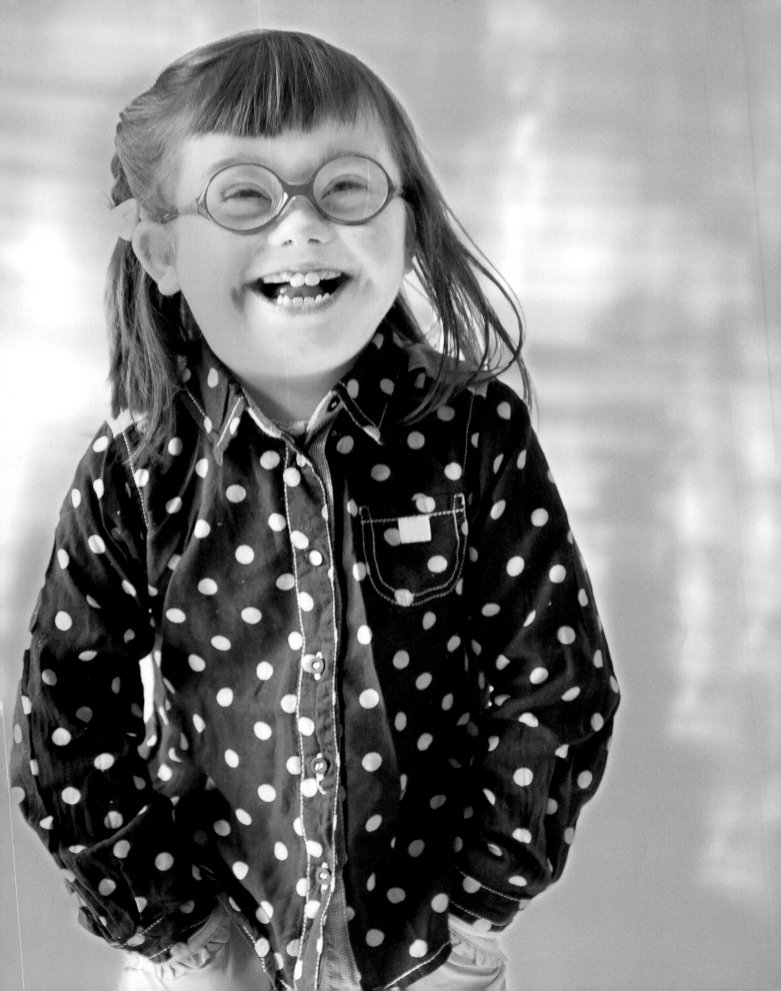

Emergency paediatrics

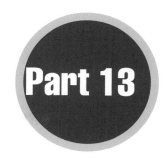

Chapters

58 Assessing the acutely ill child

Presentation of the acutely ill child

Children may become critically ill very rapidly and their survival depends on prompt recognition of the severity of their illness, appropriate life support and rapid treatment. Parents are usually able to recognize that their child is acutely unwell, even if they are not able to pinpoint the exact cause. Worried parents will often take their children to a primary care centre or present to an emergency department for an urgent medical opinion

Recognition of acute illness

It is very important that health professionals are able to rapidly identify signs of serious illness and triage children appropriately for further investigation and treatment. Fever is a very common presentation of infectious diseases and identifying warning signs or 'red flags' is important. The table below lists some features that should alert you to the severity of an acute illness:

Common presentations of an acutely unwell child

- High fever, often of sudden onset (Chapter 24)
- A non-blanching rash (septicaemia)
- Altered level of consciousness (Chapter 43)
- Severe dehydration
- Convulsions
- Anaphylaxis
- Inhaled foreign body or choking
- Acute asthma attack
- Drug ingestion (accidental or deliberate)
- Burns and scalds

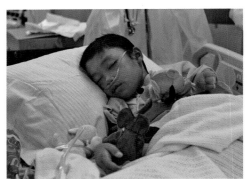

If early signs of acute illness are missed the child may eventually progress to a cardio-respiratory arrest (see Chapter 59). In children cardiac arrest usually follows respiratory or circulatory failure rather than being due to a primary cardiac problem. By recognizing these signs and treating them urgently cardiac arrest is often preventable

	Green—low risk	Amber—intermediate risk	Red—high risk
Colour (of skin lips or tongue)	• Normal colour	• Pallor reported by parent/carer	• Pale/mottled/ashen/blue
Activity	• Responds normally to social cues • Content/smiles • Stays awake or awakens quickly • Strong normal cry/not crying	• Not responding normally to social cues • No smile • Wakes only with prolonged stimulation • Decreased activity	• No response to social cues • Appears ill to a healthcare professional • Does not wake or if roused does not stay awake • Weak, high-pitched or continuous cry
Respiratory		• Nasal flaring • Tachyponea: – RR >50 breaths/min, age 6–12 months – RR >40 breaths/min, age >12 months • Oxygen saturation ≤ 95% in air • Crackles in the chest	• Grunting • Tachypnoea: – RR>60 breaths/min • Moderate or severe chest indrawing
Circulation and Hydration	• Normal skin and eyes • Moist mucous membranes	• Tachycardia: – >160 breaths/min, age <12 months – >150 breaths/min, age 12–24 months – >140 breaths/min, age 2–5 years • CRT ≥3 s • Dry mucous membranes • Poor feeding in infants • Reduced urine output	• Reduced skin turgor
Other	• None of the amber or red symptoms or signs	• Age 3–6 months, temperature ≥ 38° C • Rigors • Fever for ≥5 days • Swelling of a limb or joint • Non-weight bearing limb/not using an extremity	• Age <3 months, temperature ≥ 38° C • Non-blanching rash • Bulging fontanelle • Neck stiffness • Status epilepticus • Focal neurological signs • Focal seizures

CRT, capillary refill time; RR respiratory rate

Table from NICE guideline on feverish illness in children

Fluid loss
- Blood loss
- Vomiting
- Diarrhoea
- Burns

Fluid maldistribution
- Septic shock
- Cardiac disease
- Anaphylaxis
- Nephrotic syndrome (capillary leak)

Respiratory distress
- Foreign body
- Croup
- Asthma
- Bronchiolitis
- Pneumonia

Respiratory depression
- Convulsions
- Raised ICP
- Poisoning
- Opiates

CIRCULATORY FAILURE (SHOCK)

RESPIRATORY FAILURE

CARDIAC ARREST

Paediatrics at a Glance, Fourth Edition. Lawrence Miall, Mary Rudolf and Dominic Smith. © 2016 John Wiley & Sons, Ltd. Published 2016 by John Wiley & Sons, Ltd.
Companion website: www.ataglanceseries.com/paediatrics

Circulatory failure (shock)

Shock is used to describe a state of inadequate tissue perfusion due to an acute failure of circulation. The body responds by redistributing blood to vital organs such as the brain and the heart, at the expense of the skin, muscles and bowel. Children in shock look pale and have poor skin perfusion. Blood pressure is maintained in children by peripheral vasoconstriction, so that hypotension is a very late sign of shock. Capillary refill time, checked centrally, is a more reliable sign of circulatory failure. Normal is a capillary refill time <2 seconds.

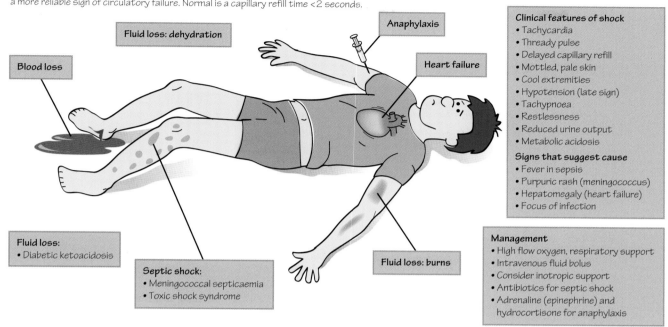

Fluid loss: dehydration

Anaphylaxis

Heart failure

Blood loss

Fluid loss:
• Diabetic ketoacidosis

Septic shock:
• Meningococcal septicaemia
• Toxic shock syndrome

Fluid loss: burns

Clinical features of shock
• Tachycardia
• Thready pulse
• Delayed capillary refill
• Mottled, pale skin
• Cool extremities
• Hypotension (late sign)
• Tachypnoea
• Restlessness
• Reduced urine output
• Metabolic acidosis

Signs that suggest cause
• Fever in sepsis
• Purpuric rash (meningococcus)
• Hepatomegaly (heart failure)
• Focus of infection

Management
• High flow oxygen, respiratory support
• Intravenous fluid bolus
• Consider inotropic support
• Antibiotics for septic shock
• Adrenaline (epinephrine) and hydrocortisone for anaphylaxis

Causes of respiratory failure

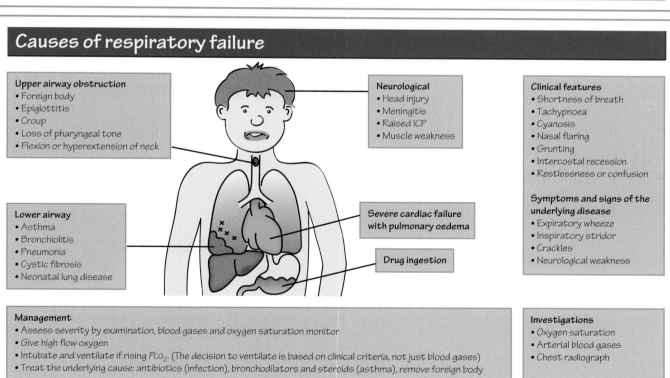

Upper airway obstruction
• Foreign body
• Epiglottitis
• Croup
• Loss of pharyngeal tone
• Flexion or hyperextension of neck

Neurological
• Head injury
• Meningitis
• Raised ICP
• Muscle weakness

Lower airway
• Asthma
• Bronchiolitis
• Pneumonia
• Cystic fibrosis
• Neonatal lung disease

Severe cardiac failure with pulmonary oedema

Drug ingestion

Clinical features
• Shortness of breath
• Tachypnoea
• Cyanosis
• Nasal flaring
• Grunting
• Intercostal recession
• Restlessness or confusion

Symptoms and signs of the underlying disease
• Expiratory wheeze
• Inspiratory stridor
• Crackles
• Neurological weakness

Management
• Assess severity by examination, blood gases and oxygen saturation monitor
• Give high flow oxygen
• Intubate and ventilate if rising P_{CO_2}. (The decision to ventilate is based on clinical criteria, not just blood gases)
• Treat the underlying cause: antibiotics (infection), bronchodilators and steroids (asthma), remove foreign body

Investigations
• Oxygen saturation
• Arterial blood gases
• Chest radiograph

Respiratory failure

Respiratory failure is defined as inadequate respiration to maintain normal arterial oxygen and carbon dioxide concentrations. Respiratory failure is obvious if the child is apnoeic or deeply cyanosed, but it is important to be able to detect impending respiratory failure and to intervene quickly. Tachypnoea >50/minute, grunting and oxygen saturation <95% in air are signs of serious respiratory distress.

Acute upper airway obstruction

Acute upper airway obstruction is a medical emergency. It can be due to infection (epiglottitis, croup) or inhalation of a foreign body (especially common in toddlers who put small objects in their mouths). Presentation is with acute sudden onset of choking, coughing and cyanosis, followed by collapse. There may be an inspiratory stridor (see Chapter 27) and marked intercostal recession. If epiglottitis is suspected, do not examine the child's throat. The management of choking is described in Chapter 59.

Septic shock

Meningococcal septicaemia is one of the most life-threatening causes of septic shock and is due to Gram-negative diplococcus *Neisseria meningitides* infection. 40–50% will present with meningitis (see Chapter 60), 40% with meningitis and septicaemia and 10% with septicaemia alone. Within hours of the onset of non-specific flu-like symptoms, a rash develops. This may initially be erythematous or petechial but rapidly becomes purpuric. Parents are advised to perform the 'glass test' (pressing on the skin with a glass beaker—see Chapter 55) to check whether any rash is non-blanching and seek urgent medical advice if positive.

Fulminant septicaemia can develop within hours, leading to endotoxin-mediated severe septic shock and coma. The case fatality rate is around 10%. Any child with purpura and a fever should be given intramuscular ceftriaxone and transferred to hospital immediately. A vaccine is now available for types A, B and C. As 20–30% of the population may be nasopharyngeal carriers of *Neisseria meningitides*, close contacts should be given rifampicin prophylaxis.

Features suggestive of meningococcal disease

Fever and a non-blanching rash, especially if
- The child looks ill.
- The non-blanching lesions are >2 mm (purpura).
- There is neck stiffness.
- The capillary refill time is ≥3 s.

Features suggestive of staphylococcal toxic shock syndrome (exotoxin mediated)

- Acute onset of high fever
- Muscle pain
- Desquamating rash
- Signs of shock.

The original site of infection may be trivial, such as a graze, or in girls may be associated with menstruation. Circulatory support and high-dose antibiotic treatment with flucloxacillin or clindamycin is required.

Neurological warning signs

Signs of an actual or impending serious neurological disorder include the following:

- Drowsiness, lethargy or other altered level of consciousness
- Severe headache, especially if associated with vomiting
- Irritability or a high-pitched cry
- Bulging fontanelle (infants)
- Neck stiffness
- Sudden onset of muscle weakness
- Any new cranial nerve lesion
- Abnormal movements
- Convulsions.

These signs should prompt a thorough search for the cause. Consider raised intracranial pressure, central nervous system (CNS) infection and whether neuroimaging with CT or MRI scan is required.

KEY POINTS

- Early recognition of impending cardiorespiratory failure is vital.
- Irritability may be an early sign of hypoxia or CNS infection.
- A non-blanching rash in an ill child should be assumed to be meningococcal septicaemia and is a medical emergency.
- An altered level of consciousness should always be taken seriously.

59 The collapsed child

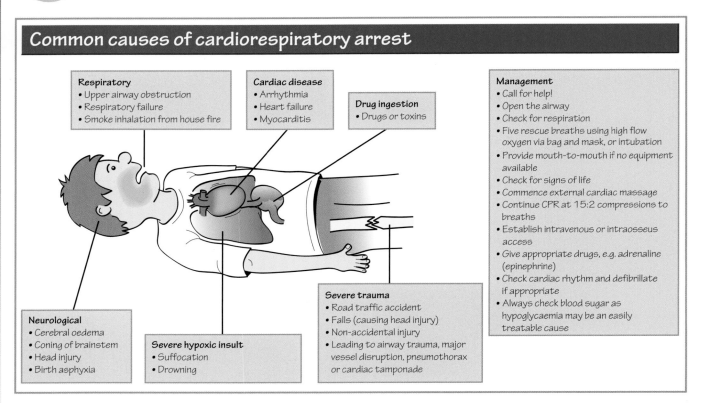

Common causes of cardiorespiratory arrest

Respiratory
- Upper airway obstruction
- Respiratory failure
- Smoke inhalation from house fire

Cardiac disease
- Arrhythmia
- Heart failure
- Myocarditis

Drug ingestion
- Drugs or toxins

Neurological
- Cerebral oedema
- Coning of brainstem
- Head injury
- Birth asphyxia

Severe hypoxic insult
- Suffocation
- Drowning

Severe trauma
- Road traffic accident
- Falls (causing head injury)
- Non-accidental injury
- Leading to airway trauma, major vessel disruption, pneumothorax or cardiac tamponade

Management
- Call for help!
- Open the airway
- Check for respiration
- Five rescue breaths using high flow oxygen via bag and mask, or intubation
- Provide mouth-to-mouth if no equipment available
- Check for signs of life
- Commence external cardiac massage
- Continue CPR at 15:2 compressions to breaths
- Establish intravenous or intraosseus access
- Give appropriate drugs, e.g. adrenaline (epinephrine)
- Check cardiac rhythm and defibrillate if appropriate
- Always check blood sugar as hypoglycaemia may be an easily treatable cause

Collapse and cardiorespiratory arrest

Not all children who collapse will proceed to a full respiratory or cardiac arrest. Causes of sudden collapse in children are listed in the following box and many of these are discussed in detail in Chapters 43 and 60. However, if basic life support is not provided immediately, a collapsed child may progress to cardiorespiratory arrest, often due to failure to maintain an open airway.

Sudden collapse in children

- Syncope (vasovagal)
- Epilepsy
- Choking
- Cardiac arrhythmia (rare)
- Factitious illness (rare)
- Hypoglycaemia
- Drug ingestion
- Anaphylaxis

Cardiac arrest is the end point of severe respiratory or cardiac failure that has either been overwhelming or has not been adequately treated. Cardiorespiratory arrest outside hospital requires rapid basic life support until skilled help arrives. In hospital, arrest should be managed by a skilled resuscitation team. As most cardiorespiratory arrests in children are secondary to hypoxia rather than due to cardiac disease, it is crucial to achieve a patent airway and adequate oxygenation using high-flow oxygen and artificial respiration and where necessary (e.g. asystole or severe bradycardia) to circulate this oxygen by use of cardiac massage.

Establishing an airway and artificial ventilation

The airway should be opened by lifting the chin and tilting the head back to a 'sniffing the air' position. In infants, the head should be in a neutral position. If there is a possibility of cervical spine injury, then the airway should be opened by the 'jaw-thrust' method, while a helper stabilizes the cervical spine. The airway should then be cleared by removing any vomit or secretions with suction. Artificial ventilation can be given by mouth to mouth or in infants by mouth to mouth and nose. After five rescue breaths, check for signs of circulation (i.e. moving, normal breathing, coughing or presence of a central pulse). If there are no signs of life, then commence cardiac massage.

Paediatrics at a Glance, Fourth Edition. Lawrence Miall, Mary Rudolf and Dominic Smith. © 2016 John Wiley & Sons, Ltd. Published 2016 by John Wiley & Sons, Ltd.
Companion website: www.ataglanceseries.com/paediatrics

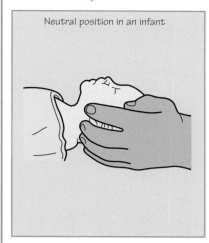
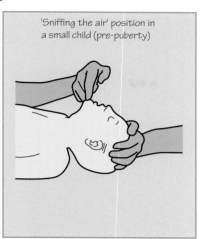
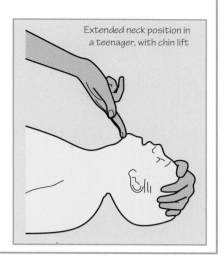

The correct airway position for children of different ages

Neutral position in an infant

'Sniffing the air' position in a small child (pre-puberty)

Extended neck position in a teenager, with chin lift

Choking

Children are at high risk of obstructing their airway with a foreign body. This is partly due to their nature (toddlers putting small objects into their mouths, older children throwing food in the air or sucking on pen tops) and partly due to the small size of the airway and the anatomy. A child's airway is conical, with the narrowest part at the cricoid ring, so objects tend to lodge in a position where they can cause complete airway obstruction. This leads to sudden onset of choking, cyanosis and collapse. Choking should be managed by encouraging coughing or in the unconscious child by opening the airway, removing any visible obstruction and performing alternating back blows and chest/abdominal thrusts to expel the obstruction. Abdominal thrusts (the Heimlich manoeuvre) should not be attempted in infants because of the risk of trauma to the liver and spleen; instead, perform five alternate back blows and chest thrusts with the child held in a head-down position. If these measures are unsuccessful, ventilation will be required via an emergency tracheostomy or cricothyroidotomy.

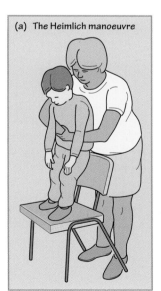

(a) The Heimlich manoeuvre

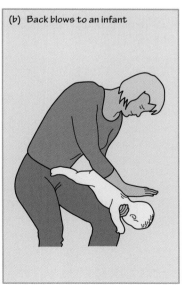

(b) Back blows to an infant

External cardiac massage

In infants, cardiac massage can be achieved by encircling the chest with both hands and compressing the lower third of the sternum with the thumbs. In young children, the heel of one hand is used

and in older children two hands are used. A ratio of 15 compressions to 2 breaths is used for all ages except *newborn* infants, where the ratio is 3:1.

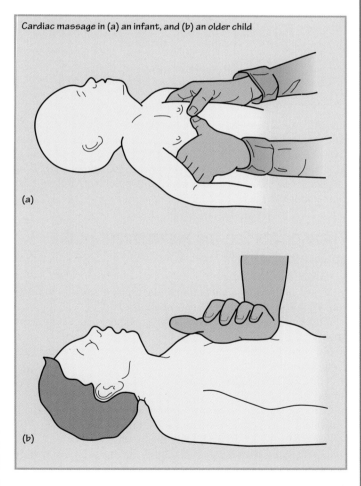

Cardiac massage in (a) an infant, and (b) an older child

(a)

(b)

If these measures are not effective, then drugs such as adrenaline (epinephrine), sodium bicarbonate and a fluid bolus may be necessary, depending on the cause of the cardiac arrest. Adrenaline can be given via the intravenous or intraosseous routes. Endotracheal adrenaline should only be used if intravenous or intraosseous access is impossible as the evidence for efficacy is not good. Defibrillation is very rarely required in paediatric cardiac arrests but is indicated for certain cardiac

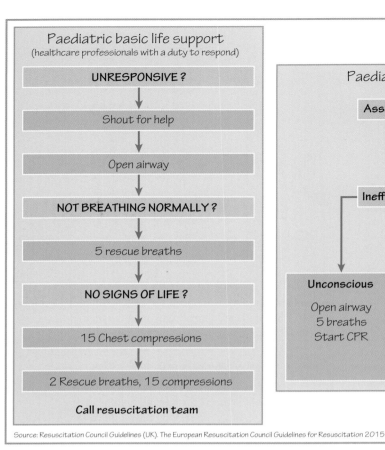

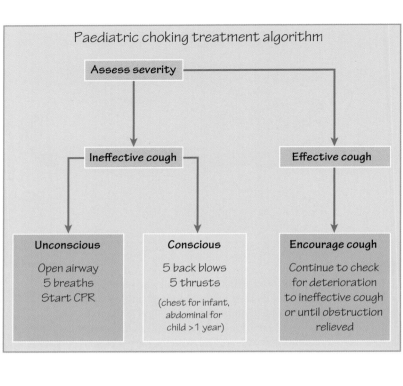

Source: Resuscitation Council Guidelines (UK). The European Resuscitation Council Guidelines for Resuscitation 2015.

arrhythmias such as ventricular fibrillation, ventricular tachycardia and supraventricular tachycardia unresponsive to drug therapy. Life-threatening cardiac arrhythmias are more common in children with congenital heart disease (post-operatively), drug ingestion (e.g. overdose of a tricyclic antidepressant) and in those with a long QT interval on the ECG.

Focal points for the assessment of the collapsed child

- Call for help immediately.
- Make a rapid assessment of the child's responsiveness—stimulate and say 'are you all right?'. Do not shake the child.
- If the child responds and is breathing with an open airway, leave them in this position and await help.
- If the child does not respond and is not breathing, proceed with basic life support.
- If the child is breathing normally but not responding to you, turn them onto their side in the recovery position.
- Continue basic life support uninterrupted until help arrives. If help has not arrived after 1 min of CPR, then go and get help.
- Apply pressure to any active bleeding points.
- Rapidly assess the neurological state by looking at pupils, posture and the level of consciousness.

- Once help arrives, or if in a hospital setting:
  - Continue basic life support uninterrupted.
  - Commence advanced life support (e.g. tracheal intubation, vascular access and administration of drugs) as indicated.
  - Commence monitoring (ECG and oxygen saturation).
  - Always check blood sugar level.
- Perform appropriate investigations and commence definitive treatment (e.g. infection screen and broad spectrum antibiotics if sepsis is suspected).
- Once the child has been stabilized, transfer to an intensive care unit for definitive care.

KEY POINTS

- Cardiac arrest is usually secondary to respiratory failure or shock.
- Upper airway obstruction is a common cause of acute respiratory failure in young children.
- Opening the airway and providing adequate oxygenation is critical.
- The technique of basic life support is a practical skill that you should acquire.

60 The unconscious child

Causes of coma

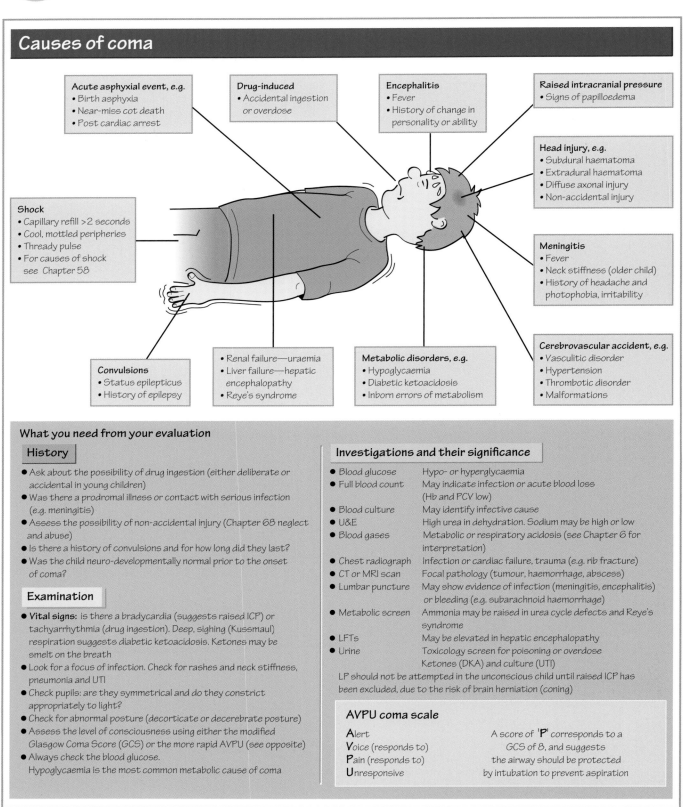

Acute asphyxial event, e.g.
- Birth asphyxia
- Near-miss cot death
- Post cardiac arrest

Drug-induced
- Accidental ingestion or overdose

Encephalitis
- Fever
- History of change in personality or ability

Raised intracranial pressure
- Signs of papilloedema

Head injury, e.g.
- Subdural haematoma
- Extradural haematoma
- Diffuse axonal injury
- Non-accidental injury

Shock
- Capillary refill >2 seconds
- Cool, mottled peripheries
- Thready pulse
- For causes of shock see Chapter 58

Meningitis
- Fever
- Neck stiffness (older child)
- History of headache and photophobia, irritability

Convulsions
- Status epilepticus
- History of epilepsy

- Renal failure—uraemia
- Liver failure—hepatic encephalopathy
- Reye's syndrome

Metabolic disorders, e.g.
- Hypoglycaemia
- Diabetic ketoacidosis
- Inborn errors of metabolism

Cerebrovascular accident, e.g.
- Vasculitic disorder
- Hypertension
- Thrombotic disorder
- Malformations

What you need from your evaluation

History

- Ask about the possibility of drug ingestion (either deliberate or accidental in young children)
- Was there a prodromal illness or contact with serious infection (e.g. meningitis)
- Assess the possibility of non-accidental injury (Chapter 68 neglect and abuse)
- Is there a history of convulsions and for how long did they last?
- Was the child neuro-developmentally normal prior to the onset of coma?

Examination

- **Vital signs:** is there a bradycardia (suggests raised ICP) or tachyarrhythmia (drug ingestion). Deep, sighing (Kussmaul) respiration suggests diabetic ketoacidosis. Ketones may be smelt on the breath
- Look for a focus of infection. Check for rashes and neck stiffness, pneumonia and UTI
- Check pupils: are they symmetrical and do they constrict appropriately to light?
- Check for abnormal posture (decorticate or decerebrate posture)
- Assess the level of consciousness using either the modified Glasgow Coma Score (GCS) or the more rapid AVPU (see opposite)
- Always check the blood glucose. Hypoglycaemia is the most common metabolic cause of coma

Investigations and their significance

- Blood glucose — Hypo- or hyperglycaemia
- Full blood count — May indicate infection or acute blood loss (Hb and PCV low)
- Blood culture — May identify infective cause
- U&E — High urea in dehydration. Sodium may be high or low
- Blood gases — Metabolic or respiratory acidosis (see Chapter 6 for interpretation)
- Chest radiograph — Infection or cardiac failure, trauma (e.g. rib fracture)
- CT or MRI scan — Focal pathology (tumour, haemorrhage, abscess)
- Lumbar puncture — May show evidence of infection (meningitis, encephalitis) or bleeding (e.g. subarachnoid haemorrhage)
- Metabolic screen — Ammonia may be raised in urea cycle defects and Reye's syndrome
- LFTs — May be elevated in hepatic encephalopathy
- Urine — Toxicology screen for poisoning or overdose Ketones (DKA) and culture (UTI)

LP should not be attempted in the unconscious child until raised ICP has been excluded, due to the risk of brain herniation (coning)

AVPU coma scale

Alert
Voice (responds to)
Pain (responds to)
Unresponsive

A score of 'P' corresponds to a GCS of 8, and suggests the airway should be protected by intubation to prevent aspiration

Coma

A child who is deeply unconscious is said to be in coma. *Encephalopathy* refers to the pre-comatose state with an altered conscious level. An unconscious child requires urgent and careful evaluation to establish the cause of the coma and to commence appropriate therapy. Whatever the cause, the airway must be protected and adequate ventilation maintained.

Meningitis

Meningitis is caused by either bacterial or viral infection invading the membranes overlying the brain and spinal cord and should be considered in any irritable child with unexplained fever. It is most common in the neonatal period but can occur at any age. The causes are listed in the following box.

> **Causes of meningitis**
>
> **Viral**
> - Mumps virus
> - Coxsackie virus
> - Echovirus
> - Herpes simplex virus
> - Poliomyelitis (if unvaccinated)
>
> **Bacterial**
> - *Neisseria meningitidis* (meningococcal meningitis)
> - *Streptococcus pneumoniae* (pneumococcal meningitis)
> - *Haemophilus influenzae* type B (now rare if immunized)
> - Group B streptococcus (in newborns)
> - *Escherichia coli* and *Listeria* (in newborns)

Viral meningitis is preceded by pharyngitis or gastrointestinal (GI) upset. The child then develops fever, headache and neck stiffness. In **bacterial meningitis**, the child is drowsy and may be vacant. Irritability is a common feature, often with a high-pitched cry, and convulsions may occur. Examination shows an ill child, with a stiff neck and positive Kernig's sign (pain on extending the legs). These signs are not reliable in young infants. Tonsillitis and otitis media can also mimic neck stiffness. In infants, the fontanelle may be bulging. A petechial or purpuric rash suggests meningococcal meningitis.

Meningitis is confirmed by a lumbar puncture (see Chapter 6), which shows a leucocytosis, high protein count, low glucose and may show organisms present. The fluid will look cloudy to the naked eye. Culture or PCR analysis will confirm the organism, but treatment should be commenced empirically as soon as the cultures have been taken.

Intravenous ceftriaxone is usually given, depending on the age of the child and the likely organism. Steroids reduce meningeal inflammation in haemophilus meningitis. Meningococcal meningitis is associated with pharyngeal carriage, and household contacts should receive prophylaxis with rifampicin. Meningococcal septicaemia is discussed in Chapter 55.

Encephalitis

Viral infection sometimes spreads beyond the meninges to infect the brain tissue itself. This is known as meningoencephalitis. The onset is often more insidious and the child's personality may change or they may become confused or clumsy before the onset of coma. Meningism is less of a feature. The lumbar puncture shows a lymphocytosis, and specimens should be sent for viral culture and PCR analysis. Herpes simplex virus or *Mycoplasma pneumoniae* may be responsible, so always ask about contact with herpetic lesions (cold sores). Treatment with aciclovir, erythromycin and cefotaxime is given until the organism is known.

In herpes encephalitis, the EEG and an MRI brain scan may characteristically show temporal lobe involvement. Prolonged treatment may be required.

Metabolic causes of coma

In the absence of trauma or infection, a metabolic cause for coma must be considered. By far the commonest metabolic cause is hypoglycaemia, and blood glucose must be measured immediately at the bedside in every unconscious child. Hypoglycaemia may be due to inadequate carbohydrate intake or excess insulin in children with diabetes mellitus, but it can also be the presenting feature in infants with inborn errors of metabolism or adrenal insufficiency. Hyperglycaemia in uncontrolled diabetes can lead to ketoacidosis with coma, though the onset is often more gradual. Diabetes is discussed in detail in Chapter 21.

Any severe metabolic derangement can cause coma, including severe uraemia (in renal failure) or high ammonia (inborn errors of metabolism such as urea cycle disorders), severe hypernatraemia or hyponatraemia. Coma can also be caused by cerebral oedema from over-rapid correction of electrolyte imbalance in severe dehydration.

Reye's syndrome

Reye's syndrome may be preceded by a viral illness such as influenza or chickenpox and is more common in winter. Although it is rare and not in itself infectious, it can be triggered by the use of aspirin (salicylic acid) during a viral illness; hence, aspirin is not recommended in childhood. The exact aetiology is unknown, but there is an initial phase of vomiting and lethargy followed by a non-inflammatory encephalopathic illness with personality change, irritability and then coma with raised intracranial pressure. Fatty change (steatosis) in the liver may lead to acute hepatic failure. Treatment is mainly supportive with aggressive intensive care treatment to treat raised intracranial pressure.

Unexplained coma

In unexplained coma, the possibility of non-accidental injury such as shaking injury must be considered. A CT brain scan and skeletal survey may show evidence of trauma and retinal haemorrhages may be present. Accidental drug ingestion or overdose, or deliberate poisoning may cause coma, and a urine toxicology screen can sometimes identify the drug. Drugs affecting the central nervous system such as opiate analgesics, alcohol and antidepressants are often implicated.

> **KEY POINTS**
>
> - Evaluate coma using the AVPU (alert, voice, pain, unresponsive) score.
> - Always check the blood glucose in coma.
> - Consider poisoning, drug overdose or non-accidental injury.
> - Altered consciousness, fever and irritability suggest meningitis, even in the absence of neck stiffness.
> - Never perform a lumbar puncture in an unconscious child until raised intracranial pressure has been excluded.
> - Consider Reye's syndrome if there has been ingestion of aspirin or recent viral infection.

61 The fitting child

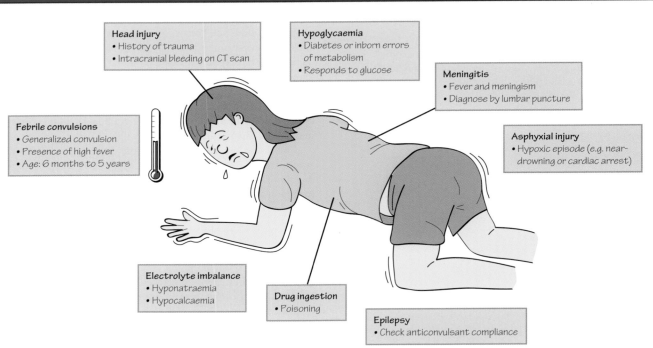

Causes of convulsions

Head injury
- History of trauma
- Intracranial bleeding on CT scan

Hypoglycaemia
- Diabetes or inborn errors of metabolism
- Responds to glucose

Meningitis
- Fever and meningism
- Diagnose by lumbar puncture

Febrile convulsions
- Generalized convulsion
- Presence of high fever
- Age: 6 months to 5 years

Asphyxial injury
- Hypoxic episode (e.g. near-drowning or cardiac arrest)

Electrolyte imbalance
- Hyponatraemia
- Hypocalcaemia

Drug ingestion
- Poisoning

Epilepsy
- Check anticonvulsant compliance

What you need from your evaluation

History
- Is there a history of previous convulsions? The child may have established epilepsy
- How long has the convulsion lasted? Seizures lasting less than 20 min are unlikely to cause brain damage
- Obtain an accurate description of the convulsion—how did it begin, was it focal or generalized? Speak to witnesses. Some parents may have video footage
- Was the child unwell or pyrexial beforehand? Could it be a febrile convulsion or part of a CNS infection?
- Is the child developmentally normal? Non-febrile convulsions are much more common in children with learning disability or cerebral palsy
- Is drug ingestion or poisoning possible? There may be an organic treatable cause for the fits

Examination
- Make sure the airway is open
- Is the convulsion generalized, affecting all limbs?
- Check the temperature
- Is there an obvious focus of infection?
- Are there signs of trauma or head injury?
- Examine the eyes—are they flickering or rolling?
- Look for signs of meningitis and check the pupils

Treatment
- Give oxygen and maintain a patent airway
- Place the child in the recovery position
- Give buccal midazolam or rectal diazepam
- Correct any metabolic disturbance
- Give dextrose if hypoglycaemia likely
- Consider IV anticonvulsants—lorazepam, phenytoin, or phenobarbital
- If in prolonged status epilepticus, thiopental infusion and ventilation may be needed

Investigations and their significance
- Blood glucose — Must always be checked in any fitting child. Can be done at the bedside
- U&E, calcium, magnesium — Hyponatraemia, hypocalcaemia and hypomagnesaemia can cause fits
- Lumbar puncture — If meningitis suspected, but beware raised ICP in prolonged fit
- CT/MRI scan — If any history of trauma or focal neurological signs suggesting intracranial lesion
- Blood and urine cultures, throat swab, CXR — To look for focus of infection in febrile convulsions
- Urine toxicology — If drug ingestion or overdose suspected

Generalized convulsions

The term *convulsion* is synonymous with *fit* or *seizure*. Convulsions are due to synchronous discharge of electrical activity from a number of neurons, usually with loss of consciousness and abnormal movements. In a generalized convulsion, all four limbs and the face are affected. Convulsions are common, occurring in 3–5% of children. They do not necessarily mean the child will go on to develop epilepsy, and many children only ever have one convulsion. However, 60% of epilepsy develops in childhood (Chapter 44). Children's brains are particularly susceptible to convulsions and the commonest trigger is the rise in temperature during a febrile illness.

Febrile convulsions

These occur between the ages of 6 months and 5 years in normal children and are triggered by fever, usually as part of an URTI, although they may also be triggered by any febrile illness. They can be simple or complex (see the table).

Simple febrile convulsion (75%)	Complex febrile convulsion (25%)
• Child age 6 months to 6 years • Single seizure lasting <15 min • Neurologically normal before and after normal neurodevelopment • Fever not due to CNS infection	• Child age 6 months to 6 years • Seizure either focal or prolonged >15 min, or many seizures occurring in close succession, or status epilepticus

Febrile convulsions should be managed by identifying and treating the source of the fever and cooling the child by undressing them and sponging with tepid water. Antipyretics such as paracetamol or ibuprofen should be given. If the convulsion persists for more than 10 min, give anticonvulsants. Status epilepticus (see below) occurs in less than 1% of febrile convulsions. Investigations should be performed to exclude serious infection, and if no obvious focus of infection is found, a lumbar puncture is indicated to exclude meningitis.

Advice to parents is very important. About one-third of children will have further febrile convulsions in future. Parents must be taught how to manage fever and basic first-aid management of convulsions. The good prognosis should be explained. Children with uncomplicated febrile convulsions are at very little risk of epilepsy. Overall, the risk of epilepsy is 2–3% (about twice the normal incidence). Prophylactic anticonvulsants don't seem to reduce the risk of future convulsions. If seizures are very frequent, a benzodiazepine can be given at the onset of seizure prior to transfer to hospital.

Management of the fitting child

Most parents who witness their child having a seizure imagine that the child is going to die and seek medical attention urgently. Children may still be fitting when they present. The most important thing is to support the airway and turn the child into the recovery position, semi-prone with the knee flexed under the chest and the hand under the head. Objects (other than an oropharyngeal airway) should not be put into the mouth. If oxygen is available, this should be given by facemask. If the convulsion is ongoing, lorazepam should be given intravenously to terminate the seizure. If intravenous access is not possible, buccal midazolam or rectal

diazepam may be used. Occasionally, some convulsions persist; this is known as status epilepticus (see below).

It is vital to check blood glucose immediately in any fitting child as hypoglycaemia is a common and rapidly treatable cause. Not all children with hypoglycaemic convulsions are diabetic; some may have inborn errors of metabolism. Once the convulsion has terminated, the child may remain drowsy or 'postictal' for some time. They should be observed carefully and kept in the recovery position until they are able to maintain their own airway. If it is the child's first convulsion, the parents will require much reassurance and will need to be taught how to manage future episodes. This will include prescribing buccal midazolam or rectal diazepam to be administered at home.

Status epilepticus

Seizures may be very prolonged and are an important cause of coma. Status epilepticus is defined as continuous seizure activity for more than 30 min or a series of seizures without a full recovery in between. Status may occur following febrile convulsions or more commonly in children with known epilepsy or with other acute causes such as trauma or metabolic disturbance. The child's airway should be opened, oxygen given and blood glucose checked. Anticonvulsant medication should be given as described below. Any child with very prolonged seizures should be monitored carefully on an intensive care unit, and urgent investigations performed to identify the cause.

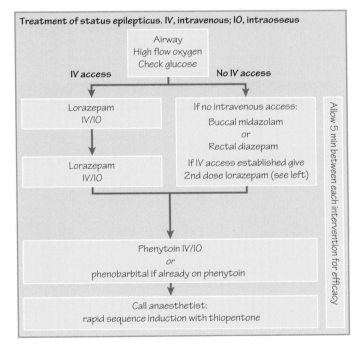

Treatment of status epilepticus. IV, intravenous; IO, intraosseus

Airway
High flow oxygen
Check glucose

IV access → Lorazepam IV/IO → Lorazepam IV/IO

No IV access → If no intravenous access: Buccal midazolam or Rectal diazepam. If IV access established give 2nd dose lorazepam (see left)

Phenytoin IV/IO or phenobarbital if already on phenytoin

Call anaesthetist: rapid sequence induction with thiopentone

Allow 5 min between each intervention for efficacy

KEY POINTS

• Febrile convulsions occur in 3% of children between age 5 months and 5 years. The prognosis is usually excellent.
• Children who are fitting must be placed in the recovery position and their airway maintained.
• Always check blood sugar as hypoglycaemia is a common and treatable cause.
• Any convulsion lasting more than 10 min should be terminated with buccal midazolam or rectal diazepam.
• Status epilepticus is fitting for more than 30 min and requires urgent treatment.

62 Injuries and burns

Accidents

Each year in the UK about 200 children are killed and 10 000 permanently injured by accidents. About 2 million children a year attend hospitals each year due to accidents. Nearly half of these have occurred in the home. Most accidents are not just chance events but are to some extent predictable and therefore preventable. As most accidents occur in and around the home, one of the main accident-prevention strategies is parental education and improving the awareness of potential hazards. Some of the common causes of accidents and their prevention strategies are listed below.

Choking
- Keep small toys away from toddlers
- No nuts for children under 5 years
- Use pens with safe tops

Road traffic accidents
This is the most common cause of accidental death in childhood. The child is usually a pedestrian or cyclist. Road traffic accidents can be prevented by reducing the speed of traffic and by educating both drivers and children
- Use child car seats and seatbelts
- Teach road safety to children from a young age
- Traffic calming schemes around schools and playgrounds
- Cycle helmets reduce the number of serious head injuries in cyclists
- Enforce speed limits by use of speed cameras
- Improve access to specialized trauma and neurosurgical centres

Drowning
- Mostly occurs in fresh water (baths, swimming pools, rivers)
- Outcome is better in very cold water due to protective effect of hypothermia
- If the child is resuscitated from a near-drowning, the outcome is usually good

Prevention
- Never leave children unattended in the bath
- Swim only where a lifeguard is present
- Fence off pools and ponds

Falls
- Fit stair gates at home
- Fit child-proof window locks
- Soft surfaces in playgrounds

Poisoning (See Chapter 63)

Burns

Every year 57 000 children in the UK attend hospital Emergency Departments with burns or scalds. Burns are the second most common cause of accidental death in childhood after road traffic accidents and account for about 90 deaths a year. Fatal burns are usually associated with house fires. Half are due to smoke inhalation and half to direct burns. Death from burns arises due to the massive fluid loss through the exposed tissues and due to infection. The severity of a burn is determined by the temperature and the duration of contact. Most skin burns are due to scalding with hot water or hot drinks

Prevention
- Caution in the kitchen
- Reduce hot water temperature to 48°C
- Install smoke detectors
- Avoid trailing flexes on kettles and irons
- Use fire guards
- Cover electrical sockets

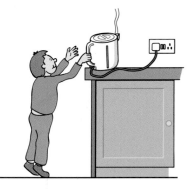

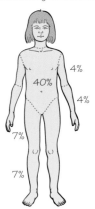

4%
40%
4%

Trunk represents
20% back
20% front

7%

7%

Management
Remove the heat source and any hot clothing immediately. Cool the skin under a cold tap and wrap the area in a clean sheet or cover with clean cling film. If there has been smoke inhalation, check for wheeze, cyanosis or respiratory distress. There may be soot in the nose and mouth. Check oxygen saturation and carboxy-haemoglobin level (in case of carbon monoxide poisoning). Give high-flow oxygen and consider ventilation. The extent of the burns should be assessed, and the percentage of the body surface area affecting full-thickness or partial thickness burns should be estimated (palms of hand = 1%). Burns affecting >10% are highly significant and intravenous fluid resuscitation will be required. The fluid management is complicated and depends on the percentage area affected. Give morphine to control pain. Full-thickness burns are less painful than partial ones. Most burns victims are now treated in specialized burns units. Skin grafting may be necessary and psychological support will be needed for the child and the family, especially if there is extensive scarring

Paediatrics at a Glance, Fourth Edition. Lawrence Miall, Mary Rudolf and Dominic Smith. © 2016 John Wiley & Sons, Ltd. Published 2016 by John Wiley & Sons, Ltd.
Companion website: www.ataglanceseries.com/paediatrics

63 Poisoning

Accidental ingestion in young children

Accidental poisoning is becoming less common as parents become more aware of the risks and drugs are sold in child-resistant containers. Accidental poisoning most commonly occurs in inquisitive toddlers, especially when they are staying in grandparents' homes where there are likely to be more medicines and household products may be stored less carefully

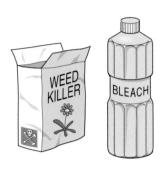

Common drugs ingested
- Aspirin
- Paracetamol
- Antidepressants

Common household agents
- Button batteries
- Disinfectants and bleach
- Weedkiller
- Paraffin or white spirit
- Dishwasher tablets

History and evaluation
- Substance ingested
- Time ingested
- Calculate maximum quantity that may have been ingested
- Inspect the product container
- Alkalie's cause more oesophageal corrosion than acids.

Examination
- What is the child's conscious level and are the pupils reacting normally?
- Check pulse and blood pressure and monitor if arrhythmias are likely
- Is there evidence in the mouth of ingestion, e.g. ulcers, or clues from the clothing, such as burns or smell?

Investigations
- Blood and urine for toxicology if the poison is not known
- Paracetamol, alcohol, salicylate or drug levels, as appropriate
- Blood glucose, especially in alcohol poisoning
- Keep the product and packaging for further analysis

Management
- Discuss with nearest poisons unit
- Where possible remove the poison. Gastric lavage should not be used routinely but may be considered if a life-threatening quantity of a drug (e.g. aspirin) has been ingested within the last hour. Lavage is contraindicated if the airway cannot be protected. Button batteries should be removed endoscopically within 2 h to prevent erosion
- Activated charcoal can absorb many drugs (e.g. aspirin, paracetamol, phenytoin, carbamazepine) but should only be given if a life-threatening quantity has been ingested within the last hour. Multiple dose charcoal therapy may be helpful in some situations
- Inducing vomiting with ipecacuanha syrup is dangerous and no longer recommended
- Give specific antidote if available (e.g. naloxone for opiates, vitamin K for warfarin)
- Supportive treatment for respiration. Monitor for cardiac arrhythmias and treat as necessary
- Advice should be given to parents on safety within the home

Intentional overdose in older children and adolescents

Agents used to overdose
- Paracetamol
- Aspirin
- Alcohol
- Drugs of abuse (e.g. opiates)
- Sedatives and antidepressants

Risk factors for overdose
- Children in care
- Emotional upset
- Child abuse or bullying
- Psychiatric illness
- Suicidal thoughts (usually rare)
- Other self-harming behaviour

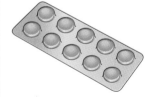 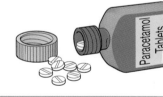

Management
- Evaluation, history and examination, as above
- Removal of poison where possible or administration of charcoal
- Aspirin remains in the stomach for a considerable time and gastric lavage should be considered
- Treatment of the toxic effects of drug, as above
- Assessment by child psychiatrist in all cases
- Consider the possibility of serious risk factors, such as abuse

Paracetamol poisoning
- Blister packs and limiting packets to 16 tablets has reduced the risk of severe poisoning
- Rarely severe enough to cause serious problems but liver failure can occur after ingestion of 20–30 tablets and is likely if >150 mg/kg of paracetamol has been ingested
- If >150 mg/kg ingested, start treatment immediately with IV N-acetylcysteine. This must be commenced within 8 h of ingestion. These antidotes can be stopped if the serum concentration falls below the treatment line
- Serum paracetamol levels should be measured 4 h after ingestion and the level plotted on a nomogram. If above the treatment level, an infusion of N-acetyl cysteine should be commenced and continued for at least 24 h. This reduces the risk of liver damage
- In significant overdoses, serial measurements of liver enzymes and coagulation times should be made to monitor hepatic function Serum urea and electrolytes should be used to monitor renal function
- The initial symptoms of nausea and vomiting usually settle within 24 h, but hepatic necrosis can occur 3–4 days later with the onset of right upper quadrant pain and later encephalopathy
- In the most severe cases (acidosis, encephalopathy or severe coagulopathy), urgent liver transplantation may be life-saving

Paediatrics at a Glance, Fourth Edition. Lawrence Miall, Mary Rudolf and Dominic Smith. © 2016 John Wiley & Sons, Ltd. Published 2016 by John Wiley & Sons, Ltd.
Companion website: www.ataglanceseries.com/paediatrics

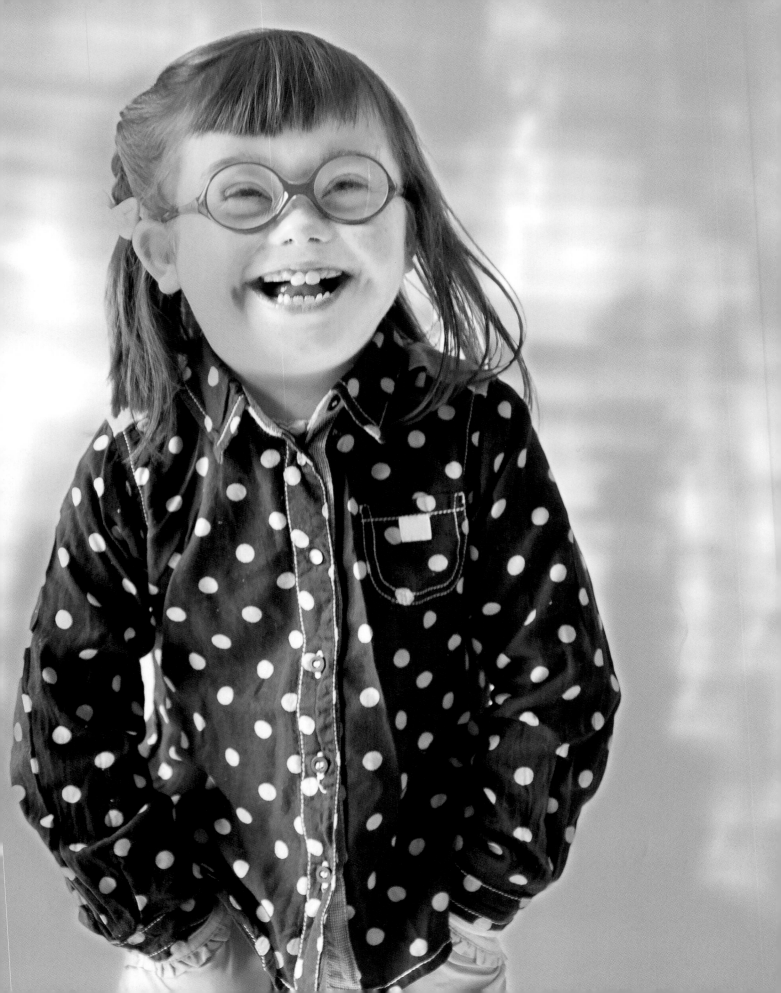

Child health in the community

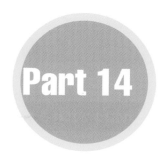

Part 14

Chapters

64 Living with a chronic illness

Living with a chronic condition

More common long-term conditions in childhood
- Asthma
- Epilepsy
- Congenital heart disease
- Diabetes mellitus
- Arthritis
- Cystic fibrosis
- Chronic renal impairment
- Malignancy
- Neurodevelopmental disorders

Factors affecting a child's adjustment to a chronic illness

The child
- The age of the child
- The age at which the illness developed. School entry and adolescence are particularly vulnerable periods
- Learning disability or physical difference can cause peer relationship problems

The illness
- Conditions with unpredictable flare-ups or recurrences can be more distressing than stable conditions than stable conditions
- 'Invisible' conditions (e.g. diabetes) may be concealed and lead to anxiety about peer group attitudes if the condition is revealed

The family
- The family's attitude and ability to function is the most critical factor in determining the child's adjustment
- Positive warm family relationships support children
- The family need to be interested and engaged in managing the illness, attending clinics, complying with treatment and seeking help when problems occur
- Successful parenting enables children to become confident, independent, positive about their abilities and resilient to challenges

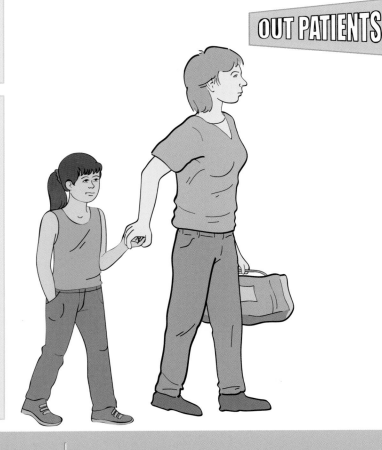

OUT PATIENTS

What you need from your evaluation

Assessment

- What is the extent of the disease and its complications in the child?
- What are the physical effects (e.g. poor growth, delayed puberty) of the illness on the child?
- How has the illness affected the child's performance at home, at school and with peers?
- What is the level of school absence?
- How has the child adjusted to the illness?
- What impact does the child's illness have on the family and its members?
- Does the child understand their illness and take responsibility for their management?
- How has the family adjusted to the special impact or burden of the illness?
- Who is acting as main carer? What support do they get?
- Has there been change in parents work or relationship?
- Have siblings had any emotional or behavioural difficulties?

Management

- Try to confine the consequences of the condition to the minimum manifestation
- Encourage normal growth and development
- Assist the child in maximizing their potential in all possible areas
- Support children and young people's emotional wellbeing. Consider support for siblings and parents. Aim to reduce the behavioural and social adverse consequences of a chronic condition

Paediatrics at a Glance, Fourth Edition. Lawrence Miall, Mary Rudolf and Dominic Smith. © 2016 John Wiley & Sons, Ltd. Published 2016 by John Wiley & Sons, Ltd.
Companion website: www.ataglanceseries.com/paediatrics

A chronic medical condition is defined as *an illness that lasts longer than 3 months, and is sufficiently severe to interfere with a child's ordinary activities*. According to the UK General Household Survey, as many as 10–20% of children experience a long-standing medical condition, with 5–10% having a moderately to severe long-term illness or disability.

The effect of chronic illness on the child

It is not only the severity and prognosis of a condition that influences how a child adjusts. In fact, there appears to be little relationship between the severity of the condition and the extent of psychosocial difficulties. Children with mild disabilities may suffer as much or more than those where the condition is severe.

Emotional, behavioural and educational difficulties are two to three times more likely than in healthy children. Low self-esteem, impaired self-image, behavioural problems, depression, anxiety and school dysfunction are all common. They may result from the child's own response to the chronic illness or relate to how parents, peers, professionals and society react.

Children's ability to perform at school can be affected, placing them at risk for becoming underachievers and failures in their own eyes and the eyes of their peers. School is often missed because of acute exacerbations, outpatient appointments and hospitalizations. Chronic illness affects social aspects of school life too. Frequent illness episodes and restrictions may exclude children from activities. Physical appearance, acute medical problems, taking medications at school and special diets all can contribute.

The effect of chronic illness on the family

When parents learn that their child has a chronic illness, they tend to respond in a way similar to experiencing a bereavement. The initial reaction is shock or disbelief, followed by denial, anger and resentment, and eventually reaching an acceptance of the situation. Clinical anxiety, depression, guilt and grief are common, particularly for mothers, who often take the major caring role. Parents relationships can suffer greater pressure and long-term relationships are more likely to break down if chronic illness affects a family.

Siblings may also be at higher risk. Anxiety, embarrassment, resentment and guilt are common, as are fears about their own well-being and the cause and nature of their sibling's health problems. Parents may be less available to their healthy children, and they may also neglect, overindulge or develop unrealistic expectations for them.

We tend to focus on psychopathology and psychosocial problems when considering chronic illness, but it is important to remember that the impact is not always negative. Some families seem to grow closer to each other and provide outstanding care for their children. The question often arises: 'How do some families of chronically ill children survive so well?'

The paediatric care of children with long-term medical conditions

Paediatric care of children with chronic illnesses needs to be holistic and go beyond clinical management alone. Time, good communication and skill are needed. This is particularly so around the time of diagnosis, and also at transition points such as starting school or during adolescence. At times, parents may need the opportunity to talk without their child being present, and adolescents should also be encouraged to be seen on their own—to talk about problems, and also to begin to be responsible for their own health care. The role of the paediatrician includes the following:

- **Counselling:** Concern and empathy can go a long way in assisting the family to make the best of the circumstances they face. It is important that the family knows that concealing a chronic condition (where that is possible) is rarely helpful as it encourages the child to believe that the illness is a secret and something shameful.
- **Education:** An important aspect of management is educating the family about the condition. This increases trust and provides the family with skills to self-manage many aspects of the condition—particularly critical in conditions such as asthma and diabetes.
- **Coordination:** Children with chronic conditions are often looked after by a variety of health professionals: consultants, therapists and dietitians, not to mention teachers and social workers. Liaison and coordination are very important as differing opinions and advice can be very confusing for the family. Specialist clinics can be helpful, especially when there is a specialist nurse to take on this role as well as offer close support.
- **Genetic issues:** Parents often have questions about genetic implications for other children, and the affected child's own chances of fertility. A genetics referral may be appropriate.
- **Support:** Chronic illness can be an isolating experience and many families do not have the support of extended family and friends. A referral to social services may be needed for advice about benefits and other services. If there are emotional and behavioural difficulties, referral for counselling may also be required. Self-help and voluntary organizations such as Diabetes UK or Epilepsy Action can be helpful and often run support groups and activities allowing families with similar problems to meet.

Involvement with school

Good liaison with school is important. Staff need to understand about the medical condition so that they can cope competently with problems. Their greatest concern is usually around acute exacerbations, but they may also need to dispense medication or understand dietary restrictions. Asking teachers to report untoward events such as symptoms or drug side effects can be helpful. A formal healthcare plan should be prepared to give instructions on the illness, emergency procedures and key contact details.

A child who is underachieving needs extra support. This may include help in making up work lost through absence or providing preferential seating in class. Teachers can be instrumental in helping children cope and integrate socially into school life—particularly important if the family is not coping well. Some children may have special educational requirements that need to be met (Chapter 66).

KEY POINTS

- Chronic and recurrent medical problems are not uncommon.
- They have a broad impact on both the child and the family.
- A holistic approach involving the whole family is important.
- Paediatric care should involve support, coordination of care and liaison with other professionals and school.

65 Living with a disability

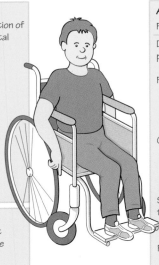

Prevalence of disability
1 in 20 children in the UK have a long term condition of which nearly half are long term neurodevelopmental problems.
- **Physical and multiple disabilities**
  Cerebral palsy
  Muscular dystrophy
  Spinal disorders
- **Severe learning difficulties**
  Chromosomal abnormalities
  CNS abnormality
  Idiopathic
  Autism
- **Special senses**
  Severe visual handicap
  Severe hearing loss

How disability presents?
- Antenatally or at birth if anomalies are present
- In the first year for motor handicaps and severe learning disabilities
- In the second or third year for moderate learning disabilities, language disorder and autism
- After cranial insults

Assessment of disability
This involves:
- A detailed assessment of the child's abilities
- Recognition of any underlying medical problem
- An assessment of the likely long-term difficulties

A Child Development Team is involved for complex difficulties

Professional	Role
Developmental paediatrician	Diagnosis of medical problems Advice on medical issues
Physiotherapist	Assessment and management of gross motor difficulties, abnormal tone and prevention of deformities in cerebral palsy Provision of special equipment
Occupational therapist	Assessment and management of fine motor difficulties Advice on toys, play and appliances to aid daily living
Speech and language therapist	Advice on feeding Assessment and management of speech, language and all aspects of communication
Psychologist	Support and counselling of family and team
Special needs teacher	Advice on special educational needs
Social worker	Support for the family Advice on social service benefits, respite care, etc.
Liaison health visitor	Support for the family Liaison with local health visitor

Management of disability

- **Giving the diagnosis:** this must be carried out in a skilled way by a senior professional
- **Medical management:** therapists' input should be provided initially at home or the child development centre, and then in nursery and school
- **Genetic counselling:** required by many families even if no obvious genetic cause is identified
- **Education in the UK:** An Education Health and Care Plan (previously Statement of Special Educational Needs) describes the education, health care and social care needs provision that must be made for a child with disabilities. Where possible the child should be integrated into mainstream school
- **Provision of services:** Social Services are responsible for preschool childcare, respite care, home help, advice about benefits and assessment for services on leaving school. Voluntary agencies may provide support and information

Living with a disability

- Parents' initial reaction to news of their child's disability is similar to bereavement; they may feel shock, fear and loss, anger and guilt. Each stage of childhood then requires further adaptation, and independence is an ongoing issue
- Schools need to be prepared for any anticipated difficulties and to accommodate physical disabilities. Staff must work with therapists to implement their recommendations. Young adult disability teams can advise about options beyond high school

Children with disabilities have complex health needs. Many of the issues described in Chapter 64 are relevant to families with a disabled child. It is important to appreciate the terminology relating to disability.

A *disorder* is a medically definable condition or disease; an *impairment* is a loss of function; *disability* refers to any restriction of ability (resulting from an impairment) and *handicap* is the impact of the impairment on the child's activities.

The distinction between disability and handicap is important. One of the aims is to minimize the handicap that results from disability. It is important to consider how people with disability are perceived by society—there are ongoing issues of poor accessibility, prejudice and discrimination affecting people with disability.

Some parents will describe their child as having 'special needs' rather than as either disabled or handicapped. This term is used by professionals in discussion with families and in the educational setting when a child may have a *Statement of Special Educational Needs*.

How disability presents?

Children with disabilities may be identified as a result of parental or professional concern. A syndrome or central nervous system abnormality may be identified in the antenatal period or at birth. Babies with neonatal problems are followed up closely as they are at high risk of disability. Deafness, motor handicaps and severe

Paediatrics at a Glance, Fourth Edition. Lawrence Miall, Mary Rudolf and Dominic Smith. © 2016 John Wiley & Sons, Ltd. Published 2016 by John Wiley & Sons, Ltd.
Companion website: www.ataglanceseries.com/paediatrics

learning disabilities often become apparent during the first year. Moderate or even severe learning disabilities, language disorder and autism may not be recognized until the child is 2 or 3 years of age, when it becomes clear that their developmental progress is not normal. Problems may arise in later childhood after acute illness events such as head injury or brain tumour.

Assessment and diagnosis of a child with a disability

Identifying the underlying medical problem is one aspect of the assessment. There is also a developmental evaluation and an assessment of how the difficulties are likely to impact on the child's family and school life. When difficulties are complex, a Child Development Team should be involved (see adjacent box).

Paediatric care

A holistic approach is needed. Sensitive support is important while parents come to terms with their child's difficulties and at each transition. Care often involves a number of professionals, both medical and non-medical, from different specialties and agencies. It can be helpful for families to have a named professional who acts as their key worker in coordinating the multidisciplinary team, for example, arranging outpatient visits to different therapists on the same day to reduce absence from school.

The diagnosis of a disability is usually devastating, and the way that the diagnosis is communicated is important, coming at the start of a long doctor–patient relationship. The session should be conducted in private by a senior doctor with both parents present. There should be opportunity for questions, with a follow-up session arranged shortly after. If a baby is born with congenital anomalies, consultation with parents should take place as concerns arise, with the baby present, sharing with the family the concerns and describing the process of making a definitive diagnosis.

Once the child's difficulties have been fully assessed, developmental therapy is required. This may be delivered in the child development centre, at home or at nursery. Once the child is in full-time school, the services are often delivered by community therapists who work with the child and advise school staff.

Provision of services

Agencies other than health are involved in providing services to the family:

- **Education services** are responsible for assessing learning difficulties, providing preschool home teaching, nursery schooling and education both in mainstream and special schools. Children who require medical treatments in school (such as drugs via gastrostomy) should have a written health care plan agreed to support staff in giving the child's treatment.
- **Social services** are responsible for providing preschool child care, relief care, advice about benefits and assessment for services

needed on leaving school. Child protection concerns also fall into their area.
- **Voluntary organizations** provide support and information for families, run play facilities, provide educational opportunities and sitting services. Some are large national agencies with numerous local branches; others are smaller groups concerned with a local issue or a single diagnosis.

The child with special educational needs

Children with special needs are educated in mainstream schools where possible. Extra help with learning and physical difficulties is provided in the classroom. This often involves a special needs assistant for the child and may also include physiotherapy, occupational therapy and speech and language therapy. Mainstream placement has the advantage of integrating children with special needs into a local peer group and encourages their inclusion in society from an early age. It has the benefit that other children learn to live alongside children with disabilities and view this as normal. However, there can be disadvantages such as large classes, less specific support and buildings poorly adapted for physical difficulties.

Special schools provide teaching in smaller classes. Staff have a greater experience of complex medical needs. The disadvantage is that children are not included in a wider social group. An alternative approach is to have specialist units within a mainstream setting.

The Education, Health and Care Plan

In the UK, the local authority is obliged to assess children who need additional provision because of severe or complex difficulties. The assessment includes reports from an educational psychologist, a paediatrician and other professionals such as therapists and the child's nursery or school. Parents also contribute information on their child's needs to the assessment and children themselves should be included if possible. It clarifies the medical needs, the educational needs, the needs for physical assistance, supervision, transport and social care to be provided for the child and family. A legally binding document is produced called the Education, Health and Care Plan. The child's educational needs and the necessary support are stated and these are reviewed on an annual basis.

Transition to adult services

There is a statutory requirement that social services make a formal assessment of a child's long-term needs as they approach adult years for those children with a Education, Health and Care Plan with complex health or disability problems. The assessment is conducted with information from health, education services, the young person and family. Transition from the long-term paediatric medical team, therapists and education setting to adult health and social care is difficult and needs careful planning. Children with severe complex needs may need residential care as adults or significant extra support to live independently. There is a need for ongoing support from specialist clinicians with expertise in adult learning disability.

66 Learning disability and autism

Prevalence
- 4 per 1000 children

Aetiology/pathophysiology
• Chromosome disorders	30%
• Identifiable disorders or syndromes	20%
• Associated with cerebral palsy, microcephaly, infantile spasms, postnatal cerebral insults	20%
• Metabolic or degenerative disease	<1%
• Idiopathic	25%

Clinical features
- Reduced intellectual functioning
- Delay in reaching developmental milestones, particularly language and social skills, in early childhood
- Often associated with:
  Epilepsy
  Vision and hearing deficits
  Communication problems
  Attention deficit/hyperactivity
  Feeding problems and failure to thrive
  Microcephaly

How learning disability presents?
- Dysmorphic features may be noted at birth
- Severe learning disability presents as developmental delay before 12 months
- Moderate learning disability often presents with delayed language in toddlers
- The diagnostic process is discussed in Chapter 3

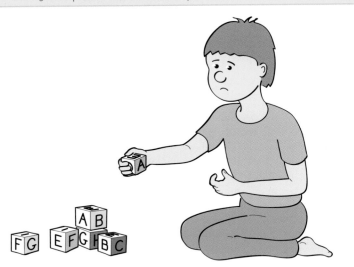

Management (needs to be multidisciplinary)

- Attempt to find underlying cause
- Early intervention and educational programmes to stimulate cognitive, language and motor development
- Attention to special educational needs, with Statement if severe
- Behavioural difficulties must be addressed
- Family support and benefits should be provided
- General paediatric care must not be neglected

Paediatric follow-up

- Developmental progress and physical growth require review
- Screening for specific associated problems in some conditions
- Behaviour is often an issue
- Liaison with other professionals is important, particularly regarding education
- The family needs support

Prognosis

- Depends on the underlying cause
- Degree of independent living relates to the severity of learning disability and the underlying aetiology

Children are said to have a learning disability when they experience significantly greater difficulty than their peers in making progress with intellectual developmental skills. Intellect overlaps with all other developmental areas, so severe learning difficulty is normally part of a pattern of global developmental delay linked with problems of mobility, communication and self-care skills.

There can be many reasons why a child may have learning difficulties. There may be a clear pathological cause such as Down's syndrome or brain injury. Learning difficulties may arise as a result of neglect in early life. In many cases, there is no clear genetic, neuroanatomical, metabolic or environmental cause that can be identified. This is an evolving area of medicine and ongoing advances in genetics and brain imaging science help understand a greater proportion of these problems.

Learning disability is termed mild, moderate, severe or profound according to the intellectual limitation and degree of independent self-care. Children and adults with *profound* learning disability are totally dependent on their carers for all activities of daily living, including self-care and feeding, and usually have very limited communication. Those with *severe* learning difficulties may learn limited self-care and simple communication skills, but will not be able to live independently. Those with *mild* or *moderate* learning disability may live independently with support.

Paediatric management
The role of the paediatrician is to assess patterns of early development that may indicate a significant future developmental problem, to diagnose the underlying cause through examination and

Paediatrics at a Glance, Fourth Edition. Lawrence Miall, Mary Rudolf and Dominic Smith. © 2016 John Wiley & Sons, Ltd. Published 2016 by John Wiley & Sons, Ltd.
Companion website: www.ataglanceseries.com/paediatrics

investigation, communicate openly with the family to ensure there is understanding of the problems and the likely future implications, to manage medical problems and to coordinate multidisciplinary developmental therapy and multiagency liaison for the child.

Growing up with learning disability

The diagnosis of severe learning disability is devastating, and families require particularly sensitive support at diagnosis and beyond. Each stage of childhood brings its own issues from starting school to adulthood. Adolescence is usually a particularly difficult time when issues related to independent living, friendships and sexuality, vocational training and care into later adult years may arise. Transition away from the well-known children's services to adult services also presents difficulties and needs planning with social care staff.

It is important to begin therapeutic input early to stimulate cognitive, language and motor development. Therapists from the Child Development Team provide advice on play activities to stimulate development and maximize function. Parents learn about methods of communication with speech therapy and alternative communication systems such as Makaton signing or visual language cards if necessary. Attendance at specialist preschool nursery can be enjoyable and promote social learning for the child. This also gives parents contact with other families.

Many children with learning disabilities are included in mainstream nursery and primary school, with appropriate help provided. Others, particularly if they have additional disabilities, may be better placed in a specialist school. Depending on the degree of disability, a Statement of Special Educational Needs may be needed (see Chapter 65). Education goals must be realistic and should include skills such as personal care, development of social behaviour and independence. On leaving school, facilities should be available for the young adult, which may include specialist accommodation and further vocational education placement.

Behavioural problems occur with greater frequency in children with developmental disabilities. This may include attention difficulties, hyperactivity (see Chapter 15), stereotypic or self-injury behaviour. Psychological help is often needed to understand difficult behaviours and advise on strategies for management. Medical problems such as eyesight, hearing, gastrointestinal symptoms, nutrition issues, seizures and acute illness need active management.

It is difficult for health staff to assess children with learning disability when acute illness occurs. A problem such as acute appendicitis can be very difficult to detect in a patient with no speech communication and limited understanding. Health staff need training in the specialist needs of people with learning disability to provide good care.

Down's syndrome (trisomy 21)

Down's syndrome is an example of a condition that causes significant learning disability with implications for long-term independent living. Down's syndrome is the commonest genetic anomaly causing learning disability. The extra chromosome is usually maternal, and the incidence of Down's syndrome increases with maternal age (1% at age 40 years).

Features include facial features of upward sloping palpebral fissures, folds of skin over the epicanthus of the eyes, a protruding tongue, flat occiput, single palmar creases and mild-to-moderate developmental delay. Associated medical problems include gastrointestinal problems (most commonly duodenal atresia),

40–50% have cardiac anomalies (most commonly atrioventricular canal defects), otitis media, squint, hypothyroidism, atlanto-axial vertebral instability and leukaemia.

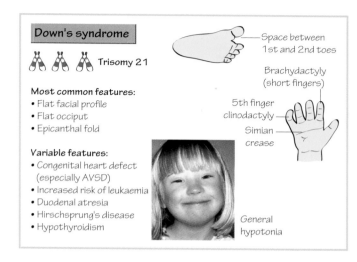

Down's syndrome

Trisomy 21

Most common features:
- Flat facial profile
- Flat occiput
- Epicanthal fold

Variable features:
- Congenital heart defect (especially AVSD)
- Increased risk of leukaemia
- Duodenal atresia
- Hirschsprung's disease
- Hypothyroidism

Space between 1st and 2nd toes

Brachydactyly (short fingers)

5th finger clinodactyly

Simian crease

General hypotonia

Fragile X

Fragile X is an important genetic cause of learning disabilities among boys. The diagnosis should be sought in any boy who has unexplained moderate or severe learning disability. Some girls carrying the chromosome have mild learning disabilities.

Autistic spectrum disorders

Autism is a developmental disorder with abnormal behaviours in three key elements:

- Poor verbal and non-verbal communication (often reduced eye contact)
- Obsessive intense repetitive interests
- Reduced imaginative play.

Autism is sometimes described as a 'mind-blindness'—an inability to relate to others, to understand that someone else might view something in a different way. There is evidence of genetic factors in a number of children with autism.

There is a broad spectrum of severity of autism. In severe autism, language development is profoundly impaired and behaviours are often extremely difficult to manage. There are a number of children with some, but not all, features of the autistic spectrum. An example is *Asperger's syndrome* in which language development is usually good, but social empathy is poor, leading to problems with peer relationships and school progress.

Specialist education support is required, and the family need support to manage difficult behaviours and communication at home and school.

KEY POINTS

- Where possible, the underlying condition should be diagnosed.
- The child's developmental progress should be monitored.
- Appropriate input should be provided in the preschool years and appropriate school placement made.
- The child and parents need a supportive framework.
- Transition to adult services needs careful planning.

67 Visual and hearing impairment

Visual impairment

A child is partially sighted if visual acuity is less than 6/18, and, therefore, educational aids such as large print books can be used. A child is defined as blind if visual acuity is <3/60, and, therefore, education can only be provided by methods such as Braille that do not involve sight.

Prevalence

One in 2500 children are registered blind or partially sighted and 50% have additional functional impairments.

Aetiology

The commonest causes are optic atrophy, congenital cataracts and choroidoretinal degeneration.

Clinical features

The eyes of visually impaired children may look abnormal or there may be unusual movements. When children are visually impaired from birth, their psychomotor development is altered. Early smiling is inconsistent and they do not turn towards sound. Reaching out for objects and the development of a pincer grip is delayed. Although early language may be normal, the development of more complex language may be slower. 'Blindisms' (eye poking, eye rubbing and rocking) may occur. Hearing deficit or severe learning difficulties are commonly associated problems.

How visual impairment presents?

In neonates, the diagnosis is suspected if cataracts, nystagmus or purposeless eye movements are present. Otherwise, it may be identified by parents or through child health surveillance. If there is any suspicion of visual impairment, an ophthalmological examination is required, which may involve visual evoked response (VER) testing.

Management

Early intervention needs to focus on developmental progress, reducing blindisms and increasing parental confidence. Expert teaching assistance for educational support is needed to advise on approach to learning, mobility and support services.

Growing up with visual impairment

Parents need advice on how to care for their child, adaptations for the home and how to provide stimulation in a non-visual way. Mainstream preschool is usually appropriate with support. Beyond this, placement depends on learning abilities and may be at mainstream school, a partially sighted unit or school for the blind. Mobility training is an important aspect of education.

Hearing impairment
Prevalence

Four per cent of children have hearing deficits. Most are mild but 2 per 1000 need a hearing aid and 1 per 1000 needs special education.

Aetiology

Most mild-to-moderate hearing loss is conductive and is secondary to otitis media. Sensorineural deafness may be genetic, may result from pre- or perinatal problems or follow a cerebral insult.

Factors that increase the risk of deafness	
Neurosensory	**Conductive**
History of meningitis	Cleft palate
Cerebral palsy	Recurrent otitis media
Family history of deafness	
Aminoglycoside treatment	
Congenital cytomegalovirus infection	

How hearing impairment presents?

Universal neonatal screening with otoacoustic emissions (OAE) is now used to identify congenital sensorineural loss. Additional audiological testing should be requested for children at risk (see above) and in any child with significantly delayed or unclear speech or where there is parental suspicion of deafness. Investigations may include brainstem-evoked responses (BSER) if the child is young or unable to cooperate.

Clinical features

Hearing impairment may manifest itself in a number of ways:

- A lack of response to sound
- Delayed speech
- Behavioural problems
- Associated problems: learning disabilities, neurological disorders and visual deficits.

Management

Grommets are inserted in children with persistent conductive hearing loss. Hearing aids are fitted for sensorineural deafness, and early speech therapy is needed to develop communication. Cochlear implant surgery has transformed the outcome for children with severe sensorineural deafness. Genetic counselling is advisable.

Growing up with hearing impairment

Parents need to learn to communicate with the child, which may include sign language. Moderately deaf children can attend mainstream school. Severely deaf children require specialist education in a hearing unit attached to a mainstream school, or at a special school for the deaf. Deaf children have a higher risk of psychological developmental disorders.

Paediatrics at a Glance, Fourth Edition. Lawrence Miall, Mary Rudolf and Dominic Smith. © 2016 John Wiley & Sons, Ltd. Published 2016 by John Wiley & Sons, Ltd.
Companion website: www.ataglanceseries.com/paediatrics

68 Neglect and abuse

Types of abuse and neglect

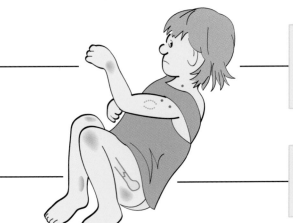

Emotional abuse
- 'Frozen, watchful' appearance
- Expressionless face, wary eyes
- Abnormally affectionate to strangers

Sexual abuse
- Anogenital bruising and tears if acute
- Pregnancy, sexually transmitted diseases
- There may be no physical signs

Non-accidental injury
- Bruises of suspicious shape or site
- Burns and scalds
- Bites
- Hidden head injuries
- Suspicious fractures

Neglect
- Unkempt dirty appearance
- Sores
- Uncared-for nappy rash
- Failure to thrive

What you need from your evaluation

History

- **How was the injury incurred?** Characteristically, the explanation is unconvincing, does not match the injury and there is a delay on obtaining medical advice. It is particularly suspicious if young not-yet-mobile infants have been injured
- **Past medical history.** Ask about previous injuries
- **Development and behaviour.** Both are affected by neglect and abuse
- **Social history and family history.** Find out who is in the home and who cares for the child. Abuse is more likely where there are changes in partner. Other professionals (e.g. health visitors and nursery nurses) can often provide extra details

Investigations and their significance

As the implications of non-accidental injury are so serious, rare medical causes of excessive bruising or fragile bones must be ruled out

• Photographs	Useful for further consultation and evidence in court
• Full blood count, coagulation studies	To rule out haematological causes of excessive bruising
• Skeletal survey (radiographs)	Certain fractures (of ribs, spiral fractures and metaphyseal chips in the long bones) and fractures at various stages of healing are particularly suspicious
• Pregnancy test and cultures (in sexual abuse)	The finding of sexually transmitted disease is strong corroborative evidence (and requires treatment)
• CT scan	May be needed to assess for intracranial injury (subdural haematoma) in infants with concern about physical injury

Physical examination

- **General appearance.** Are there signs of neglect? Is the child particularly wary or over-affectionate towards the examiner?
- **Growth.** Plot measurements and weight and compare with previous measurements. Abused and neglected children often fail to thrive
- **Injuries.** Many non-accidental injuries have a characteristic appearance. Multiple injuries are suspicious, particularly if sustained at different times
  - **Bruises:** Bruises, except on toddlers' legs, may be suspicious. The pattern may indicate how they were acquired. The age (identified from colour) may help in refuting an implausible explanation
  - **Burns and scalds:** Inflicted scalds are classically symmetrical without splash marks. Inflicted cigarette burns cause deep circular ulcers
  - **Bites:** The dental impression can be used forensically to identify the perpetrator
  - **Bony injuries:** Clinical evidence of fractures may be found
- **Neurological examination.** Retinal haemorrhages are a clue to subdural haemorrhage, which can occur when a baby is shaken
- **Signs of sexual abuse.** If sexual abuse is suspected, the genitalia and anus must be examined by an experienced paediatrician. Signs may be overt, such as bruising and tears, or subtle. The absence of signs does not refute the diagnosis

Paediatrics at a Glance, Fourth Edition. Lawrence Miall, Mary Rudolf and Dominic Smith. © 2016 John Wiley & Sons, Ltd. Published 2016 by John Wiley & Sons, Ltd.
Companion website: www.ataglanceseries.com/paediatrics

Overview

Children are dependent on their carers for their physical, emotional and developmental needs, their supervision and safety. It is hard to understand that adults can harm children—yet this occurs commonly. Abuse is typically carried out by family members or friends who have close contact with children. Health professionals need to understand the different presentations of child abuse and how to work with agencies to safeguard children.

How does child abuse present?

Child abuse can present in many ways. Some of the more common scenarios are:

- A parent or teacher seeks help following an episode of abuse which the child has disclosed.
- Families present a child to primary care or the emergency department with non-specific signs of illness or injury. Evaluation reveals inconsistencies in the history, background social risk factors or physical signs that indicate abuse.
- Physical signs of abuse are detected during routine contacts.
- Abused children may have emotional or behavioural problems such as poor mood, anxiety, poor social interaction, attention problems, aggressive behaviours and sexualized behaviours.

Physical abuse

Physical injuries are usually inflicted when adults lose emotional control while caring for babies and children. Risk factors include parental stress, substance abuse, poor social support and situations where parents have suffered abusive experience in their own childhood. Injuries can occur with premeditation such as deliberate physical punishment. Injuries may range in severity from minor bruises to fatal brain or abdominal injury. Injuries may recur over an extended period of time, through years of childhood. A child who has suffered a minor abusive injury is at risk of a future severe injury.

Any type of injury may have an abusive cause, and there may be many different mechanisms including punching, slapping, kicking, biting, hitting with an object, abdominal trauma, fractures, shaking, burns, scalds, asphyxiation and poisoning.

Factors that indicate abusive injury include the following:

- Carer conceals injury
- Delay in presentation for medical assessment of injury
- Unusual or inconsistent history of mechanism of injury
- Multiple injuries
- Different age injuries
- Some specific injuries are typical of abuse
- Previous social concerns
- Child discloses abusive injury.

Some injury patterns are more highly suggestive of abuse:

- **Bruises**: distinctive shapes such as bite marks, multiple bruises in young babies, unusual sites on the body
- **Burns**: cigarette burn, immersion hot water scald injuries
- **Fractures**: young babies, multiple fractures, different age fractures
- **Shaken baby pattern**: subdural haematoma brain injury with retinal haemorrhages and skeletal fractures.

Neglect

Neglect is inadequate care that can result in serious harm to a child. Basic care is to provide food, warmth, clothing, hygiene, dental care and immunizations, and to seek medical attention for an illness. Parents should act to protect children from harm by injury. Basic care involves good parenting behaviours including establishing boundaries relating to children's behaviour and a healthy lifestyle of diet, exercise and activity.

Neglect and failure to thrive

Some young children fail to thrive with poor nutrition. Good infant feeding requires a good emotional interaction during the feed. Parents need to be responsive to the child, manage periods of difficulty and seek advice if there are problems. This can be impaired if parents have poor models of parenting, social stresses, mental health problems or substance abuse problems.

Children can present with problems of faltering growth, acute illness and developmental problems. If admitted to hospital, these babies often show rapid weight gain. Catch-up growth may occur, but brain development may be disrupted. Subsequent emotional and educational problems are common.

Emotional abuse

Attachment is the close emotional bond that binds families—the relationships in which children learn skills for future relationships and independence. Quality of attachment depends on quality and consistency of parent–child interaction.

Children suffer emotional abuse if exposed to persistent or severe ill-treatment with dysfunctional parental responses such as rejection, excessive punishment, isolation, scapegoating, manipulation or overprotection. Emotional abuse also includes giving children inappropriate responsibilities and allowing children to witness harmful adult actions such as domestic violence.

The consequences of emotional abuse are profound. Children fail to learn normal emotional responses. They may develop problems in empathy, self-esteem, resilience and independence. There is usually significant emotional abuse in all forms of physical abuse, sexual abuse and neglect.

Sexual abuse

Sexual abuse is inappropriate sexual behaviour involving a child such as exposing a child to pornography, sexual touching, involvement in sexual acts, vaginal, oral or rectal intercourse. Perpetrators are most commonly family members or acquaintances. Perpetrators befriend ('groom') children to create situations of close contact. Perpetrators use threats to discourage children from disclosing abuse and may give children drugs or alcohol.

Sexual abuse is disclosed if a child talks about what has happened. An abused child may demonstrate inappropriate sexual language or behaviour in their play. Abuse may be suspected from a pattern of soft tissue trauma (mouth, anus or genitalia) or infection. Abuse can cause non-specific illness symptoms or behavioural problems. If children feel safe, they may be able to tell a trusted adult relative or teacher that someone has hurt them. Staff need to be able to talk to children in a way that lets them disclose what has happened through open and supportive questions.

Sensitive, skilled medical management is required. General examination and anogenital examination with a colposcope is performed to document injuries and obtain photographic and forensic evidence. Following sexual abuse, physical signs are commonly absent.

Medical care with advice on emergency contraception, sexually transmitted infection screening and post-exposure anti-retroviral drug treatment may be needed.

Victims of abuse need future safeguarding and follow-up psychological support to address the emotional harm of the abuse.

Child sexual exploitation

It is increasingly recognized that some young people suffer sexual abuse, which is perpetrated by groups of adults who identify vulnerable young people and abuse them over a period of time, with sometimes multiple abusers. Unsupervised use of the Internet can expose children to risk in this area. Child sexual exploitation should be considered by staff in health, education, social care and the police services if they see young people who seem to be in regular contact with adults, which is putting the young people at risk of harm. Adults can use extreme emotional pressure to force young people to take part in sexual activity that they do not agree to and this can be repeated over many occasions.

Factitious or fabricated illness

There are situations where adults present children for medical investigation with illness symptoms or signs that have been fabricated. This can lead to extensive medical investigation that can physically and emotionally harm the child. There are complex reasons for these behaviours—possibly a form of inappropriate care-seeking behaviour.

Medical investigation

A full skeletal survey radiography series is performed in infants where there is concern about previous physical abuse. Brain imaging and ophthalmology review are performed to investigate for shaking injury.

From the medical assessment, it is usually possible to differentiate between abusive injuries and rare disorders that predispose to fractures or brain injury.

Blood tests to exclude haematological problem such as coagulation or platelet disorder may be performed in children with bruising injuries.

Screening for sexually transmitted infection, pregnancy and forensic testing may be performed following sexual abuse.

The safeguarding process

Professionals must report incidents that raise concern to the statutory authority with responsibility for child welfare. In the UK, it is the local authority social services department that will investigate a situation of concern. It is best practice to keep families informed at all stages of the process and communicate clearly why actions are being taken.

Medical assessment is part of the investigation of a concern. Careful documentation of the history (including the child's own words), examination and medical investigation is essential. The paediatrician gives an opinion on the features in the history and examination findings. Background information is shared with other professionals such as health visitors, nursery nurses, social workers, the GP and school. This gives a picture of the risk factors in the family and any previous concerns. A multi-agency case conference meeting is held to review the combined assessments, decide the level of risk and agree how to protect the child.

If a child is at risk, then a safeguarding plan is put in place with key professionals to work with the family and monitor the future welfare of the child. In many situations, it is possible for the child to remain in the care of their family. However, some children are at risk of serious harm with background factors that cannot be resolved. In the most serious cases, a court may need to consider whether the child should be removed from the family by court order and looked after by the local authority, usually in foster care. Children in long-term care have better outcomes if permanent adoption into a new family can be arranged.

KEY POINTS

Characteristics of non-accidental injury:

- Injuries in very young children
- Explanations that do not match the appearance of the injury and that change.
- Multiple types and age of injury.
- Injuries that are 'classic' in site or character.
- Delay in presentation.
- Disclosure by the child.

69 Adolescent issues

Adolescence is the time between childhood and full maturity and is when growing-up occurs. It is a time of great physical, psychological and social change, and can be a time of considerable stress for adolescents and their parents

Physical changes
- Growth spurt occurs—may feel 'gangly'
- Secondary sex characteristics develop:
  - pubic hair
  - facial hair and testicular enlargement in boys
  - breast enlargement in girls
- Voice deepens in boys
- Girls undergo menarche and become fertile
- Acne may develop
- Gynaecomastia may develop in boys

'Tasks' of adolescence
- Establish sense of identity
- Achieve independence
- Achieve sexual maturity
- Take on adult responsibility
- Develop adult thinking

Psychological problems
- Eating disorders
- Depression
- Self-harm
- Overdosing on medicines
- Suicide

Psychological changes
- Develop insight
- Able to use abstract reasoning
- Develop logical thought
- Able to reason morally, often leading to questioning of parents and awareness of social injustice in the world
- Search for independence
- May be emotional turmoil and conflict
- Experimentation and risk-taking behaviour

Health issues
- Risk taking behaviour increases risk of injury in road traffic accidents
- Risk of injury or exploitation if drug or alcohol use
- Sexual health and contraception
- Deliberate self harm is common in adolescence
- Eating disorders
- Challenges of managing any long term conditions
- Issues of consent

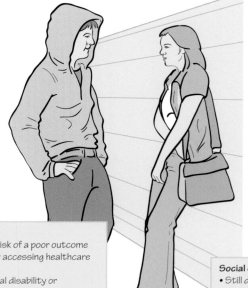

Health destructive behaviour
- Alcohol
- Smoking
- Drug use
- Substance abuse
- Accidents
- Unsafe sex
  - sexually transmitted disease
  - unwanted pregnancy
  - teenage pregnancy
- Harmful eating behaviours

Vulnerable adolescents
Certain groups of adolescents are at particular risk of a poor outcome through adolescence and may also have difficulty accessing healthcare They include:
- Those with chronic illness (e.g. diabetes), physical disability or learning difficulties
- The homeless and unemployed
- Victims of physical, emotional or sexual abuse
- Those who are pregnant
- Some ethnic minority groups
- Those with poor family support or looked after children

Social change
- Still dependent on parents financially and for housing
- Greater freedom and flexibility
- Self-motivation and self-discipline expected by school
- Sexual interest and activity increases; most experience some form of sexual activity
- Face leaving school and moving to higher education, work, financial independence or unemployment

Approach to the adolescent
- Adolescence is generally a time of life when illness is rare
- Partly because of this, healthcare facilities for adolescents are poor, often falling between paediatric and adult care
- The low rate of contact with doctors means health promotion must be delivered to the adolescents in accessible ways such as drop in clinics in schools and communication via text (SMS) message
- Adolescents may be concerned about confidentiality when seeing their family doctor Drop-in clinics can offer immediate advice on health issues, counselling for emotional and personal problems and contraceptive advice
- The way in which health professionals treat adolescents is important

How to treat adolescents
- Take time to listen
- Ask what they understand by the idea of the discussion being confidential. After this then add your view so you understand each others expectations of the discussion
- Show respect for their emerging maturity
- Allow them to express their concerns
- Avoid making judgemental statements
- Respect the need for privacy—offer to see them without their parents

Paediatrics at a Glance, Fourth Edition. Lawrence Miall, Mary Rudolf and Dominic Smith. © 2016 John Wiley & Sons, Ltd. Published 2016 by John Wiley & Sons, Ltd.
Companion website: www.ataglanceseries.com/paediatrics

The HEADSS screening questions to prompt adolescents to discuss personal issues that impact on health and wellbeing

-H = Home and environment
-E = Education and Employment situation
-A = Activities such as social interests, sports
-D = Drugs and alcohol use
-S = Sexuality
-S = Suicide ideation or depression feelings
These are sensitive areas to discuss and staff need training in how to communicate effectively.
Example of non-threatening questions-
"Who lives at home with you, how do you get along with them?"
"When you go out with friends do some people use drugs, smoke or drink? Do you ?"
"Are you involved in a relationship? Have you had an experience where someone did something to you that you were not comfortable with or disrespected you?"

Adolescent harmful health behaviours

Adolescence is a time of increasing independence for young people away from parental supervision. It is normal for young people to experiment with their choices. There are often difficulties for families in communicating about these issues.

Smoking, drug and alcohol abuse

Smoking often starts in adolescence and can become a life-long dependency.

Many teenagers experiment with drug use. Young people need age-appropriate support to manage substance abuse.

Harmful drinking behaviours often begin in adolescence. There is a risk of injury through accident, vulnerability to sexual assault and coma.

Accidents

Road traffic accidents are the leading cause of death in this age group. Alcohol and failure to wear seat belts or crash helmets increase the risks.

Self-harming

Drug overdose is a common cause of admission to hospital in adolescence. This is often a response to a stressful situation linked to family or peer relationship problems and reflects vulnerability and difficulty getting effective support. Self-harming can also manifest as deliberate soft-tissue cutting. Young people who self-harm should be seen acutely by mental health professionals to assess level of risk and to arrange ongoing support.

Sexual health issues
Menstrual complaints

Amenorrhoea is often physiological as periods may be very irregular or scanty for months after the onset of menarche. Stress can disrupt periods. Eating disorders and chronic illness can cause amenorrhoea. Pregnancy should also be considered as a cause.

Menorrhagia (heavy periods) and *dysmenorrhoea* (painful menstrual cramps) are common in the first few years after menarche. Treatment options include prostaglandin synthetase inhibitors (e.g. mefenamic acid) to reduce bleeding or the combined oral contraceptive pill to regulate the cycle.

Polycystic ovary syndrome can present in adolescence with the combination of amenorrhoea, obesity, hirsutism and acne.

Unsafe sex

Many adolescents have higher risk-taking sexual behaviours. Provision of accessible school-based sexual health services can help by giving confidential health information and improving uptake of contraception and testing for sexually transmitted diseases. Young people are at a higher risk of sexual assault from peers and older adults with a greater risk following drug or alcohol use.

Teenage pregnancy

Some 40% of sexually active teenage girls become pregnant within 2 years. There are increased perinatal risks for the mother and for the baby. Early support to young mothers and their children is important in improving their long-term outcomes.

Abortion

One-third of teenage pregnancies are managed by termination of pregnancy. There may be reluctance to seek help, sense of guilt and fears about confidentiality, so there is a clear need for sensitive support.

Contraception

Less than 50% use contraception at the time of first having sex. Information and ready access to contraception are important to reduce the rate of unplanned pregnancy and protect against sexually transmitted infection.

Sexually transmitted diseases

Chlamydia, gonorrhoea and herpes are prevalent in the community and increasingly seen in adolescents. HIV is also a risk. Screening for chlamydia by urine polymerase chain reaction (PCR) test is offered at school sexual health clinics.

KEY POINTS

- Adolescence is a time of rapid physical, psychological and social change.
- Adolescents learn independence but are at risk of harmful risk-taking behaviour.
- Eating disorders are common and need expert management.
- Health workers need to find novel ways of engaging with adolescents, especially vulnerable groups.

70 Sudden infant death

Sudden infant death and acute life-threatening events

Aetiology
- Most common cause of death in infants >1 week
- Normally previously well babies, sometimes with minor cough or cold
- In 20% an unexpected cause is found at post-mortem

Risk factors for sudden infant death
- Lying prone to sleep
- Prenatal and postnatal smoking
- Parental drug or alcohol use
- Co-sleeping with parent in bed or chair
- Soft mattress and over blanket wrapping
- Male sex

Examination
- Found collapsed
- Pale and mottled
- Bradycardia
- Hypotension

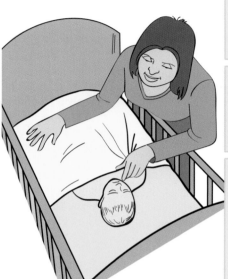

Management of acute life-threatening events
- Cardiopulmonary resuscitation (CPR)
- Admit for observation and investigation
- Train parents to administer CPR
- Home apnoea monitor may relieve anxiety but is of no proven benefit

Investigations
- Blood sugar
- Infection screen
- CXR and barium swallow
- ECG monitoring
- Metabolic screen

Differential diagnosis
- Infection
- Gastro-oesophageal reflux
- Neurological abnormality
- Hypoglycaemia
- Cardiac arrhythmia
- Inborn error of metabolism
- Suffocation
- Non-accidental injury

Acute life-threatening events and SIDS

Sudden infant death syndrome (SIDS) is the sudden death of an infant with no apparent pathological cause on post-mortem. It is commonly known as 'cot death' since typically the death occurs overnight in the baby's cot. It is vital for the family to have a thorough investigation of the sudden death. A detailed case investigation needs a combined approach by a senior paediatrician, social services and police professionals. There is review of the history and clinical examination findings, examination of the scene of death to consider any environmental risk factors and a later meeting to review post-mortem results. It is very important to involve the family in this process to give as full an explanation as possible of the events and what can be understood about their child's death.

Sometimes, infants are found in a collapsed state, not breathing and looking grey or mottled, but can be successfully resuscitated. This is referred to as an acute life-threatening event (ALTE) or as 'near-miss cot death'. All of these cases need careful medical investigation to try to establish a cause.

SIDS is the commonest cause of death (40%) in infants after the first week of life. The rate varies in different countries, but in the UK it is currently 0.45 per 1000. The exact aetiology remains unknown and is probably multifactorial. A triple-risk model has been proposed (see the following box), which may explain the fact that SIDS peaks between 2 and 4 months, and 90% occur before 6 months of age.

Triple-risk model

- A vulnerable infant with inherent problems of cardiorespiratory control (e.g. the premature infant)
- A critical period of development (changes in arousal, sleep–wake patterns and metabolism)
- External environmental stressors (e.g. prone sleeping, cigarette smoke, temperature and infection)

In the UK, the incidence of SIDS has fallen by over 50% as a result of the 'Back to Sleep' campaign, which started in the early 1990s (see in the following box), which advises that babies should be put to sleep on their backs, at the foot of the cot, not over-wrapped or overheated. This followed research that established that there is an eightfold increase in SIDS if the child sleeps in the prone position and a twofold risk in the side-lying position. Other risk factors include cigarette smoke in the home, parental alcohol intake and co-sleeping. There is some recent evidence that keeping the baby in the parents' bedroom (but not bed-sharing) and the use of a dummy (pacifier) may be associated with a reduced risk of SIDS. A small number of what initially appear to be SIDS cases may be due to non-accidental injury with atypical history or findings of injuries on post-mortem. In the UK, the 'Care of the Next Infant' (CONI) project can provide support to families who have suffered a sudden death in infancy to try to reduce the small possibility of recurrence through advice about risk factors, regular monitoring

Paediatrics at a Glance, Fourth Edition. Lawrence Miall, Mary Rudolf and Dominic Smith. © 2016 John Wiley & Sons, Ltd. Published 2016 by John Wiley & Sons, Ltd.
Companion website: www.ataglanceseries.com/paediatrics

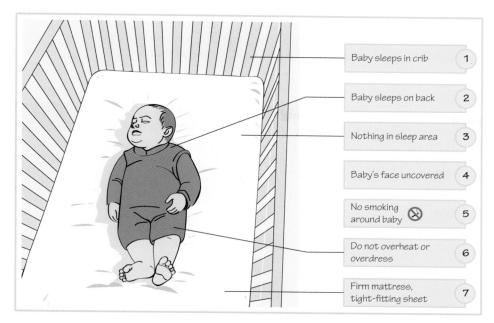

1. Baby sleeps in crib
2. Baby sleeps on back
3. Nothing in sleep area
4. Baby's face uncovered
5. No smoking around baby
6. Do not overheat or overdress
7. Firm mattress, tight-fitting sheet

check-ups and resuscitation training. The use of breathing alarm (apnoea) monitors is controversial, but some parents find them reassuring.

Sudden unexpected death in childhood (SUDIC) is a broader category where a child has died unexpectedly from any cause. It is best practice to review all such deaths (e.g. road traffic accidents and acute catastrophic infection) through a multi-disciplinary approach, so health protection agencies can learn lessons and also to provide as full an explanation as possible to the family.

Acute life-threatening events

A large number of infants are admitted to hospital following an apparent ALTE. This may be from an obvious cause such as choking on a bottle feed to unexplained apnoeic episodes or even a 'near-miss cot death', where the child has been successfully resuscitated. All these infants need careful evaluation and usually a period of observation and monitoring in hospital. In difficult cases, prolonged cardiac, respiratory, oxygenation and some-times video analysis may be necessary to establish the sequence of events. Common causes include gastro-oesophageal reflux, infection (e.g. RSV bronchiolitis) and choking. Inborn errors of metabolism, seizures and cardiac arrhythmias are more unusual findings.

Parental support must be offered. There is controversy over the role of apnoea monitors, but they may provide parental reassurance in selected cases.

The 'Back to Sleep' campaign

- Place the baby on its back to sleep.
- Do not smoke in the house. Try not to smoke during pregnancy.
- Put the baby in the 'feet to foot' position in the cot, with feet touching the foot of the cot and the head uncovered. This aims to prevent the baby slipping under the covers.
- Do not sleep a baby on a pillow or cushion. Do not use padded cot sides.
- Use a firm mattress.
- Do not let the baby get too hot or cold. Use a sheet and layers of blankets appropriate for the temperature rather than a duvet. Keep room temperature at 16–20 °C.
- Do not sleep in the same bed as the baby if you smoke, have taken alcohol or drugs or are very tired. Never sleep on a sofa with your baby.
- Seek medical advice if your baby seems ill.

For further details, see http://www.fsid.org.uk.

KEY POINTS

- SIDS is the commonest cause of death in infancy outside the neonatal period.
- Following the advice of the 'Back to Sleep' campaign can dramatically reduce the risk.
- Acute life-threatening events (ALTEs) need careful evaluation as they may be a precursor of sudden death in infancy.
- SIDS has a multifactorial aetiology, which is the subject of ongoing research.

71 Ethics, research and consent

Ethics, research and consent

There are many situations in paediatric medicine that involve ethical questions. Ethics are the moral values that people hold, which enable them to understand whether a judgement is right or wrong. These values usually start to develop from the early experiences of childhood and continue to develop right through into adult years. The values involve a sense of consideration for others, the law, personal conscience, religious beliefs, cultural beliefs and personal experience.

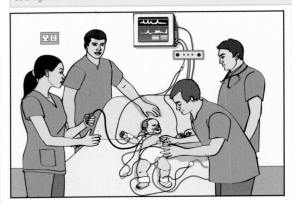

Cornerstones of medical ethics
- Autonomy (self-determination)
- Non-maleficence (not doing harm)
- Beneficence (doing good)
- Justice (fairness and equality)

Important concepts that guide ethical decisions in critical care:
- **Human rights—the right to life**: There are different views on whether life must always be sustained, but there is a general view that life must be respected. There are some situations where the vast majority of people would agree that prolonging life at all costs is wrong (such as following diagnosis of brain death) and the law will support a decision to stop treatment and allow death to occur.
- **Acts of commission and omission**: The difference between a decision that actively ends life and a decision to withhold or discontinue intervention that is prolonging life
- **Quality of life**: Most people believe this is important and is significantly impaired if:
  - life is dependent on invasive medical support
  - there is chronic distress or severe impairment of consciousness.

Consent, autonomy and confidentiality

In general, treatment should always be given with a patient's consent. However, this is not always possible with young children. Children are unlike adults in that other people (usually parents) are legally allowed to make decisions on their behalf. If children are under a court order then the court, social worker or guardian may have to make decisions about consent that are felt to be in their best interests.

Very young children are not able to understand or communicate a decision, so their parents or carers act as advocates in agreeing to treatment. Usually, there is no conflict of interest, but this is not always the case. A parent may hold a view that is different from that of the healthcare team—they may wish to prevent a specific life-saving treatment being given, despite medical advice. There are also some situations where parents may disagree with a request to withdraw life-sustaining treatment. Usually such disagreements can be resolved through sensitive communication or by offering an independent second opinion, but occasionally it is necessary for doctors to ask a court to give a judgement.

As children get older, they should be more involved in decisions about their care. It is best practice to seek consent from children as well as their parents. It is generally believed that young people are best supported by involving their parents in issues relating to their health. However, there may be situations where the young person is reluctant to involve a parent, and this may be harmful if they then fail to seek medical care. An example of this is an adolescent girl who seeks contraception but is fearful that the doctor will inform her parent. If the doctor considers that the young person is mature enough to understand the implications of a treatment, then the parent does not have to be informed. This level of competence is sometimes referred to as 'Gillick competence' after a legal test case ruling in the UK. If a doctor believes a treatment is life saving and is in the patient's best interest, then they should provide that treatment even if consent is not available.

Justice and equality

It is vital that we treat patients and families without prejudice. Many people in society have extra protections in law including racial, religious and ethnic groups and those with disability. Doctors need to ensure that where feasible, translation services are used if communication with patients or families is difficult. Equality of access to healthcare is an important concept in many health systems and this includes making sure that expensive treatments are available where there is evidence of an improvement in quality of life, but equally that limited resources aren't used to provide treatments of little proven benefit. These difficult judgements are decided in the UK by the National Institute for Clinical Excellence (NICE).

Ethics in critical care—withdrawal of intensive care

It is not always clear whether it is right to start, or to continue, intensive life-support. If a baby is born at the very limit of prematurity (22–23 weeks gestation), then some people would consider it wrong to proceed with intensive care given the extremely poor chance of survival. If a child has severe chronic ill health with no cure available, then it may be wrong to pursue repeated episodes of intensive care. If a child has severe brain injury, then it may be right to withdraw ventilator support to allow it to die. It is important to anticipate these situations in advance. There are situations where this can be discussed beforehand with the family, and if appropriate with the child.

These decisions are very difficult and require doctors to work together with families to ensure that families have full understanding of the issues of prognosis, pain and suffering and potential quality of life if treatment is continued. It is important that all members of the medical and nursing team are able to raise any concerns and any disagreement is resolved. Palliative care and end-of-life care are discussed in Chapter 72.

KEY POINTS
- Ethical decisions usually do not need to be made rapidly—there is usually time for full consultation
- It is usually wrong to make decisions that conflict with the views of parents
- All relevant staff members must be involved in discussions before a decision is made
- A child who is mature enough should be involved in ethical decisions
- Adolescents may receive treatment without parental knowledge, provided they are deemed mature enough to appreciate its consequences
- Where dispute persists between clinical staff and parents, the courts should be asked to make a final decision

Paediatrics at a Glance, Fourth Edition. Lawrence Miall, Mary Rudolf and Dominic Smith. © 2016 John Wiley & Sons, Ltd. Published 2016 by John Wiley & Sons, Ltd.
Companion website: www.ataglanceseries.com/paediatrics

Research and evidence-based medicine
Clinical research

Clinical research is fundamental to the ongoing development of paediatrics and to ensure that our patients receive the most effective evidenced-based treatments. Various types of study are used. The gold standard for assessing the efficacy of a treatment is the randomized controlled trial (RCT) where a group is randomly allocated to receive the treatment (intervention) and another group acts as control. The control group may receive a placebo (inactive treatment) or the current standard treatment. All other aspects of their care should be the same. The outcomes of both groups are analysed, preferably by researchers who are 'blinded' to which treatment they received.

Different types of research study and their uses.

Study design	Methodology and rationale
Case–control study	Compares a group with the disease against a matched control group. Often use to look retrospectively at aetiology or risk factors for a disease or outcome
Cohort study	A defined group is followed prospectively to assess their outcomes. May or may not have a control group. Used to determine prognosis and long-term outcomes (e.g. of prematurity). The best cohorts are based on an entire geographical populations
RCT	Used to compare two treatments or a new treatment with standard care. May be single- or double-blinded (where both assessor and participant do not know which treatment they received). Used to eliminate bias as much as possible when comparing treatments
Registers and surveys	Used to assess longer term outcomes of new treatments once they are in common use, and to assess rare conditions in the population (e.g. congenital anomalies)
Systematic reviews and meta-analyses	These studies take the outcomes of several RCTs, and use statistical methodologies to combine them. This has the advantage of pooling the number of participants to allow narrower confidence intervals but the studies must be of similar design

Evidence-based medicine

Evidence-based medicine tries to bring the evidence from research trials into everyday practice by making it accessible and easy to interpret. Paediatric health professionals should develop the ability to critical appraise research papers and decide if their conclusions are valid.

Ethics of research involving children

A research ethics committee must approve all research projects, and participants (or their parents) should give fully informed written consent before they enter a clinical trial or receive experimental treatment. Patient information leaflets should be easily understandable, and age appropriate. Perceived difficulty with consent together with a fear of adverse outcomes having life-long consequences in children has impeded research in children, especially research involving medicines. However, this means many drug treatments used in childhood have not been formally tested in that population, but results have been extrapolated from adult studies. This is in itself unethical. Now all new drug treatments in children must be tested in children. Taking part in a trial will usually be of benefit to future patients more than to the participant themselves, but there is evidence that (in general) participants in clinical trials receive improved care compared with non-participants. This may be due to use of standardized protocols or greater scrutiny of their care by the research team.

Landmarks in paediatric research

- **Immunizations:** Haemophilus influenza B (HiB) and rotavirus vaccines have significantly reduced the number of children admitted to hospital with serious infections.
- **Respiratory distress syndrome (RDS) in preterm infants:** The widespread use of antenatal corticosteroids and early surfactant therapy in babies has improved survival and outcomes in preterm babies.
- **Back to sleep:** Research showing that putting babies to sleep on their backs reduced sudden infant death syndrome has led to a dramatic reduction in cot deaths.
- **Leukaemia:** Research into chemotherapy protocols for acute lymphoblastic leukaemia (ALL) has improved the survival from less than 50% to more than 90%.
- **HIV transmission:** Research that led to optimization of antiretroviral therapy in mothers has reduced mother to child transmission of HIV from 25% to less than 2%.

A forest plot—comparing probiotics with control for the prevention of necrotizing enterocolitis (NEC) in preterm babies.

Study or subgroup	Probiotics Events	Total	Control Events	Total	Weight (%)	Risk ratio M-H, random, 95% CI
Al-Hosni 2012	2	50	2	51	2.9	1.02 [0.15, 6.96]
Bib-Num 2005	1	72	10	73	2.6	0.10 [0.01, 0.77]
Braga 2011	0	119	4	112	1.3	0.10 [0.01, 1.92]
Fernando-Carrocera 2012	6	75	12	75	12.5	0.50 [0.20, 1.26]
Huang 2009	0	95	3	98	1.2	0.15 [0.01, 2.81]
Kitajima 1997	0	45	0	46		Not estimable
Lin 2005	4	217	14	217	8.9	0.29 [0.10, 0.85]
Lin 2008	7	180	20	187	15.3	0.36 [0.16, 0.84]
Manzoni 2006	1	39	3	41	2.2	0.35 [0.04, 3.23]
Mihatsch 2010	2	93	4	90	3.8	0.48 [0.09, 2.58]
Oncel 2013	8	200	10	200	13.0	0.80 [0.32, 1.99]
Proprems 2012	12	550	24	550	23.0	0.50 [0.25, 0.99]
Rouge 2009	2	45	1	49	1.9	2.18 [0.20, 23.21]
Samanta 2009	5	91	15	95	11.4	0.35 [0.13, 0.92]
Total (95% CI)		**1871**		**1884**	**100.0%**	**0.45 [0.32, 0.62]**
Total events	50		122			

Heterogeneity: Tau^2 = 0.00; Chi^2 = 9.03, df = 12 (P = 0.70); I^2 = 0%
Test for overall effect: Z = 4.84 (P < 0.00001)

Each line represents an individual study. The confidence intervals often cross the line of equality, indicating a non-significant result. The risk ratio is represented by the blue box.

The kite symbol shows the overall effect. As this is to the left of the line it shows that the overall effect favours the intervention (probiotics) compared with control.

72 Palliative and end-of-life care

Palliative and end-of-life care

Philosophy

Paediatric palliative care is the active care of the child with a terminal illness—physically, emotionally and spiritually. Family support is a central element. The aim of palliative care is to help children, young adults and their families to optimise the quality of their lives, rather than focussing on extending its duration.

There is a misconception that palliative care only involves end of life care. Palliative care can begin at the time of diagnosis of any life limiting condition and continue alongside active treatments. There is a move towards parallel planning: 'hoping for the best and planning for the worst'

Clinical aspects of palliative care

Symptom control

- Pain
  - Appropriate choice of analgesia-can include opiates
  - Appropriate route of administration—liquid medicine or lozenges for oral drugs and subcutaneous route for infusions can be useful
- Nausea & vomiting
  - Review medications (side effects)
  - Choose anti-emetics
  - Consider jejunal feeds
- Seizures and spasms
  - Anticonvulsants and sedatives
- Agitation
  - Sedatives (benzodiazepines) may be help. Treat hypoxia with oxygen

Holistic care

- Support for the child and family's psychological and emotional needs can be provided by a variety of people
  - Spiritual and religious leaders
  - Psychologists and counsellors
  - Social workers
  - Palliative care nurses and care staff
  - Play therapists
- Ensure financial support and benefits are in place
- Practical support about issues that arise when a child dies—registering the death, organ donation, funeral arrangements, who to tell and how
- Bereavement support for the family will need to continue for some time after the child has died
- Remember that hospice and hospital staff may also need emotional support

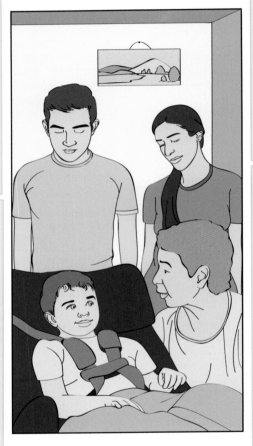

Nutrition

- Special feeding support may be needed—good nutrition can alleviate discomfort. Even at the end of life, feeding and hydration should be considered if the child appears thirsty or hungry to alleviate distress
- Providing tasty freshly cooked nutritious meals tailored to the child's needs will help. Many children's hospices have their own chef
- Consider Gastrostomy or Jejunostomy feeds if long term (the latter can help with vomiting)
- Ice-lollies and lozenges can help with nausea

Care planning

- An MDT approach is required to coordinate care between
  - hospice
  - local community nurse
  - school
  - paediatrician
  - family doctor
- Remember with very rare conditions the parents often become experts in the disorder. Their opinion should be listened to
- Need for palliative care should be anticipated and addressed early
- A 'care plan' should be shared with all professionals and the family
- Limits of treatment agreements should be agreed with the family—e.g. what degree of emergency treatment or resuscitation is appropriate?
- Anticipate events—parents need to know who to call if child dies at home. Ambulance service need to know what to do if they are called

Conditions

A significant number of children with neurodegenerative, cardiac, metabolic and genetic conditions require palliative care. Over 80% of children receiving palliative care do not have a diagnosis of cancer. There are many conditions that can fit under the umbrella of palliative care but these can be broadly classified in to four categories:

Category	Conditions
1	There is a curative option but this may fail, e.g. cancer
2	There are treatments to prolong life but premature death is inevitable, e.g. cystic fibrosis.
3	No curative option, palliative care may extend over many years, e.g. Batten's disease
4	Irreversible non-progressive conditions likely to lead to premature death, e.g. very severe brain injury

Paediatrics at a Glance, Fourth Edition. Lawrence Miall, Mary Rudolf and Dominic Smith. © 2016 John Wiley & Sons, Ltd. Published 2016 by John Wiley & Sons, Ltd.
Companion website: www.ataglanceseries.com/paediatrics

Palliative care is one of the newer emerging specialties in paediatrics. Much palliative care can be performed by local doctors and nurses with support from specialist palliative care team. Care needs to be flexible, fitting around the child and their family. Often the local doctor will have a long-standing relationship with the family. It is important that contact is maintained with the local hospital and the family doctor so that community and acute services can be accessed.

Referral to palliative care services

It can be difficult to decide when to refer a child for palliative care. A clear discussion with the family is needed with an explanation that this does not mean that you are giving up on their child. Considering parallel planning is very helpful. Most families who have been referred to palliative care services are very grateful for the support they experience and often wish they had been referred sooner.

Hospices

In most areas of the UK and in many other countries, there are hospices for children, teenagers and young adults, providing respite. This can often involve the whole family going to stay for a short break. Hospices need to be designed so that children and young people in wheelchairs can access all areas and have adapted gardens and outdoor activities. Play therapists, music therapists and chefs are integral to the working of a hospice.

Hospices also provide symptom control stays. This gives the family a break and allows treatments to be carefully tailored to the individual.

Symptom management

It can be helpful to write a care plan that gives some background about the child and the most appropriate way to manage their symptoms. It can include information for professionals about what to do when the child becomes unwell. Families should keep a copy of the plan at home to show to their GP, ambulance service, and hospital. It can include, where appropriate, a 'do not resuscitate' plan (can be called an "extent of treatment plan"), if this has been fully discussed and agreed with the child and family, for actions to take in event of cardiopulmonary arrest or need for intensive care. Pain, nausea, vomiting, seizures and spasms are common symptoms that are managed in palliative care.

Pain

It is important to try and work out what is causing the pain – e.g is it bone pain, visceral pain or muscular pain?

If children have communication difficulties, it is important to consider hidden pain from sites such as teeth, hips, urine infection.

There are many ways in which analgesics can be given. Liquids and tablets are commonest, but lozenges, nasal/buccal administration and patches are also available.

There can be anxiety amongst health professionals about the use of morphine in palliative care patients and the risk of respiratory depression. However, if morphine is titrated appropriately for pain, then it is safe.

Feeding

It is very common for children in palliative care to need some form of support for their feeding, which may be in the form of oral supplementary drinks, nasogastric tube or feeds given via gastrostomy. Dietician support is helpful.

Psychological and spiritual aspects of care
Social interaction

Regular social contact with other children or young people is essential. Usually, this means support to attend school as much as possible.

Psychological support

Psychological support is needed for the children and young people and also their families through working with clinical psychologists through palliative care and in bereavement.

Spiritual support

Spiritual support can be provided by faith leaders if the family are religious. Many people are not religious but have a sense of spirituality. Spirituality is linked to personal identity and the meaning of being human—the 'self' as different to the physical body, how people connect emotionally with others and with their environment. At a time of crisis, distress can involve a challenge to beliefs. Hospice staff have training in understanding spiritual needs and giving support.

End-of-life care and bereavement

Paediatric palliative care includes end-of-life care. It is important that their preferred place of death has been discussed with the families and child, where appropriate and as much as possible is done to facilitate their wishes. It is important to be clear how distressing symptoms will be managed.

There may be anxiety about hastening death by giving sedatives such as opioids and benzodiazepines. The doctrine of 'double effect' is recognized; the risk of hastening death is acceptable if the intention is to control distressing symptoms when the patient is clearly in the process of dying.

After death

Most children's hospices have a refrigerated bedroom, where the child's body can be cared for until the funeral. Often families of children who have died have been caring for them for a long time and they need time to adapt. They often say that having time after their child's death in the hospice is invaluable. It allows families to grieve at their own pace. Support is provided for practicalities such as planning for funerals. Siblings will need support.

Bereavement support may also need to be provided for months or years following death. Families' responses to bereavement can be very different and whilst each is an individualized reaction, most people experience predictable 'stages' of bereavement:

- Denial followed by acceptance that the loss is real.
- The pain of grief.
- Adjustment to life without the person.
- Gradually spending less emotional energy on grieving and directing it towards something new (moving on).

> ### KEY POINTS
>
> - Palliative care can begin as soon as a diagnosis has been made.
> - Palliative care needs to be holistic, addressing all the child's needs, not just pain control.
> - Care must be coordinated between all the care givers and health professionals involved with the child.
> - End-of-life care is only a small part of palliative medicine, but a vitally important part for the families who will have lasting memories.

Index